The International Behavioural and Social Sciences Library

DELINQUENT AND NEUROTIC CHILDREN

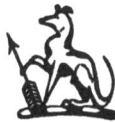

I0042301

TAVISTOCK

The International Behavioural and Social Sciences Library

CHILD DEVELOPMENT
In 9 Volumes

DELINQUENT AND NEUROTIC CHILDREN

A Comparative Study

IVY BENNETT

Routledge
Taylor & Francis Group

LONDON AND NEW YORK

First published in 1960 by
Tavistock Publications (1959) Limited

Published in 2001 by
Routledge
2 Park Square, Milton Park, Abingdon, Oxfordshire OX14 4RN
711 Third Avenue, New York, NY 10017

First issued in paperback 2014

Routledge is an imprint of the Taylor and Francis Group, an informa business

British Library Cataloguing in Publication Data
A CIP catalogue record for this book
is available from the British Library

Delinquent and Neurotic Children
ISBN 0-415-26397-2
Child Development: 9 Volumes
ISBN 0-415-26506-1
The International Behavioural and Social Sciences Library
112 Volumes
ISBN 0-415-25670-4

ISBN 13: 978-1-138-86739-0 (pbk)
ISBN 13: 978-0-415-26397-9 (hbk)

IVY BENNETT

M.A., Ph.D.

Delinquent and neurotic children

A COMPARATIVE STUDY

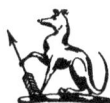

TAVISTOCK PUBLICATIONS

First published in 1960
by Tavistock Publications (1959) Limited
2 Park Square, Milton Park, Abingdon,
Oxon, OX14 4RN

To the Memory of
Dr. Kate Friedlander

CONTENTS

FOREWORD

Psychology is an old art but a new science.

The Delphic exhortation, 'Know Thyself', foreshadowed the need to know how our mind works: how our mind is affected by circumstances and conditions and how it can develop and master itself and so surmount such difficulties.

This treatise on delinquents and neurotics by Miss Bennett is a valuable addition to our knowledge. It will contribute materially to the more successful understanding of difficult children, especially in the sphere of mother and child relationships.

It is very necessary in what is a new science to lay good foundations by the precise use of terms, even if these present certain difficulties for the layman at the moment. Once terms carry the same connotation for all interested parties, discussion becomes easier and more fruitful. In order that precise terms may come into common use, careful classification of cases, with examples and explanations, is very necessary.

Miss Bennett has rendered signal service and in doing so pays a just tribute to that remarkable woman Dr. Friedlander. I had the privilege of collaborating with Dr. Friedlander as her Chairman in the establishment of the Child Guidance Service of whose foundation years this book provides some record. We were pioneers and met all the difficulties of prejudice and lack of understanding which a new venture of this kind inevitably has to face.

It was Dr. Friedlander's scientific and at the same time normal and practical outlook which persuaded me of the value of such a Child Guidance Service. I stress the value of a thoroughly normal outlook, because too many unscrupulous charlatans have misled and exploited the public.

Certainly we are still groping and casting our soundings in unknown waters; mistaken approaches have and will continue to be made. By painstaking analysis and the sorting of cases we shall, however, gradually make progress in alleviating or illuminating certain factors which lead to child delinquency.

There are dangers. One lies in reducing the individual to a type and then jumping at some general conclusions. Another, in regarding the child as a clinical case instead of a personality. The greatest danger, however, lies in the belief some people have that everything in a child can be explained.

I do not think that the inner self—the conscience—the soul of a child, call it what you will, is ultimately capable of analysis and classification, though the damage which has been done to it may be.

A lily may flourish in a dungheap; a saint be raised in the most unlikely surroundings. We are not, however, in our day-to-day problems concerned with these miracles of Providence.

Our task is to try to mitigate the welter of unhappiness which antisocial and delinquent children bring to others as well as to themselves.

We are grateful, therefore, for this book and for the author, who, with integrity of thought, patience, and intelligent analysis, sorts the false from the true and presents us with the facts necessary to probe further into the mysteries of the mind.

EVELYN EMMET, J.P., M.P.

ACKNOWLEDGEMENTS

I am indebted to the British Council for a research scholarship for three years between 1946–9 which made the practical work of collecting data for this investigation possible.

I am grateful to Sir Cyril Burt, formerly Professor of Psychology at University College, London, for supervision of part of this work as a doctoral thesis, and especially for his help in planning the research lay-out and the statistical sections. I am immensely indebted to Miss Grace Rawlings, also of the Psychology Department, University College, London, for numerous discussions, practical help, and advice over a long period in the early part of the work, and for her extensive collaboration in the major part of the routine psychometric work.

I would like to express very great gratitude to the Council and Clinical Directors of the rural district Child Guidance Service concerned for permission to use research data obtained from the Clinic records and for various practical arrangements which made this possible. I am most of all grateful to the late Dr. Kate Friedlander for her psychiatric collaboration, for drafting with me the original plans for this work as a supplementary investigation to that published in her own volume, *The Psycho-analytical Approach to Juvenile Delinquency*, and for her very great help throughout the conception of the thesis.

I am indebted to Dr. Anna Freud, Dr. Ilse Hellman, the late Professor J. C. Flugel, and the late Dr. Julia Mannheim, for preliminary discussions on the theoretical aspects and plan of the research, and for various suggestions related to details of psycho-analytic theory which were incorporated into the general procedure and acknowledged elsewhere.

Most of all I am deeply grateful to the sixteen individual members of the staff of the Child Guidance Service without whose continued help and cooperation this research would not have been possible. In the interests of preserving the anonymity of their small patients, the team of psychiatrists, psycho-analysts, educational psychologists, child psychotherapists and psychiatric social workers who formed the staff of the three clinics during the period when this study was in progress have not been named. I would like to place on record my personal indebtedness to each of them and to express my thanks for their valuable help in so many ways throughout the preparation of this work. I am grateful to them for discussions, both individually and in staff meetings and case conferences at the three clinics, of my plans of procedure and the meaning of the terms and definitions used in this research. I would like to acknowledge also their help in the collection of dossiers of information about each case studied, and permission to have access to scientific records of their treatment interviews. I am also grateful for lengthy and illuminating discussions upon individual cases and for 'free trade in ideas' in discussions that were held in the clinics, in special interviews, over meals, in pauses between cases, in correspondence extending over many years, over special scientific papers, and after hours in the clinics at night. I am especially grateful for the help, time, and patience put into this work by the secretaries of the three clinics.

I am also grateful to Mr. A. Lubin, formerly of the Maudsley Hospital, London, for advice in the statistical section of the work and to Mrs. A. Hackel, Mrs. M. G. Taylor, and Mrs. Mervyn Mills for clerical and editorial assistance. I am most especially indebted to Dr. F. J. Knobloch for his very great help on psychiatric and methodological questions, for his sustaining interest and the belief in this work which gave it birth.

I am greatly indebted to my colleague, Miss Anneliese Schnurmann, for her kindness and painstaking care in reading the original manuscript of this work and for the many helpful suggestions she has made.

I am above all grateful to the small patients themselves, whose unhappy stories stimulated our thinking and gave rise to so much compassionate labour.

*   *   *

Acknowledgement is due to William Heinemann for permission to reproduce the passage from *The Brothers Karamazov*, by Feodor Dostoevsky, translated by Constance Garnett, which appears on p. xiii.

London, 1958   I. V. B.

Aloysha. 'Boys . . . Let us make a compact, here, at Ilusha's stone that we will never forget Ilusha and . . . let us always remember how we buried the poor boy at whom we once threw stones . . . and afterwards we all grew so fond of him . . . in the first place, we will remember him, boys, all our lives. And even if we are occupied with most important things, if we attain to honour or fall into great misfortune—still let us remember how good it was once here, when we were all together, united by a good and kind feeling which made us, for the time that we were loving that poor boy, better perhaps than we are . . . perhaps you won't understand what I am saying to you, because I often speak very unintelligibly, but you'll remember it all the same and will agree with my words some time. You must know that there is nothing higher and stronger and more wholesome and good for life in the future than some good memory, especially a memory of childhood, or home. People talk to you a great deal about your education, but some good, sacred memory, preserved from childhood, is perhaps the best education. If a man carries many such memories with him into life, he is safe to the end of his days, and if one has only one good memory left in one's heart, even that may some time be the means of saving us. Perhaps we may even grow wicked later on, may be unable to refrain from a bad action, may laugh at men's tears and at those people who say, as Kolya did just now "I want to suffer for all men", and may even jeer spitefully at such people. But however bad we may become—which God forbid!—yet, when we recall how we buried Ilusha, how we loved him in his last days, and how we have been talking like friends all together, at this stone, the cruellest and most mocking of us—if we do become so—will not dare to laugh inwardly at having been kind and good at this moment! What's more, perhaps, that one memory may keep him from great evil and he will reflect and say, "Yes, I was good and brave and honest then!" Let him laugh to himself, that's no matter, a man often laughs at what's good and kind, that's only from thoughtlessness. But I assure you, boys, that as he laughs he will say at once in his heart, "No, I do wrong to laugh, for that's not a thing to laugh at".'

'That will be so, I understand you, Karamazov!' cried Kolya with flashing eyes.

The Brothers Karamazov, from Book III, The Epilogue, Ch. III— 'Ilusha's Funeral. The Speech at the Stone'—by Feodor Dostoevsky, 1880 (translated by Constance Garnett).

PART ONE

THE RESEARCH PROBLEM

CHAPTER I

Historical background

The developing spirit of humanity in educational theory in the eighteenth century, as represented by the doctrines of Locke and Rousseau, contrasts sharply with the harshness of then current laws and punishments relating to petty delinquency and minor deviations from social standards of conduct. The presence of beggars, the cruelties of the workhouses, the neglect of unwanted children, the severity of parents and teachers, and the high rate of child mortality were commonplaces that caused little concern. Yet from this background sprang the new concept of childhood that was developed in the latter part of the nineteenth century, with its basic reforms, and carried on with greater impetus in preventive, educational, and remedial programmes in our own time.

During the latter part of the nineteenth century, legal procedures for dealing with child offenders were patterned directly on those applied to adults, and punishment, including even the death penalty, was meted out in accordance with the 'crime'. Today, society's former acceptance of the barbarities of the reformatories has given way to a belief in re-education and psychological treatment. The successful employment of these facilities, however, depends more than ever on human skill. A high degree of psychological understanding is required, as well as the maximum flexibility in social machinery, for directing the individual offender or sufferer to the treatment best suited to him, whether it is psychological or psychiatric treatment, institutional training, or some change in environment. A great deal of wasted effort still goes into unsatisfactory cases, due not so much to inadequate facilities for treatment as to their misapplication. The establishment of greater precision in our psychological understanding of the causation and development of maladjustment will possibly prove more important in the future than the invention and multiplication of remedial measures and new types of 'treatment'. All these latter aim, in effect, at giving the child a new kind of human relationship to replace that which has contributed so greatly to the thwarting or distortion of his development in the past.

A survey of the main lines of the development of psychological understanding over more than half a century of delinquency research might be divided, for convenience, into three main periods, (a) 1890–1920, (b) 1921–35, (c) 1936–50. A review, in loose chronological order, of some of the main topics on which research into childhood maladjustment has been focused will reveal the main purposes behind the present investigation.

(a) 1890–1920

Healy occupies a dominant position in the first quarter of this century, at a time when conventional psychiatry was still absorbing the effects of Kraepelin's drive towards order and organization among the disputed diagnostic entities of the day, and when the psychology of the normal child had received little systematic study. Prior to the establishment in 1909 of Healy's 'Juvenile Psychopathic Institute', with plans for a programme of research on delinquents in Chicago, no such clinic existed. Witmer had attempted to add psychological tests to the routine physical examination in his clinic for retarded children at the University of Pennsylvania, and Goddard had used similar laboratory methods. Healy's pioneer researches tended to grope after some biological explanation of delinquency, e.g. his studies into the inheritance of criminalism, or into the nature of the 'born criminal'. Only with his massive textbook on the juvenile delinquent (1915a), based on the study of 1,000 juvenile court cases (mainly adolescent recidivists) did he begin to demonstrate the intricate and complex interweaving of psychological causal factors in the development of the offender. Healy's permanent achievements are due largely to his departure from speculation and theorizing and to his adoption of systematic empirical methods, allied with a psychodynamic approach (derived mainly from Freud's early teachings) that was still far from gaining acceptance in the fields of psychology and psychiatry. His pioneering work is of greater

4

significance because he included among his techniques the tools of academic psychology and social work, and called upon the cooperation of juvenile court officers, juries, lawyers, and staffs of educational centres. He laid great emphasis on the individual case approach, on individuality in treatment, and on the quantitative nature of the differences between the normal, the neurotic, and the delinquent child. He also had to forge new methodological tools for empirical research in genetics and psychodynamics, and he made a strong plea for the early treatment of offenders and for a genuine attempt to treat causes, not symptoms, whether mental or environmental.

Healy's collection of facts about large numbers of delinquents demonstrated the necessity for teamwork research on a long-term basis. He was also one of the first strongly to emphasize the fundamental importance of the 'family drama' and its infinite ramifications in the emotional life of young children. Healy's work was nevertheless largely limited to questions of aetiology, diagnosis, and prognosis in delinquency, and treatment was at first thought of as little more than a matter of social manipulation allied with frank talks between worker and child. The value of the frequent extensive policies of removal from home and placement in various other settings, particularly orphanages and institutions, has been seriously questioned in more recent years.

An early over-emphasis on feeble-mindedness as a primary cause of delinquency, rather than as an abetting or predisposing factor, as in Goddard's (1915) historical collection of material relating to mental deficiency and criminality, proved an unproductive line of inquiry. Glueck's study (1918) of criminals admitted to Sing-Sing Prison, which found a high proportion of the inmates suffering from some kind of mental disorder, did much to secure public recognition of the part played by psychological factors in criminal behaviour.

Another prominent name among the early pioneers in research on delinquency and crime was that of W. A. White, who was a leader in the movement for revolution in the organization of mental hospitals in the United States between 1890 and 1930. This reform he describes as having been overdue since the inmates of the Salpêtrière were released by Pinel in 1793. In the face of continued opposition, White introduced the principle of non-restraint for the insane, and vigorously condemned the death sentence for offenders who were not responsible for their actions even though not technically insane according to the McNaghten Rules. His great achievements were in educating the public with regard to insanity and the criminal law. White (1923) advocated individual psychiatric study as well as legal care for most offenders, and urged the recognition by the courts that criminality may be a psychologically conditioned reaction and that problems of responsibility and punishment should be reviewed in that light.

White came to accept the basic tenets of psycho-analysis, and in 1919 published a textbook on the mental hygiene of childhood. This early statement of many of the principles of moral and social education now embodied in the teaching and therapeutic work of child guidance clinics formulated some of the basic psychological problems involved in the emotional relationship between parent and child. Two of his major conclusions were, first, that the child is possessed of a developing sexuality and, second, that the stresses and strains of family life can have either a disruptive or a productive effect on the child's character. He recommends, for an improvement in the parent-child relationship, a fuller recognition of these factors and of the asocial, amoral, and primitive nature of a small child's unguided impulses. He accepts the Freudian doctrine that these primitive instincts, rechannelled and sublimated, will grow into respect, understanding, and sympathy, and the capacity to make the mutual concessions that render human society possible. Infancy is the period when these fundamentals of character and social life are laid down. In a later publication, White (1926) offers a summary of the principles of character formation and submits that in many ways neurotics are highly moral persons, i.e. their conflicts are moral conflicts that have arisen on the way to socialization, whereas delinquents have preserved their primitive instincts (like the savages) in an unsocialized and often crude form.

Meanwhile, Freud's early papers on hysteria (1893a, 1893b, 1896, 1905b, 1908a, 1909a), on anxiety neurosis (1894, 1895a), and on phobia and obsessional neurosis (1895b, 1907, 1908b, 1909b,

1909c, 1913) had reorientated psychiatric thinking about these conditions. He had put forward his theory of the part played by sexuality in the aetiology of the neuroses (1898, 1905, 1905a, 1908a), and his theories about homosexuality and the perversions became widely known (1905b, 1919). His publications on repression and the unconscious (1915b and c), on dream analysis (1900, 1913), on infantile neuroses (1909b, 1918), and on the transformation of instincts (1915a, 1915b) aroused strong opposition. In 1915, Freud described three special character types, which he terms 'the exceptions', 'those wrecked by success', and the 'criminal from a sense of guilt'—which pointed the way for deeper researches on the subject of the psychopath, the neurotic character, and other deviant types. Jung and, to a much lesser degree, Adler offered alternative theories of the aetiology of the neuroses, while more temperate students of 'conscious' psychology (e.g. Suttie, W. I. Thomas, *et al.*) put forward other formulations of the basic human drives, such as the 'need for companionship', 'need for security', 'need for adventure', which if thwarted were thought to lead to antisocial conduct.

By the end of the second decade of this century, and after the fifteen-year period of fundamental contributions of high quality dominated by Healy and White, most psychologists who had worked with juvenile offenders, and many legal and medical writers as well, were agreed about certain basic concepts, themselves almost revolutionary at the time, that form the groundwork for much of the research carried out by the next generation. The social consequences of mental disease and of mental defect were beginning to be widely understood, and many new ideas and new publications gave to psychology and to psychiatry a special impetus after the end of the 1914–18 war. Among these concepts was a conviction that many criminals are not responsible for their deeds but are comparable to sick persons, and should therefore be treated as patients or re-educated, rather than punished. Emphasis was consequently placed on the responsibility of society for individual offenders, on the need for more hospitals instead of prisons, and on indefinite confinement rather than sentence. It was recognized that the causation of delinquency must be sought in an intricate complex of factors—psychological, physical, social, and economic—and stress was placed on individual studies and on detailed and elaborate techniques of taking case histories. Society was held responsible for various environmental circumstances thought to foster delinquency, such as bad companions, lack of healthy leisure pursuits, bad housing, and overcrowding. Delinquency was slowly recognized as a social problem the causes of which lie in the forces that tend to disrupt society as well as in the failure of the normal socialization and education processes in the individual. Varying emphasis was placed on the importance of the home, the school, the community, the Churches, and various recreational facilities in the prevention of delinquency. Under the impetus of the work of Healy, White, Thomas, and others, the juvenile court began to exchange its policing and punitive role for a more constructive and remedial one. Certain other social problems, such as illegitimacy, truancy, vagabondage, prostitution, divorce, and the rise in frequency of crimes committed at adolescence, were approached for the first time from a psychological viewpoint. It was becoming increasingly recognized that the determinants of juvenile delinquency penetrated deeply into the social and emotional life of home and community, and that the problem was not one to be solved by any simple unitary solution, since delinquency itself is not a single isolated problem, but a symptom of a general weakness or conflict within the fabric of society.

(b) 1921–1935
In the 'twenties and 'thirties a number of major attempts were made at the reform and re-education of delinquents according to psychological principles. One of the most successful of all reported experiments in the re-education of delinquent youth was carried out by Anton Makarenko in attempting to deal with the gangs of vagabond youth who ran wild in Southern Russia in the years following the 1917 Revolution. Makarenko examined and then discarded current 'advanced' educational theories that advocated kindliness and lack of restraint verging on indulgence, and emphasized only the hard-won knowledge derived from actually living with mainly illiterate and savagely delinquent youth, and taking responsibility for their physical and mental

re-education. He found that the children did not show much respect for a person who was only kind and fondled them.

'What most attracted them were high qualifications, assured and exact knowledge, intelligence, art, capable hands, and unfailing readiness for work. You could be as curt as you liked with them, and exacting to the point of captiousness; you could ignore them even if they were hanging on your arms; you could be quite indifferent to their likes and dislikes, but if you were brilliant and successful in your work, in your knowledge, there was no need for anxiety: they were all on your side and would never let you down. And it made no difference what your abilities were: whether you were a carpenter, agriculturalist, smith, teacher, or motor driver.

'On the other hand, no matter how kind you were, how amusing in your conversation, how good and friendly, how "sympathetic" you were in work and play, if you were associated with failures and breakdowns, if at every step it was evident that you did not know your business, if everything you did ended faultily, you would never win anything but their contempt . . .' (Makarenko, 1936, p. 236).

The basis for the success of Makarenko's work lay in his profound belief in all types of children and individuals; in his provision of a relationship of tolerant and infallible friendship and of a model or ego-ideal commanding respect from the whole group; in his reliance on group pressure to mould desirable socialized habits and achieve community standards of conduct; and in his considerable emphasis on integrating the life of his delinquents with that of the community as a whole, using this as a natural part of the educational medium. Makarenko, like Aichhorn and those workers who have reported success in dealing by unorthodox methods with groups of thousands of homeless children in post-war Europe,[1] was always willing to transgress conventional regulations, whether to promote the children's welfare or to convince the individual delinquent that he was really on his side. A technique for achieving the latter aim has been described more fully by Biddle (1933), Aichhorn (1936), and Hoffer (1949).

[1] Hauser, R. (1948a) and in private communications.

In attempting to understand, in its historical setting, the fundamentals of Makarenko's achievement, it is important to remember two points. Makarenko worked first through the provision of the fundamental nurtural requirements of food and shelter, which most of his youthful bandits and beggars completely lacked. Moreover, working within the framework of an authoritarian ideology, he was able to offer to youth a positive role in a new society. Makarenko fought for and gained recognition for his boys and girls in Communist youth organizations, and having built both inner and outer values for his children he watched them develop realistic life-goals, while maintaining himself in their eyes as a model Communist fighting with selfless devotion for the advancement of society.

In 1925 came three classic contributions of major importance for the study of delinquency and possibly for the pyschological understanding of many other forms of human conduct. It is interesting that these came from three different countries and from three distinct currents of psychological thought, yet some of the conclusions were by no means dissimilar. In 1925 Aichhorn published in Vienna his *Verwahrloste Jugend;* in the same year appeared Burt's *The Young Delinquent,* in England, and Healy and Bronner's *Delinquents and Criminals: Their Making and Unmaking* in the United States.

Aichhorn's work was based on a rich collection of psychoanalytic studies, but he placed his main emphasis on character education and continually bore in mind that those who work with dissocial youth are primarily educationists. He stressed that the new-born babe is a primitive non-social being who becomes civilized through social experience and an appropriate training, without which it will not fit into our social order and is likely to come into conflict with society. With the delinquent child (Aichhorn, 1936, p. 7 ff), 'our work as remedial educators begins when an educational emergency arises, that is, when the usual educational measures have not succeeded in developing in the child or youth the social capacity normal for his age level. In purpose our work does not differ from education in general, since both attempt to fit the child for his place in society'. Aichhorn is primarily concerned with methods for achieving this aim and in particular with the application of psycho-analytic principles to the educational problems involved.

Aichhorn stressed that the form of the actual delinquent act may provide no clue to the nature of the psychological disturbance of which it is an expression. His method of re-education involved first an understanding of the psychic processes motivating the dissocial behaviour. He then aimed at the establishment of a home situation in which the emotional situation could be manipulated until a genuine relationship between the therapist and even the most incorrigible delinquent had been formed. Only on the basis of this deep emotional tie, Aichhorn believed, could genuine re-education towards better social behaviour or improved educational performance be achieved. What followed the establishment of the desired transference relationship was the same process that occurs in the rearing of every child, i.e. that of identifying with the parent-figure and incorporating his ideals.

Aichhorn, like Makarenko, was ingenious in finding means to create, heighten, or exploit an emotional situation, which he used both for the purposes of catharsis and for overcoming the child's defences by eliciting from him a deep emotional response. He thus used the transference to perform quite another task from that undertaken in the treatment of neurotics. He aimed at a definite achievement, consisting of a real character change and the 're-trieving of that part of his development which is necessary for a proper adjustment to society' (ibid., p. 234). Like Makarenko, he judiciously made use of the 'moment of surprise', in which, by some sudden manipulation of the emotional situation, he completely reversed the delinquent's situation and so gained a tactical advantage. Biddle (1933) quotes an occasion on which Aichhorn gave a meal and shelter to a miserable and penitent boy after a runaway that Aichhorn himself had secretly contrived; and describes an interview with a plausible and attractive deceiver that Aichhorn terminated thus: 'I see you wish to play a game of cat and mouse—that is quite all right. But I will be the cat and you can be the mouse. Good morning.' The psycho-analyst, Aichhorn maintained, has to prove himself superior to a certain type of narcissistic delinquent on his own ground in order to gain his genuine confidence and admiration.

Aichhorn describes a group of 'aggressive' delinquents who are shackled to those in authority by bonds of hatred and negative emotion, courting punishment to allay unconscious guilt, and whose psychic structure remains fixated at the early level of obtaining satisfaction through inflicting and receiving pain. In dealing with this type of delinquent, Aichhorn found it necessary to evolve a different method, which undermined their psychic structure and deprived them of the accustomed gratification of punishment. This then led to the possibility of a redistribution of psychic energy and a 'freeing of libido' for direction into a new and real emotional tie. Aichhorn's description of his social experiment in successfully re-educating twelve of the most incorrigible delinquents, the violence and destructiveness of whose behaviour had withstood all previous attempts at 'reform', ranks together with Makarenko's formidable undertaking in the Gorki Colony. Both Aichhorn and Makarenko have given full importance to the influence of socio-economic and cultural factors in fitting the delinquents' lives once more into the pattern of the society against which they had formerly rebelled; and allowing them to live out their frustrated hunger for pleasure before a slow development of ideal-formation, adapted to the reality principle, can gradually and surely begin to take place.

Healy and Bronner's *Delinquents and Criminals* (1925) marks the end of the first period of the authors' long and fruitful collaboration since the establishment of the Judge Baker Foundation Clinic in Boston in 1917. *Delinquents and Criminals* was the report upon 'a study in outcomes'. The authors compared and estimated the success of their work with groups of children in two cities during the period between 1909 and 1914 whose subsequent histories had been traced over several years. The results of this study were interesting in that bad heredity, in general, appeared to contribute little to crime. Healy and Bronner found that delinquency is an acquired form of behaviour and the problem of its causation largely an environmental one. They placed little emphasis upon physical factors, and found very little evidence to show that malnutrition, physical stigmata, developmental deviations, or physical defects contribute to delinquency. The authors stress the role of mental conflicts and the individual emotional background of misbehaviour in the aetiology of delinquency, and they reassert their earlier finding that punishment does not serve as a deterrent to delinquent behaviour. The comparison by treatment results revealed in Chicago 'a disconcerting measure of failure' but greater success was revealed in Boston where considerable use had been made of child placement in supervised homes, well followed up after a thorough study of the individual case.

Sir Cyril Burt's *The Young Delinquent* (1925) is a classic among psychological studies of the delinquent and has formed a model for generations of research workers in the various forms of behaviour disorder and childhood maladjustment. Burt's research gathered together many of the trends evident in previous research both in England and the United States, and gave systematic organization and statistical support to data investigated over a broad area of the child's life. His findings are of great importance both for educational practice and psychological theory. Burt emphasized the importance of the home life and social influences for the growing child, and spared no amount of labour in the quest for more exact and reliable research methods. He stressed the need for studies in the early development of delinquent cases rather than later studies of the emotionally hardened recidivist for whom apprehension and diagnosis frequently occur too late to be of help. Burt brought to his investigations the aid of extensive psychological tests of the intelligence, the emotional life, and the will (morality) of delinquents.

Burt found himself in agreement with Healy that the older theories of crime causation were too simple and that there are countless causes of crime. One may expect to find different reasons for different cases and a multiplicity of causative factors in any one case—Freud's 'over-determination'. Burt stressed that the emotional and moral conditions of the family are more important than the intellectual, physical, or material ones. He found that 26 per cent of the cases came from 'vicious homes' and over 60 per cent from homes where discipline was too weak or too severe (Burt, 1925a, p. 2 ff.). Burt investigated with scientific thoroughness the adverse social surroundings of juvenile offenders, but maintained that these were never sufficient in themselves to account for crime and that some hereditary weakness of intelligence or temperament is usually to be discovered in the child who gives way to bad external influences. He found that 'nearly half of the juvenile offenders examined were distinguished by a profound and widespread instability of the emotions' (Burt, 1925, pp. 507 ff.).

By the late 'twenties, the study of delinquency and criminality had attained recognition as the domain of experts in psychology, psychiatry, law, and sociology, and the understanding of many problems was enriched by a combination of these disciplines. Sociologists became interested in many problems of the child, and such studies as that of W. I. and D. S. Thomas (1928) presented a broad picture of the varieties of childhood maladjustment existing in contemporary society. Interest at this time seems to have fallen away from the delinquent *act* labelled as theft, truancy, and so forth, towards an attitude that considers delinquency as a symptom of the failure of the normal interaction between individual and society, and as an indicator of profound disharmony within society.

During the 'twenties and early 'thirties the psycho-analytical study of children assumed an importance of its own and began to complement the study of neurotics in psycho-analytic research (Hug-Hellmuth, 1913, 1921a, 1921b; Flugel, 1921; Klein, 1923, 1924, 1927, 1932; Freud, 1924; M. N. Searl, 1924; Aichhorn, 1925; Anna Freud, 1923, 1927, 1931, 1936; Glover, 1927; Ferenczi, 1929, 1931; Isaacs, 1929, 1933a, 1933b). Psycho-analysts turned only secondarily, however, to a dynamic formulation of the problems of crime. Reich (1925) broke new ground with his study of the 'impulsive character' and its various anti-social manifestations. Alexander and Staub (1931) attempted a statement of psycho-analytic doctrine in terms of criminal behaviour but without the support of convincing clinical data, and accepting the assumption that the same general principles and unconscious mechanisms underlie the behaviour of both delinquents and neurotics. Such a formulation, although interesting and provocative of thought, remains in many ways baffling and incomplete. In the following years a wider range of clinical work with delinquents cast doubt upon this ready explanation and many psycho-analysts found their 'orthodox' methods unsuitable for

14

delinquents, since they failed to make a strong enough transference to carry them through the difficult psychic tasks the patient must be ready to undertake in psycho-analysis (Glover, 1926; Schmideberg, 1935). Also, the delinquent himself did not suffer as others around him did from his troublesome behaviour, and therefore had little motive for wanting to change or be 'cured' of behaviour with which he felt quite satisfied. Psycho-analysts who have worked with delinquents and criminals have, in recent years, become more open-minded about adapting the techniques and methods of psycho-analysis to meet the special problems presented in the treatment of the non-neurotic delinquent. The result has been a theoretical and technical yield of very considerable interest, and, although this knowledge comes slowly from long-term psycho-analytic studies of criminals, intensive and prolonged observation upon individual cases has provided material for a theory of 'latent delinquency' or predisposition to delinquency, the development of which is distinct from, if sometimes over-lapping with, that of neurotic development.

By the middle 'thirties a considerable measure of agreement had been reached about certain concepts in delinquency research. There was unanimous agreement about the multiple causality of crime and the need for early ascertainment of delinquent tendencies (Healy, 1915a, 1917; Burt, 1925; Gordon, 1928). The part played by the 'delinquency fostering milieu' had been described in broad terms, and various re-educational programmes and social reforms gained strong support (Burt, 1925; Healy and Bronner, 1925; W. I. and D. S. Thomas, 1928; Levy, 1932b). A picture of the physical and mental characteristics of the offender had been drawn, including the delinquent's tendencies towards subnormality of intelligence and emotional instability (Burt, 1925; Healy and Bronner, 1925, 1936). Less importance had been given in this period to questions of constitution, and more emphasis was placed upon the environment, personality, and education of the offender (Shaw, 1929, 1930). Delinquency was described not as a single type or special reaction but as a way of life pervading the whole behaviour of the individual. The importance of the repercussions of early emotional (and especially repressed) experiences in later development was increasingly understood (Freud, 1915d; Healy,

1917; Stekel, 1925, 1929; Healy and Bronner, 1929; Alexander, 1930; Alexander and Staub, 1931). There could be seen the gradual understanding and acceptance of the decisive roles played by guilt, aggression, hostility, insecurity, rejection, and frustration in antisocial conduct (Stekel, 1929; Ferenczi, 1929; Levy, 1932b; Tiebout and Kirkpatrick, 1932; Ackerley, 1933; Healy, 1934). A new concept began to emerge of the chronic delinquent as a disfigured, distorted, 'scarred', or warped personality—a psychological or social cripple rather than a mentally sick or diseased person (Freud, 1905, 1915d; Reich, 1925; Alexander, 1930; Bartemeier, 1930; Karpman, 1929, 1933; Alexander and Healy, 1935).

In the period 1920 to 1935 a number of psychological studies were presented of which the results are inconclusive and difficult to assess. Many of these were made under poorly controlled conditions upon inadequate samples, and their results contradicted each other to a bewildering degree. Insufficient attention to methodology, inadequate definition of problems, and confused terminology probably account for some of these contradictions. Other studies were carried out at a high scientific level, and their results repeatedly verified by subsequent research. A number of investigations have increased our knowledge about the conditions of normal children's behaviour, but many more have been based upon observations of heterogeneous maladjusted groups, in which the results might apply equally well to the causation of neurotic as of delinquent behaviour. Research into problems of causation in contrasted pathological or deviant groups had, in this period, scarcely begun.

The penetration of psychological thought into the related specialized fields of sociology, economics, jurisprudence, education, social anthropology, and literature produced a stimulating effect upon studies of many socially aberrant types. More and more it was recognized that few problems can be solved by 'lumping all delinquents together as constitutional defectives' (Simey, 1949), and that juvenile delinquents constitute a very heterogeneous group. At least three different types of delinquent had been isolated for special study and their clinical pictures described. These were (a) the *dull or handicapped delinquent* (Burt,

1925); (b) the *neurotic delinquent* (Stekel, 1925; Reich, 1925; Aichhorn, 1925; Gordon, 1928; Levy, 1932b; Healy, 1917, 1934 *et alia*); and (c) the *'psychopathic' delinquent* (Reich, 1925; Glover, 1926; Karpman, 1929, 1933; Alexander, 1930; Bartemeier, 1930; Wittels, 1937). During this period the establishment of a number of journals concerned with mental health and with childhood maladjustment, such as the *American Journal of Orthopsychiatry*, offered opportunity for the publication of detailed special studies aimed chiefly at the exploration of minor problems. A research microscope was slowly being turned on the social and psychological problems of juvenile delinquency that had hitherto been approached as a whole, only in unfocused, macroscopic fashion

(c) 1936–50

The succeeding fifteen years yielded a voluminous literature upon delinquency and associated problems. Advances were made from the three inter-related approaches of psycho-sociological, psychiatric, and psychodynamic studies. Much of this research has not yet been coordinated with, or absorbed into, earlier theories, but the major part of it has been built upon, or extended from, foundations that were well laid in the preceding thirty years. Many of the investigations reviewed in the following rather sweeping historical survey have been imbued with concepts taken, directly or indirectly, from psycho-analytical theory; other investigations have been strictly 'objective' in approach. There is, however, an increasingly large number of research workers prepared to undergo the training and discipline necessary to obtain a grasp of some of the basic principles of both psychological fields. It has been interesting to observe how far investigators with widely divergent opinions, working from entirely different aspects of the psychological field, have slowly begun to describe similar observations, e.g. on aberrant sexual behaviour, on the influence of institutional rearing, and on 'susceptibility to delinquency'.

Foremost among the sociological contributions are the works of Shaw (1938), Shaw and McKay (1942), Carr-Saunders, Mannheim and Rhodes (1942), and Mannheim (1948, 1949), whose researches into the localities and social and environmental

17

circumstances of delinquency have provided a ground-plan for further research of fundamental importance. This represents what Mannheim, in his interesting smaller-scale local study, *Juvenile Delinquency in an English Middletown* (1948), has called only a first step in an advance towards scientific understanding of delinquency in its sociological setting, seen as one problem-aspect of community life, closely interlocked with many others. A collaboration of many sciences must be brought about before this sociological picture can be complete.

Increasing recognition has been given in recent years to the importance of taking into account psychodynamic factors, as well as social and physical conditions, for an understanding of the individual delinquent. An understanding of deep emotional factors (such as reactions to rejection or over-protection, jealousy, guilt, hostility, and all degrees of family disharmony) in the causation of delinquency, has become less a matter for a speculative 'cult of the Unconscious', and more and more a matter for observation in the stages of the child's early development—especially at times of minor breakdowns of adjustment. Increased knowledge about psychodynamic factors and an accumulation of observations by those skilled in recognizing their manifestations have greatly enlarged the scope of psychological investigations (Cf. Mannheim, 1942; Glover, 1944, 1947). This trend has led to research on the influences of the emotional relationships between parent and child and between parent and parent in the shaping of the child's personality (Silverman, 1935; Lowrey, 1936; Burlingham and Freud, 1942, 1943; Friedlander, 1947) and studies on special topics like maternal over-protection and sibling rivalry (Levy, 1932a, 1936, 1939, 1943; Vollmer, 1946). A number of very interesting studies have been carried out upon aberrant sexual behaviour and the authors appear to be unanimous in finding the sex offender to be neurotically disturbed and, without exception, in grave need of psychiatric help. Perverted sexual behaviour has been shown to be inextricably connected with the general personality and delinquency pattern of the offender, and other misdemeanours have been frequently found to originate in the same cause, related to the child's cultural milieu and to disturbances in his psycho-sexual development (Freud, 1905; Healy,

18

1917; Burt, 1925; Shaskan, 1939; Frosch and Bromberg, 1939; Waggoner and Boyd, 1941; Bender and Paster, 1941; Wortis, 1939; Benedict, 1939; Mead, 1931, 1935, 1949). Investigations upon cases of childhood suicide, usually supposed to be rare (Menninger, 1933; Zilboorg, 1937), and suicidal or self-destructive preoccupations and attempts in children (Bender and Schilder, 1937) have tended to show these to be rooted in unconscious instinctual expressions, in which aggressive tendencies are turned against the self in reaction to unbearable situations. These situations usually arise from the deprivation of love and in guilt-laden aggressive fantasies directed primarily against those who deny the child love.

An increasing number of studies have been concerned with the impoverishment and stunting of general personality growth consequent upon certain specific experiences in early childhood, as observed in the lives of delinquents and other 'problem' children. Representative of this group are studies of maternal rejection in infancy (Ferenczi, 1929; Newell, 1934, 1936; Levy, 1937; Rosenheim, 1942; Lippman, 1937, 1943); of the role of early traumatic experiences (Lander, 1941; Lowrey, 1940b; Lindner, 1944); and on the influence of institutional rearing (Lowrey, 1940b; Bender, 1943; Goldfarb, 1943, 1944, 1945, 1947, 1949). Observations concerning the specific influence on the child's social development or separation of the child from the mother during the first five years of life, or of the absence or lack of a permanent mother-person in the child's early years, have been corroborated in various ways by Aichhorn (1925); Lowrey (1940b); Burlingham and Freud (1942, 1943); Bender (1943); and Bowlby (1940, 1944, 1951).

Other important studies have been concerned with the development of the conscience, and, on the basis of the groundwork for a psycho-analytic theory of conscience development laid down by Freud (1914, 1917), psycho-analytic workers have made manifold observations (both clinically and in direct observations on child development) of far-reaching significance on this fundamental aspect of character formation (Aichhorn, 1925; Reich, 1925; Burlingham and Freud, 1942, 1943; Bender, 1943; Goldfarb, 1945; Greenacre, 1945, 1948; Karpman, 1948b). These studies have shown the strength and reliability of the conscience to be directly dependent upon the strength and number of the child's early love relationships, and the weakening of the earliest emotional ties to be reflected in a corresponding weakness in the super-ego or conscience. It would appear possible to subdivide the growth and development of the mental structure termed the super-ego (or group of super-ego functions) into various stages, and to assess the type and the degree of severity of disturbances that may occur in the development of these respective functions at different age levels in relation to the presence or absence of various (inner and outer) psychological conditions.

The psychodynamics and specific aetiology of a number of neurotic symptoms that take a delinquent form (e.g. violent aggressiveness, restlessness, stealing, truancy, running away, 'pseudologia fantastica') have been studied in detail by a number of psycho-analytic writers, and their more easily recognizable clinical forms have been described in detail (Tiebout and Kirkpatrick, 1932; Lippman, 1937; Alexander, 1938; Macdonald, 1938; Menaker, 1939; Yarnell, 1940; Riemer, 1940; Lowrey, 1941; Andriola, 1946; Greenacre, 1944; Levy, 1944; Deutsch, 1947; Friedlander, 1947, et alia). Several authors have noted the high frequency of enuresis among delinquents and have claimed to establish a relationship between delinquency and persistent enuresis (Alexander and Staub, 1931; Goodman and Michaels, 1934; Mowrer and Mowrer, 1938; Michaels, 1938; Michaels and Goodman, 1939; Michaels, 1940; Goldman and Bergman, 1945). Michaels found the highest percentage of enuresis in rejected and neglected children and the lowest in over-protected children, and he felt that just as there has been shown to exist a special type of neurotic delinquent, so also there may be a special type of 'persistent-enuretic delinquent'. Most authors are in agreement in regarding enuresis as an expression of some fundamental disorder of the personality (of which the delinquency itself may be only another expression) and as a persistent instinctual act, a kind of anachronism or 'psycho-biological infantilism' (Alexander and Staub, 1931) that has resisted the restrictions of instinctual activity that education would involve.

Many investigations, foreshadowed by the early clinical

observations of Healy and Burt, have verified and further extended our knowledge of the influence of home life, of immediate family influences, of the broken home, of defective discipline, of unhappy and unsatisfactory home atmosphere, and of many types of intra-psychic conflict (Levy, 1932b; Healy and Bronner, 1936; Bowlby, 1944; Banister and Ravden, 1944, 1945; Rose, 1949; Collis and Poole, 1950; Stott, 1950; Glueck and Glueck, 1934 *et alia*). Psychological studies for more than twenty-five years have emphasized that the motives for delinquency are bound up with human feeling and human experiences within the family. Defective family relationships, traumatic experiences, conflicts between parents over the handling of the child, unhappy marital relationships, lack of affection for the child or outright rejection, and inconsistency in ways of handling the child—these may exert a profound influence upon the whole of his future life. Evidence that the quality and vicissitudes of the child's psychological relationships and experiences within the family in his earliest years profoundly affect his social and emotional development can no longer be ignored. Research into the nature of the delinquent child's infantile experiences has shown that events in his early social environment prove highly significant for an understanding of his later social behaviour. A most valuable review of researches from selected sources that deal with the specific influence upon social development of one major factor, namely, maternal deprivation in the early years, has been an important contribution by Bowlby (1951).

A number of writers have emphasized that delinquents are not a homogeneous group, but include various sub-types. Schmidl (1947, p. 157), upon the basis of Rorschach experience with juvenile delinquents, maintains that '. . . there is no basis for the assumption that, so far as personality make-up is concerned, juvenile delinquents are a homogeneous group. On the contrary there is every reason to believe that we are dealing with a number of different types'. Karpman (1939) denies that there is such a thing as a 'delinquent type of personality', but rather holds that there are many personalities that *may* be delinquent and in each of these personalities the delinquency expresses a different problem. There may be nothing in common between them except the label of delinquency, just as there may be nothing in common between four mental defectives of the same I.Q. or, in the analogy suggested by Stott (1950), between four patients all of whom show symptoms of fever. The term 'delinquent' constitutes in no way a psychiatric or diagnostic entity in the proper sense, but gives a description of certain types of behaviour found in many recognizably different personality types. This contention appears to warrant a great deal more serious attention than it has on the whole received in the planning of delinquency research to date.

The neurotic type of delinquent act (i.e. that of the kleptomaniac, the pyromaniac, or of certain types of sex offender, and others) has received a great deal more spectacular publicity than have most other types. However, since Freud's analysis (1915d) of certain special character types (i.e. the 'exceptions', 'those wrecked by success', and the 'criminal from a sense of guilt'); since the insistence by Healy (1915a) and many others on the curious feature of much delinquent conduct that punishment does not act as a deterrent; since Reich's analysis (1925) of the 'impulse-ridden character', which opened up the enormous field of psychoanalytical research into the psychopath or the 'neurotic character' (Glover, 1926); and since the steady evolution and accumulation of the body of knowledge comprised within the term 'psycho-analytic ego-psychology', it has become increasingly difficult to draw the line between what can be regarded as neurotic (i.e. the neurotic symptoms of the 'pure' or classical neuroses in the strict sense) and a large group of conditions that bear a definite aetiological relation to them. These are the many types of characterological disturbance and emotional behaviour that spring from obscure and complex unconscious motivation, e.g. the so-called 'neuroses of fate' (see Freud, 1922; and Fenichel, 1945), in persons who have never shown signs of a neurotic conflict resulting in symptoms. Among the latter must be included much behaviour characteristic of defective social adjustment and many histories of long-standing aggressive and antisocial conduct. The shifts in theoretical emphasis concerning these conditions have exerted considerable influence upon our thinking both about the psycho-therapy and about the different kinds of re-education required by various types of delinquent (Aichhorn, 1925; Powder-macker, Leves, and Touraine, 1937; Friedlander, 1949a, *et alia*).

Levy (1932b) carried the attempt to distinguish between various types of delinquency a little further when he made a distinction between 'milieu delinquency' arising directly as a reaction to environmental pressures (the 'delinquency-fostering milieu'), and delinquency arising out of the nature of the individual personality. He found that the delinquent act may arise in many ways: it may be a release for aggression; it may be a disguised and symbolic neurotic symptom the motives of which are hidden through repression; or it may solve an emotional conflict. Neurotic delinquency, he thought, arose from unsuccessful attempts to prevent expression of natural impulses. In neurotic delinquency there is a discrepancy in the general social family setting, frequent lack of ordinary motivation and the patient gives nothing but irrational explanations of his conduct. Whereas in milieu delinquency the environment is held to create the delinquency in the patient, in neurotic delinquency the patient creates the delinquency in the environment in order to solve his problem.

The time now appears to be overdue for a separate study of some of the types of delinquency hitherto grouped together wholesale, and there is evidence that certain forms of non-neurotic delinquency should, rightly, be studied separately and contrasted with problems of neurotic symptoms in young offenders. To illustrate some of the types of delinquency that have, in a more or less haphazard and empirical way, emerged as loose, overlapping groups in the heterogeneous literature on delinquency during the past sixty years, the following might be listed. This is not intended to represent a logical or theoretically consistent classification, but merely a list of types of delinquents who have been studied, whose symptom pictures have been recognized, and whose needs appear to be different.

1. The dull or handicapped delinquent has been shown by almost all major psycho-social and sociological studies to represent a high proportion of delinquency cases, and many of these come from poor homes in the lower social classes.[1] These are the children

[1] Most of the cases in such studies were Juvenile Court cases.

whose innate constitutional, hereditary, intellectual, and temperamental endowment, and limited ego-development mark them off as weaker than their more fortunate fellows and less able to withstand pressure from both outer (environmental) and inner (instinctual) sources.

2. Certain delinquents, among them the more hopeful cases, appear to be potentially normal children lacking adequate social training. They show no great emotional disturbance and respond quickly to suitable changes in the environment allied with training in social values. These might be thought of as 'normal children in search of a normal environment' who have somehow lost their way along the road to normal social adjustment. The more extreme cases in this group might merge with the milder cases in section 4.

3. Adolescent delinquents who show no history of misconduct prior to puberty, whose problems cannot be considered apart from their special adolescent difficulties and needs, and who, given suitable handling and a good environment, are also potentially normal.

4. The delinquent from the 'vicious home' (Burt, 1925) or the 'delinquency-fostering milieu' (Levy, 1932b) where the child is offered faulty models of social behaviour and adopts the delinquent code of his family or neighbourhood 'as naturally as he learns his mother-tongue' (Levy, ibid).

5. The secondary antisocial conduct disorders, i.e. in children whose delinquent or uncontrolled behaviour is secondary and reactive to an organic condition, like epilepsy, encephalitis, etc.

6. The 'deprived' delinquents. This section includes the large group of children who find their way easily into a delinquent way of life *'faute de mieux'*, as a result of chronic deprivation in the formative years, such as institution-rearing, haphazard upbringing, or in some cases by gross neglect. These are children whose defective social behaviour must be considered as only one part of

the general personality picture they present of arrested growth (Lowrey, 1940b; Bender, 1943; Bowlby, 1944, 1951; Goldfarb, 1943, 1944, 1945, 1947, 1949).

7. The neurotic delinquents. Although recognized by a great number of authors to form a group of delinquents whose anti-social conduct is determined by unconscious motivation (and therefore not subject to influence by ordinary environmental methods of treatment), the category of 'neurotic delinquent' is itself a heterogeneous one. It is vague and only loosely comprehensive, with boundaries that are by no means easy to draw. Delinquent symptoms that are neurotically determined occur only relatively rarely in their 'pure' (or most morbid) forms, whereas unconsciously determined antisocial behaviour related to some form of neurotic character disorder is found only too frequently among delinquents who have been studied intensively in psychotherapeutic treatment. Such behaviour might be expected to exist most characteristically in cases of mixed origin, i.e. where neurotic tendencies are to be found allied with a 'weak ego' or defective character structure. There are many types of delinquent behaviour that can be recognized as arising from neurotic tendencies, and of these the following types appear to have received most consideration in the literature.

(a) The isolated and usually stereotyped 'ego-alien' delinquent act which arises as the typical 'compromise' solution to an unconscious neurotic conflict in an otherwise socially well-adjusted personality (e.g. the stealing of the true kleptomaniac).

(b) The 'criminal from a sense of guilt', the nature of whose unconscious 'need for punishment' with its controlling influence upon behaviour was first described by Freud (1915d, 1922).

(c) The behaviour of the passive-effeminate type of delinquent boy whose outspoken aggressive behaviour is in the nature of a violent defence against unconscious instinctual temptations and at the same time a provocation of the type of treatment he unconsciously wishes to receive. This type of delinquent behaviour—violent in its extremes—has been vividly described by Aichhorn (1925), Alexander (1938), Macdonald (1938), and Menaker (1939).

(d) Antisocial behaviour associated with some of the various types of neurotic character disorder as described by Aichhorn (1925), Alexander (1938), Fenichel (1945), and in numerous other psycho-analytic publications. This sub-section is usually regarded as overlapping the following group, but some theoretical formulations include both types under the same heading. The difference between the delinquents included in this section and psychopathic delinquents is considered by some psycho-analysts to be a question of the degree and severity of character deformation involved rather than a difference in the fundamental nature of the psychodynamic conflicts themselves.

8. Psychopathic delinquents. This type is both the least understood of all juvenile delinquents and the most resistant to treatment. Formerly referred to as the 'morally insane' or 'moral imbeciles', the classification of psychopath has been recognized by certain psychiatric schools but not by others. A large number of clinical writers use the term rather indiscriminately as a 'waste-paper basket' category to which are relegated a host of miscellaneous conditions characterized by an inability to form love relationships with any person, and by moral, emotional, and possible constitutional defects about which we know very little. There appears to be very little disagreement, however, about the clinical picture of this type of delinquent, as described (in various terminologies) by Aichhorn (1925), Karpman (1941, 1947, 1948a), Henderson (1939), Slavson (1943c, 1947), Bowlby (1944), Greenacre (1945), and many others. Karpman (1948a) has recently attempted to bring some order into the chaos of our thinking about this type of chronic and hardened recidivist by contrasting him with other non-delinquent types of psychopath, and relating both to psychoanalytic formulations about neurosis and psychosis. He prefers to delete the word 'psychopathy' altogether and to speak instead of 'anethopathy', thus emphasizing the failure in the ethical sense. He offered a diagnostic division into two chief groups:

(a) *Secondary or symptomatic anethopathy*, which would include about 85 per cent of the psychopathic personalities, and denotes psychopathic personality resulting from, or symptomatic of, a basic neurosis or latent psychosis which is the cardinal reaction.

26

(b) *Primary or idiopathic anethopathy* where the psychopathic behaviour cannot be traced to psychogenetic factors because they
either are lacking or are so deep-seated as to be impossible to discover by present psychological techniques. Karpman further
divided the group of primary anethopaths into two large divisions: (i) the aggressive, predatory type who are active, energetic,
and often socially harmful; and (ii) the passive, parasitic type, who
are the spongers on and victims of others in a passive way. In the
treatment of both types, Karpman places emphasis not so much
on the concept of cure for a disease as on that of correction of a
deformity.

9. The psychotic delinquents. This group includes those juvenile
delinquents whose misbehaviour is thought to arise from psychotic or pre-psychotic illness both in its gross forms and in the milder
cases involving psychotic or pre-psychotic complications.

An attempt to construct a list of delinquent types about which
our knowledge is so fragmentary is obviously a lamentably
unsatisfactory one. My personal view is that the persisting tendency to think from the behavioural and descriptive end of a
psycho-social process (i.e. the delinquent act) has been a mistaken
one, and that in future it will be less relevant to ask why a particular child is delinquent than to seek safeguards in our social life
against the multifarious and well-known forms of arrested growth,
family disruption, psychological or social deprivation, psychopathology, or human neglect, any of which, alone or in combination, might be expected to give rise to faulty social adjustment.
What form—delinquent or neurotic—this maladjustment takes
will diminish in importance, and the term 'delinquency' may
cease to hold any scientific meaning. In the meantime a more
general recognition of the common subdivisions among our
socially maladjusted children might form a more workable basis
for the operations of clinics and welfare agencies, as well as those
of the courts, in the care of and provision for society's weaker and
more ill-adapted juvenile members. Some such division (however
rough and ready from the theoretical point of view) when allied
with greater diagnostic care should serve to bring some preliminary order into the confused problems of the treatment of

antisocial disorders and help to avert the waste of the community's resources inherent in inappropriate use of existing social services.[1] Moreover, a body of knowledge is now available that shows that the treatment of different types of delinquent should follow along different lines; provides guiding hypotheses as to which method (parole, probation, psychotherapy, institutional treatment, foster-home placement) is applicable to each type; and indicates those that, according to the present limits of our knowledge, are not likely to respond at all to ordinary methods. Inconsistencies in the application of remedial education appear to arise mostly from the lack of a refined diagnostic system, and from the even more basic requirement for a consistent guiding theory about the fundamental needs of the human young.

Psychological observers who have worked with delinquents in a therapeutic or remedial capacity have almost unanimously attached fundamental importance to the role of *consistency and continuity in the education and training of the child*, both in matters of discipline (Burt, 1925; Healy and Bronner, 1936; Friedlander, 1947), and in the parents' personalities and their methods of dealing with the child's emotional and instinctive manifestations (Freud, 1915a; Aichhorn, 1936; Burlingham and Freud, 1942, 1943; Friedlander, 1947). Consistency over a long period should be a primary consideration, and trial-and-error approaches that switch without substantial reason from one method to another, and conditions that involve frequent moves from one foster-home or institution to another, should be avoided at all costs.

The problem of delinquency is, at bottom, that of dealing with uncivilized aggression beyond the control of society and often beyond the individual's own control. Many alternative reformulations have been made about the role of aggression in instinctive, family, and social life.[2] These studies remain inconclusive and serve more to open up new problems and to show the fundamental significance of the study of aggression for the understanding of delinquency—and indeed of normal life—than to solve urgent

[1] Willock (1949) in his *Mass Observation: Report on Juvenile Delinquency* has calculated that the number of *reconvictions* of delinquents discharged from Borstals ranges from 41 per cent to 56 per cent.

[2] See the Report of the Proceedings of the International Congress on Mental Health, London, 1948, edited by J. C. Flugel.

practical clinical problems involving primitive and unsocialized aggression. Some of these problems and their influence on group behaviour must, it would appear, await illumination from advancing research in social psychology and cultural anthropology as well as in psycho-analysis. During the decades between the wars, and since the outbreak of the Second World War, the focus of attention has been shifted from problems of sex, even in the wide meaning that Freud gave to the term, to problems of aggression. In this change of focus, psycho-analysts, and the general public as well, have given unbalanced emphasis to one aspect only of Freudian theory (Anna Freud, in Flugel, 1948). Freud did not hold that the many phenomena of social life could all be explained by an increased understanding of psycho-sexuality alone—nor that all social behaviour could be explained by the nature of aggressive impulses. Freud stated, in fact, that they could *not* be explained in such simple and unitary fashion, and that neither sexual nor aggressive instincts can be directly observed in their original, primitive forms in civilized life. A blending, fusion, and diffusion of both sexual and aggressive impulses takes place and is always present in the emotional sub-strata of community living. The success or failure of this blending and balance determines the varied nature of social life, both in its positive and constructive and in its negative and dissocial forms.

Healy evaluated the contributions of psychiatry to the understanding of delinquency in the following summing-up (Healy, 1949, p. 318): '. . . psychiatry in unearthing the varied dynamic backgrounds of delinquent impulses has disproven the existence of any great major causes of delinquency. In the individual case it looks for constitutional factors and into family relationships, conscience formation, experienced hurts, inner conflicts, non-use of special aptitudes, and all the thousand-and-one roots of attitudes and personality structuring . . . (but) . . . for psychiatry there is no 'either or'; its data are multi-valued . . . for the delinquent, delinquency is one way of coming to terms with reality—his reality.'

The following pages present an account of a research project designed in its original form jointly with the late Dr. Kate Friedlander but carried to practical fruition solely by the present writer.

Our fundamental aim was to make a comparison, critical for our theoretical understanding of later social maladjustment, of the divergent routes taken in emotional development by neurotic and delinquent children from their early years. We believe that some understanding of this difference is essential to the appropriate and successful application of remedial measures either for treatment or for prevention of these conditions. Much of the confusion and controversy about the merits of different techniques in education or in therapy appears to be merely the inevitable outcome of lack of clarity in our grasp of these fundamental theoretical issues.

CHAPTER II

The plan of research

INTRODUCTION

The aim of this investigation is to study and compare the character and case histories of delinquent and neurotic children, in an attempt to isolate certain features of their behaviour and emotional development as seen against the background of their home and social conditions. The opportunity will be taken to compare this research, carried out on subjects drawn from a rural community, with previous studies carried out on urban groups.

In the history of child psychology, as in the history of biology and medicine, advances in the understanding of human life and behaviour have resulted from two different but complementary lines of approach, and sometimes both methods have been brilliantly combined. The first method is to study in detail one individual and the infinite variations of his behaviour; the second is to study the behaviour of a number of individuals under uniform or deliberately varied circumstances. The first is usually described as the clinical method and may be applied to a long-term study of one or a few individuals whose growth is so acutely abnormal that certain of its features are more clearly recognizable than in normal development; or to the study of embryological problems where the conditions determining future growth can be isolated and studied *in statu nascendi*.

The aim of the clinical method is to gain understanding of the course of healthy growth and development as well as of the progress of disease and the interruptions or deviations in development. The second, or quantitative method bases findings upon carefully controlled observations on large numbers of cases against which certain hypotheses have been tested, yielding results which may be verified and subjected to quantitative analysis.

The aim of this method is to establish a quantitative statement of observed conditions from which a prediction of further observations may be made in given circumstances.

In the study of personality, both clinical and quantitative methods have been used separately and to supplement each other. The clinical method explores the speculative and descriptive borders of scientific knowledge and may produce interesting hypotheses which can be incorporated into the body of psychological science only after thorough testing by quantitative methods. This in turn establishes what are the normal or average conditions for a large number of individuals, and shows how the tendencies and averages of large groups are influenced by certain variables. In the study of aberrant behaviour of the types commonly included under the terms 'delinquency' and 'neuroticism', a combination of both methods is indispensable.

During the last fifty years, greater public awareness of many forms of psychological instability has helped to bring the problem of juvenile delinquency into the focus of scientific research, and since the two world wars reports of the alarming increase in juvenile delinquency and adult crime have stimulated the investigation of personality and emotional problems, particularly in the case of the very young. It is from work in this field that one may hope for fuller understanding of why children become neurotic or delinquent, as well as for the greatest social return from preventive and remedial programmes. Since the time of Ignatius Loyola lip-service has been paid to the idea that the decisive influences on the development of personality are those of a child's earliest years. Yet in legal and educational practice more emphasis has been placed on the adolescent's present environment and opportunities than on examining the facts about his early years. It would be more logical to direct our greatest efforts to finding out what leads to delinquent and neurotic behaviour and then making sure that infants are as far as possible brought up in conditions that avoid this. Loyola's formulations about early education have subsequently been re-stated by Freud, Aichhorn, Susan Isaacs and other psycho-analysts, and by a host of others who have been responsible for educating difficult children. Research during the past half-century has steadily lowered the age limit at which the root causes of later disturbances are to be looked for. Emphasis was shifted from the adolescent to the school-age child, from the pre-school child to the infant; and much research is at present directed to influences operating during the earliest months of life, even including the intra-uterine period. The old concept of the supposed 'innocence' of young children has been supplanted by a deeper understanding of the child's nature and psychological needs. The salutary observations and writings of Anna Freud and Susan Isaacs, and of many who worked with evacuated children in war-time hostels, have helped towards a better understanding of the primitive nature of much of a young child's unchecked behaviour, and paved the way for a more realistic conception of the function of early education as a basis for the socialized development of the individual.

The study that follows is based on the writer's fairly long experience in the teaching and practice of experimental psychology combined with psycho-analytic training and practice; the approach owes much to both disciplines. One of the reasons for undertaking it was to show that certain types of psycho-analytic data can be verified by statistical methods, a fact that has frequently been denied in certain academic quarters. It is my hope in this way to contribute towards a better understanding between psycho-analysis and academic psychology. Objective studies based on psycho-analytic concepts are yielding increasingly positive results, and more of such verificatory studies should be undertaken to facilitate communication not only between the various schools of psychology but also between the social sciences. I hope to show that the body of psycho-analytic knowledge about children's development may give direction and point to the planning of research according to the strict standards of experimental psychology and that the many difficulties involved in such collaboration can be overcome when there is genuine cooperation and interchange of thought between a large number of workers trained in the two different disciplines, providing the researcher has a thorough-going understanding of pyscho-analysis.

The psycho-analytic formulations underlying my account of this research, while derived largely from the works of Freud, Aichhorn, and Miss Anna Freud, were originally worked out

33

with Dr. Kate Friedlander, whose untimely death in 1949 ended our collaboration. We owe to her one of the first attempts to make a systematic statement of the psycho-analytical knowledge relating to juvenile delinquency (Friedlander, 1947). Some of the hypotheses that were tested in our project were expressly formulated to confirm or disprove by statistical methods some of the theoretical and aetiological concepts presented in her book. She does not claim that psycho-analysis can do more than explain certain manifestations of delinquency and emphasizes that the cooperation of all the relevant disciplines, including sociology and penology, is essential for research in this field. Basing her observations on the Freudian theory of emotional development, she describes the typical delinquent in terms not of illness or pathological development but of deformation or faulty character development which does not require individual psychotherapy so much as a special kind of emotional re-education of the type developed by Aichhorn (1936) or Slavson (1943c, 1947). She makes certain distinctions between types of upbringing responsible for delinquent as opposed to neurotic development; for instance, she has never, she says, found the same degree of inconsistency in the handling of primitive instinctive drives in the history of neurotic patients as she found in the histories of delinquents. She suggests a classification of delinquents separating the psychopaths, sex perverts, and neurotics from the typical delinquent, basing her system on a recognition of the varying degrees of 'antisocial character', underlying weakness or disturbance in ego-control.

Such considerations as these underlay the research carried out in a selected English rural Child Guidance Service. This service was founded in 1945 by Dr. Friedlander, in accordance with her plan (1943, 1946a) for a child guidance service providing for the application of psycho-analytic theory and experience to problems of diagnosis, treatment, and prevention of psychological disorders, and in addition for educational work in the community. All the staff had had considerable experience in psycho-analytically orientated child guidance work and most of them had had a psycho-analytic training. Thus, in contrast to other services, all workers shared a similar approach to psychological problems.

34

Psychotherapeutic treatment of varying lengths and intensities was available for all cases, and some of the children I studied had been seen over two or three years in regular interviews, many of them from fifty to a hundred times and even more. I had access to detailed records of all diagnostic and treatment interviews, and I attended case conferences over a number of years as a part of my routine work in the child guidance clinics.

When I began my research in 1946, I found that a serious approach to the problems of diagnosis, classification, and recording-systems was already being made by the staff of the three clinics. A weekly inter-clinic meeting was held by the Director for the discussion of administrative matters and for teaching and research. My own search for standards of diagnosis and terminology in the initial stages of the project coincided with similar researches by the staff so that we were able to work together and take joint decisions as to the methods to be used. Criticism of existing methods or any suggestions I made about, for instance, details of record-taking were examined and willingly followed up, while my long period of work with a highly trained staff helped me to realize the limitations on many finer points of our present-day research techniques.

Any study involving a manipulation of data obtained from an assessment of human behaviour will stand or fall by the scientific care with which individual observations or personality diagnoses are made, and nowhere is this more important than in studies of maladjusted children, where all too often diagnosis is made in a crude and unscientific manner, with snap judgements in two or three categories only, and with no sound theoretical basis for the classification. In the present study samples of delinquent and neurotic behaviour are compared in the hope that the conditions common to both, or conspicuously present in one and absent in the other, may be brought sharply into contrast in relation both to each other and to what is known about normal children. It must be emphasized from the outset, however, that it is the delinquent group that forms the more special subject of study and that the 'neurotic' group is in some ways regarded as meaning 'non-delinquent' or serving as a contrast to the delinquents. (The difficulties of selecting a satisfactory group of normal children as a

35

'control' group are referred to later, p. 50). The hypotheses to be tested are on the whole hypotheses about the aetiology of delinquency, and specific references to neurotic development are only secondarily included. This limitation is essentially one of size and scope and I envisage an approximately parallel investigation into the aetiology of neurotic behaviour. In so far as it provides a 'contrast' group, not a norm or standard, the neurotic group can be regarded as a 'control' group for the delinquents. While this latter term is usually reserved for a comparable group of normal cases, justification for comparing delinquents and neurotics or, as is frequently done, neurotics and psychotics, can be found when it is remembered that the control-group technique is essentially a substitute for experiment when conditions cannot be experimentally controlled (Mannheim, 1940), and permits of extension, within certain limitations, to two pathological groups.

Fifty delinquent and fifty neurotic children selected from over a thousand cases examined by the Child Guidance Service were the testing-ground for hypotheses taken both from statistical and psycho-sociological studies of delinquency and from psycho-analytic theories about character-formation. It was not the primary aim of our project to discover new data or even to invent new hypotheses; rather we aimed at an empirical examination of factual data by a combination of quantitative and clinical methods, which, while making full use of the psycho-analytic approach, would approximate as far as possible to the rigid standards required by experimental psychology.

THE PLAN OF RESEARCH

THE MATERIAL: CHILD GUIDANCE CLINIC CASES

The fifty delinquent and fifty neurotic children on whom our research was carried out were selected from a total of the first thousand cases examined in a selected rural Child Guidance Service during the years from 1946 to 1949. The cases were drawn in fairly even proportions from the three clinics in the service (each of which serves both town and country areas) and were considered to be fairly representative of the child population referred to the service.[1] There were in all about 20,000 children in the county, and the child guidance clinics, situated in three large towns, are open to all children up to the age of eighteen living in the area. No fees are charged, and children of all social strata have easy access to the clinics regardless of income or type of school attended. Their economic level ranges from that of poor 'problem' families to that of professional people and wealthy county families. The county at the present day is primarily devoted to agriculture, and there is a minimum of the social and economic problems found in crowded industrial towns. The background of the cases was extremely varied, children coming to the clinics from rural districts, agricultural villages, and seaside towns, as well as from urban centres.

The three clinics in the Child Guidance Service were organized to work as a unit in all important respects. The staffs met regularly for weekly case conferences and for scientific meetings which ensured that as well as having a common theoretical approach all used the same methods. In all matters concerning diagnosis a standard procedure was established for the three clinics, and a diagnostic assessment could only be reached after consideration by the psychiatrist, educational psychologist, psychiatric social worker and psycho-analyst or child psychotherapist in conference together upon the child. An important advantage was that I was at no time obliged to make my own decision about diagnosis, aetiology, or presence or absence of pathology. A psychiatric decision was, without exception, made by the 'psychiatric team', and throughout the whole research cases could be referred back to them for elucidation of doubtful points.

Since the methods of classifying childhood maladjustment used by different clinic services vary considerably, the system of diagnostic categories used in the Child Guidance Service is briefly described below.[2] It was worked out by Dr. Kate Friedlander and her staff during several years of team research work and after repeated experiments with various adaptations of the systems

---

[1] See *Table I*, p. 233, for sources of referral.

[2] This list of diagnostic categories is taken from the 1947 Annual Report of the senior psychiatrist of the Child Guidance Service.

developed by the Judge Baker Foundation and the Jewish Board of Guardians in the United States and the Institute for the Scientific Treatment of Delinquency in London.

Group I. Primary behaviour disorder. In this general group belong children who present problems like feeding difficulties, thumb-sucking, bed-wetting, difficulty in separating from their mothers, the milder forms of sleep disturbances, phobias of animals or other irrational fears, general restlessness, unhappiness and so on. These symptoms usually represent an exaggeration or prolongation of difficulties normally encountered during the various phases of a child's emotional development. For example, nightmares and fears which may occur commonly enough at certain stages in the early development of normal children would be placed in this category, whereas the same conditions occurring with great severity in an older child might be classified as neurotic tendencies.

Frequently these difficulties are caused by inappropriate handling during one or other developmental phase. To give greater flexibility in diagnosis three additional sub-groups may (or may not) be added, according to whether the clinical picture remains simple or is complicated by definite tendencies towards neurosis or delinquency, or both:

(*a*) Primary behaviour disorder with neurotic tendencies;
(*b*) Primary behaviour disorder with delinquent tendencies;
(*c*) Primary behaviour disorder with neurotic and delinquent tendencies.

In these sub-groups would be placed children showing distinct tendencies towards maladjustment that are not yet sufficiently pronounced in severity or in 'spread' throughout the whole personality to constitute a fully-developed neurosis, or a well-established and habitual delinquent behaviour pattern, or mixed types of behaviour involving some degree of both of these.

Group II. Secondary behaviour disorders. This term is used if the above difficulties occur as the outcome of an organic disease, such as meningitis, encephalitis, epilepsy, etc.

Group III. Primary antisocial conduct disorder. This category includes children who from very early ages are disobedient and unmanageable at home, who lie, steal, pilfer, stay out late at night, run away from home, are incorrigible and beyond control, or who in other ways show behaviour and attitudes towards their environment that could eventually lead to a violation of the law. To this category two sub-divisions may be added to distinguish mixed or borderline cases.

(*a*) Primary antisocial conduct disorder with neurotic tendencies;

(*b*) Primary antisocial conduct disorder with possible psychotic trends.

Group IV. Secondary antisocial conduct disorder. In this group are placed those cases where a history of delinquent behaviour as described above is thought to be the outcome of an organic illness, e.g. epilepsy, encephalitis, etc.

Group V. Neurosis. Under this heading are placed the comparatively small number of children and adolescents who present the outspoken picture of a classical neurotic illness such as hysteria, obsessional neurosis, anxiety hysteria or phobia. In the delinquent children in Groups III and IV the conflict between the child and his environment gives rise to behavioural and emotional disturbances; but in the neurotic child the conflict has become psychically internalized and its roots are unconscious.

Group VI. Adolescent disturbance. Two types of problem are frequently seen in adolescence. First, a group of extreme cases of emotional and behavioural disturbance to which even normally stable boys and girls are prone. Second, cases where a predisposition to mental instability had already existed in earlier years. In such children there may be a phase in puberty or adolescence where a boy or girl behaves in an abnormal way, e.g. has obsessional habits or hysterical fits, or is antisocial in conduct. Others who are even more severely disturbed may show signs of a deep depression or behave in bizarre ways. Only a very careful study

39

of the child's history can reveal whether the disturbance is appearing for the first time in puberty, or whether it has existed for a number of years but has become more pronounced during adolescence. In the first case, but not in the second, the child would be placed in this group. To this simple group may be added three sub-divisions where the form taken by the disturbance has been carried towards one or other extreme:

(*a*) Adolescent disturbance with neurotic tendencies;
(*b*) Adolescent disturbance with delinquent tendencies;
(*c*) Adolescent disturbance with possible pre-psychotic trends.

Group VII. Psychotic illness. In this group are placed the rare cases of definite psychosis and pre-psychotic illness in children, and cases thought to involve psychotic or pre-psychotic complications.

Group VIII. Organic disturbance. In this section is placed the relatively small number of cases seen in child guidance clinics where a behaviour disturbance is created by, or is secondary to, a constitutional weakness or an organic disease, e.g. chronic invalidism, diseases of the brain, hormonal disturbances, hyperthyroidism, Frohlich's disease, encephalitic symptoms, etc.

Group IX. Cases in which the diagnosis is not yet established. These are cases where the diagnosis has for one reason or another not been established by the time the case is withdrawn or closed. This group includes the many cases seen in child guidance clinics where the data available are for various reasons insufficient for the establishment of an adequate diagnostic assessment.

Group X. Intellectual backwardness. In this group are placed the intellectually subnormal, and dull and backward children whose disturbance does not belong primarily in one of the former groups, i.e. children who are intellectually rather than emotionally handicapped. Several secondary divisions are possible in this group but do not concern us here.

Group XI. Normal children. Normal children are sometimes brought to the clinics, not because of a real disturbance, but because the mother herself may be worried or has had no experience or knowledge of the behaviour of a small child at a certain developmental level. Occasionally, too, cases are found where a basically normal child has been placed in unsuitable or unusual circumstances to which he has reacted with temporarily difficult behaviour; or where the parent is in reality very disturbed and the child is not.

Agreement on the theoretical principles[1] underlying the use of the terms 'neurotic' and 'delinquent', and the addition of subdivisions to the foregoing groups, allowed for the finer differentiation of types according to the basic psychological tendencies *underlying* behaviour disturbances, and for a good deal of flexibility in their use. They also allowed for the amount of over-lap which is invariably found in individual borderline cases, e.g. a case of primary behaviour disturbance of delinquent type in a very dull adolescent girl might appropriately be classed in both Group VI (c) and Group X. Used in this way, and informed by an underlying theory about neurotic and antisocial character development, the diagnostic system was found to offer not only a workable basis for research in many directions within the clinics, but tentative lines of reference for a quantitative approach to some of the problems of delinquency. It first of all threw into focus the diagnostic confusion surrounding the use of the terms 'delinquent' and 'neurotic' with reference to behaviour problems of mixed psychological origin. It also offered the possibility of clarifying some of the obscurities in those sociological and statistical studies on delinquency which group together under the general heading of 'delinquency' a heterogeneous collection of recognizably different personality types.

PROBLEMS OF TERMINOLOGY AND DEFINITION

Before this system was put into operation throughout the service, diagnoses upon a number of sample cases were worked out in relation to the clinical pictures, including aetiology, and the definition of terms relating to specific disturbances. A study was made

---

[1] The school of psycho-analytic theory referred to throughout this book has been described with detailed reference to juvenile delinquency by Dr. Kate Friedlander in her book *The Psycho-analytical Approach to Juvenile Delinquency*, 1947.

of their place in the diagnostic system as seen in relation to Freudian psychological theory. Many subsidiary problems were also dealt with in the staff conferences and scientific meetings, and practical arrangements were made for the collection of data. I was able, with the interest and support of Dr. Friedlander, to present in these inter-clinic meetings an outline of the plans for research and from time to time to bring problems for elucidation or general discussion. The earlier talks with the staff were concerned with standardizing the meaning and usage of terms and establishing criteria for the effective use of the system of diagnostic categories. Later discussions dealt with how best to select the paired delinquent and neurotic groups to be contrasted, and with problems of aetiology in individual cases. Finally, the formulation of the hypotheses to be tested by this investigation was discussed, and owed much to the cooperation of the whole staff.

Ample time was taken over these preliminary discussions, since it is obviously impossible to examine *all* the psychological and sociological factors in the lives of all the children in a group of any size, and careful thought was given to the opinions of many experienced workers in the field about what goes to make a child delinquent or neurotic. A number of specific suggestions offered by members of the staff were included among the conditions examined. Some theoretical issues raised and practical decisions reached in these meetings are discussed later.

Delinquent Behaviour

An essential preliminary to the selection of cases for the project was to define delinquent behaviour. As Burt (1925), Alexander (1935), Friedlander (1947) and others have shown, all children have delinquent impulses to overcome. There is probably nobody who has not, at some time or other, committed some minor misdemeanour that is basically delinquent. Friedlander has pointed out that if the behaviour of two-year-old children left without supervision in a nursery were reproduced by adults, it would without question be termed antisocial behaviour. The small child is without shame, disgust, or pity; has no wish to be clean or to be clothed, and has no regard for the demands or for the desires of other people. Untended toddlers may be selfish, cruel, dirty, reckless and even savage in their behaviour towards each other. 'What is surprising' she writes, (1947, p. 13) 'is not that the small child is not socially adapted, or that he has impulses which are antisocial, but that the antisocial impulses so freely expressed at this early age, are tamed in a comparatively short time.' In a very few years the majority of toddlers have become socially adapted, but in a delinquent child a disturbance in his adaptation to socially accepted habits and behaviour leaves much of his antisocial behaviour unmodified.

Of all the problems of child development with which a child guidance clinic has to deal, delinquency more than any other is an environmental problem. Much delinquent behaviour will improve with a change to a more suitable environment and if this is maintained over a sufficient period the so-called delinquent behaviour will often disappear. This will depend, however, on many factors, especially on how far 'upstream' in his delinquent career the child is caught. In certain cases when the child is firmly set in antisocial or delinquent ways, he will not respond to ordinary changes in the environment. Some children have been found to be unchanged by long periods of so-called remedial education.[1] (See Case No. 49, Daisy.)

In very young children the prognosis is good if re-education can be carried on over a long period, e.g. for three or four years with the same person, whether with the probation officer, the foster-parents, or with a wise hostel staff. With older children who are confirmed delinquents genuine remedial treatment or re-education is much more difficult, but Aichhorn and Slavson, among others, have demonstrated that this is not impossible even with the most hardened cases.

For the purposes of our project we did not necessarily consider a child delinquent if he had committed only one theft or other antisocial act, or if he showed one persistent symptom. Stealing from home, for instance, particularly stealing food, is so common an occurrence among carefully investigated cases that it cannot be taken as a serious indication of a delinquent character. The child's behaviour must be examined in the light of his history and of other character traits, e.g. whether he can fit into a group of

[1] Cf. Willock, 1949.

his equals and obey the rules which make social life possible. It was not, however, considered necessary for a child to have behind him a long list of apprehended 'crimes' or a court charge of delinquency for him to be termed delinquent. There are many delinquent children, possibly the greater number, who never come before the juvenile courts, and there are some children charged before the courts who are not delinquent at all. A boy may be brought before the courts, for instance, as a member of a gang of young offenders. His behaviour, on the face of it delinquent, possibly arises from problems on the neurotic level involving submissive, passive-effeminate tendencies towards other boys. Without the gang on whom these tendencies have been focused, he may be able to withstand, as do the majority of normal boys, most of the ordinary temptations of a boy's life, while his neurotic tendencies find their outlet in other ways.

We therefore described a child as delinquent only when the 'crimes' for which he had been brought to the child guidance clinic or juvenile court had been considered in the light of the following factors: (1) other symptoms of maladjustment; (2) the history of his social development; (3) the onset and duration of his difficulties at the time of referral, i.e. whether these were deep-seated or merely adolescent difficulties or temporary reactive problems; (4) other character traits such as his ability to adapt his behaviour to the basic rules of social life without persistently reacting against the inevitable mild frustrations of family, school and elsewhere; (5) his ability to postpone immediate personal satisfactions, not necessarily antisocial in themselves, in favour of higher social aims; (6) the nature of his impulses themselves; (7) observations of his reactions, either in the past or during an experimental period, to various changes in his environment. Of these we considered that the most important favourable reactions were his ability to make a friendly and enduring relationship with one or more of the persons caring for him, and his ability to conform satisfactorily to the standards of conduct of his group, without resorting to antisocial or socially disruptive behaviour.

We discussed, from both practical and theoretical viewpoints, the earliest age at which a child might be considered to be delinquent, and we finally fixed on an age lower than that usually

44

accepted by writers on delinquency. We regarded a child as delinquent if his behaviour had been antisocial in many ways over a considerable period of time; and when he had failed to develop an independent moral code with the normal degree of control for his age group in guiding and restraining his actions. In psychoanalytic terms, a child could be called delinquent if he continued to show extreme forms of antisocial behaviour after he had entered the latency period, somewhere between the ages of 5 and 8. The cases in this study include children who had shown a history of outspoken delinquent behaviour since the age of four or five.[1] There are five cases of children between five and seven who had failed to reach the appropriate social habits and behaviour for their age and who already showed a definite break with social requirements, and there are ten cases of children between the ages of seven and nine who can clearly be termed *delinquent*, using the term to mean 'manifest' rather than 'latent' delinquency in the sense suggested by Aichhorn.

We only used the foregoing considerations as a guide, and in each case the final diagnosis was determined by the total picture of the child's personality and behaviour in response to his environment. On the whole, younger children presenting a picture of mild and recent delinquency without neurotic complications and responsive to environmental changes, were diagnosed under *Group I* (b) (primary behaviour disorder with delinquent tendencies), and these were not included in the present study. Cases with a long-standing history of delinquency which showed little or no neurotic involvement, had failed to respond to reasonable environmental changes, and for which assessments were unfavourable in most of the foregoing fields, were diagnosed under *Group III* (a) (primary antisocial conduct disorder) and these form the bulk of the delinquent cases in this study. The percentage of delinquents in whose behaviour neurotic manifestations play a part is rather high, but there are only a few well-defined types where the delinquent action can be regarded as a neurotic symptom, i.e. as an expression of an unconscious conflict. More frequently the antisocial behaviour is influenced by neurotic ten-

[1] A case in point is that of Peter (Case No. 2). This case has been described more fully by Dr. Friedlander in her paper 'Latent Delinquency and Ego Development', 1949a.

dencies which are slight and insufficient to explain a long history of delinquent acts, the motives for which are, in many cases, usually conscious. As far as it was possible to diagnose these cases, and within limits imposed by the number of cases available, children whose delinquency had a definite neurotic motivation were excluded from the present investigation, as also were all borderline and doubtful cases.

Neurotic Behaviour

An easier task than that of finding a satisfactory definition of delinquent behaviour was to find agreement among psychiatrists on the commonly accepted meaning of neuroses as illnesses of the mind that lead to the formation of psychogenic symptoms. We again adopted the policy of using an 'operational' definition, i.e. of classifying the cases according to the symptoms and behaviour displayed. Children were regarded as neurotic who showed certain behaviour manifestations commonly called neurotic symptoms, such as severe irrational fears, phobias, anxiety, inhibitions, hysterical or obsessional symptoms and so on. Only a relatively small number of children or young persons present an outspoken picture of a fully developed neurosis. Neurotic tendencies in a very definite form can, however, be recognized from early years in certain cases, just as they can be recognized in adults who suffer from neurotic difficulties, but owing to favourable circumstances never reach the point of a neurotic breakdown. In the present study only those cases were included which in the opinion of the psychiatric team showed the presence of a definite neurosis or of pronounced and long-standing neurotic tendencies.

Symptoms of fear and anxiety are commonly described by psychiatrists as the core of every neurotic condition. Neurotic fear and anxiety are present in typical cases as the indicator of an unconscious disturbance, and in many cases as its outcome also. A description of neurotic behaviour in children must therefore be a description of behaviour indicating either severe anxiety itself, or ways of fighting anxiety, or derivatives from these.

Children whose neurotic difficulties took a predominantly delinquent or violently aggressive form were excluded from the present study. Doubtful and borderline cases were also excluded,

THE PLAN OF RESEARCH

unless complete agreement was finally reached among the child guidance clinic staff, either through prolonged observation or in psychiatric treatment, that the child's disturbed behaviour pattern was unconsciously determined and therefore definitely neurotic.

PRELIMINARY STUDY

As a preliminary 'pilot study' (carried out in 1948) all cases referred to the three child guidance clinics during the first eighteen months after their opening, and upon which a psychological examination had been completed, were studied. These amounted to approximately 600 cases, coming under all diagnostic headings. From this first pool an examination was made of all cases falling into the following categories:

Group III. Primary antisocial conduct disorder (i.e. without apparent neurotic or pre-psychotic tendencies).

Group VI (b). Adolescent disturbance with delinquent tendencies (only those cases in which the delinquent tendencies were pronounced were included in this group).

Group V. Neurosis.

Group I (a) Primary behaviour disorder with neurotic tendencies (i.e. cases in which the neurotic tendencies were definite and pronounced).

At this point a careful check was made and all obviously doubtful, borderline or mixed cases were suspended. The lists of cases falling into the above groups were then divided and referred back to the clinic staffs for confirmation of the ratings 'definitely delinquent' or 'definitely neurotic' respectively. When borderline cases on which unanimous agreement could not be reached were rejected, a total remained of 194 cases in these two groups. These were provisionally termed *Preliminary Group I:* Delinquent Children, and *Preliminary Group II:* Neurotic Children. The average age and intelligence (Stanford-Binet I.Q. scores) of these

47

preliminary cases was then computed, and the two groups compared.[1] It was found that the delinquent child, who tends to be less intelligent than the normal child (Burt, 1925), is also likely to be older, and his difficulties will probably occur at a later age than those of the neurotic child. These tendencies were the same for both sexes.

These preliminary findings presented an initial problem for the planning of the present investigation. Since a significant difference was found between the age and intelligence level of the two groups, a comparison of the typical delinquent with the typical neurotic child would have involved comparing children of different ages and different intellectual abilities. The aim of the study, however, was to compare children of like ability at the same development level who had clearly taken *either* the neurotic or the delinquent line of development. It was therefore decided, in the final sample subsequently chosen, to exclude all delinquent children with intelligence lower than that of the least intelligent of the neurotic children (I.Q. 79), and all neurotic children with intelligence higher than that of the most intelligent delinquent (I.Q. 139).

FINAL SELECTION OF CASES

The next important consideration was the amount of information available about each case and this was found to vary considerably. A grading system was worked out according to the completeness of the data, and all the delinquent and neurotic cases were graded on the following scale:

A. Cases where treatment had been undertaken and satisfactorily terminated, i.e. a case where remedial treatment or psychotherapy had been successfully carried out and the case followed up. Such cases were often seen at regular interviews over a period of one to three years.

B. A current or incomplete treatment case where similar remedial treatment or psychotherapy had been undertaken and was well advanced, or had been carried on for a considerable period before being for some reason terminated.

[1] See *Tables* 2, 3, and 4, Appendix 1.

C. Cases where a full diagnostic examination had been undertaken and there was a full social history, an account of recommendations and disposal, and follow-up notes. Cases where treatment had consisted entirely of environmental manipulation or replacement and supervision were included here. Cases where this was allied with intensive psychotherapy were included under A or B.

D. A diagnostic case with a full social history but where certain psychiatric information or developmental data were for various reasons incomplete or unsatisfactory.

E. Cases where data were insufficient, e.g. the case had been withdrawn for certain reasons; the social history was incomplete; intelligence tests had not been undertaken, or the examination had for some other reason been very brief.

By the end of 1949 it was possible to examine a larger pool of approximately 1,000 cases seen in the three county clinics and from this the groups in the present study were drawn. It was decided to discard all delinquent children graded D or E so that the final selection of fifty delinquent children was made from cases that had been fully investigated from the psychiatric point of view. In many cases a record of treatment interviews was available; in others, information was available about observation periods, placement in hostels, home supervision, probation records, foster-home placements, and other remedial measures or vocational guidance undertaken with the child. In the case of neurotic children it was decided to discard all those rated C, D or E, leaving only cases that had been under psychological treatment for a considerable time. Full treatment notes, progress reports, and where treatment had been terminated, closure summaries and follow-up records, were therefore available for all the fifty neurotic children who were finally selected for study. These decisions considerably reduced the number of cases available, but were felt to be important, since finer observations on questions of character development are impossible unless cases have been studied in detail over a long period.

With these considerations in view details of the research pool of cases were represented graphically, and the graphs were

49

searched for fifty pairs of neurotic and delinquent children, determined by the same diagnostic procedure used in the preliminary study, and now matched for sex, age, and intelligence. A 'pair' consisted of a delinquent and a neurotic child of the same sex; between whom there was less than two years difference in age; less than ten points difference in I.Q. on the revised Stanford–Binet Intelligence Scale; and whose cases had been adequately investigated by the above standards. Twenty pairs of girls and thirty pairs of boys were selected by this method. Where several mates were possible for one child, the case was decided according to the completeness of the data available and the similarity of family circumstances.

Information about the fifty delinquent and fifty neurotic children who were finally selected for detailed investigation is given in the case history summaries contained in Part III.

LIMITATIONS IN THE MATERIAL

(a) Comparison with Normal Children
Throughout the first year of this research an attempt was made to find a third group of fifty normal children to be matched with the delinquent and neurotic groups. This attempt, however, proved discouraging and had to be abandoned. Although I was prepared to carry out tests of intelligence, to obtain educational and medical reports, and to take social histories of children in schools or from another normal population, there was no possibility of obtaining comparable psychiatric reports on normal children. Such a task is beset with difficulties, as Preston and Shepler (1931) have shown.[1] Nor was it possible to obtain data from prolonged observation or repeated interviews with the mothers of normal children that proved to be of such great importance in the other groups. Experienced clinicians and psychia-

---

[1] Preston and Shepler found that many types of behaviour commonly regarded as abnormal occurred fairly frequently in normal children. Of 100 'normal' children examined by them, approximately, one-third of the cases showed symptoms that would, by ordinary standards, mean referring them to a child guidance clinic. The authors conclude: '... the important fact from this study seems to be not that the problem patient showed peculiarities of behaviour in childhood, but that he did not succeed in eliminating them at some point in his development' (p. 253).

tric social workers are well aware that many of the items sought in a detailed and intimate history of a child's life are not disclosed by the mother or father during the initial interview. This is not necessarily due to lack of parental cooperation. The items may genuinely not be remembered, and in any case it is hardly surprising that information about traumatic experiences or family secrets, vitally important in a child's development, can be hidden or 'forgotten' until it is laboriously unearthed in a long series of interviews. Examples of this have been described by Bowlby (1949) and may be found in the records of almost any child guidance clinic.

An attempt made to find a control group from among the cases diagnosed as 'normal' in the child guidance clinic records had also to be abandoned, since it became clear that such a sample was too limited and comprised a highly selected group of 'normal' children.

(b) The Problem of Unknown Data

There were two aspects of this problem. First, the information about the child's inner life obtained from psychotherapeutic interviews was less complete for delinquent than for neurotic cases, since the problems of the treatment of delinquency are less understood. The kind of psychotherapeutic treatment available in a child guidance clinic is not usually suitable for delinquents; they frequently require long-term re-educational programmes which, even if planned and supervised by the psychiatrist, must be carried out in hostels, with probation officers or foster-parents or others. In many cases it was too early to assess the outcome of the measures recommended, and owing to the shortage of suitable homes and psychiatric hostels for maladjusted children, many delinquents could only be given interim support and guidance until such time as the recommendations of the clinic could be carried out.

Second, there was a marked difference, which when tested statistically was found to be significant, between the amount of data on the child's history available for each group. Detailed information about the delinquents was frequently unobtainable, and such facts as could be gathered were often vague, scrappy and not easily verifiable. The data on the neurotic children, on the other hand, were usually very full and well-organized and could be checked from many sources. It was found several times that a rather pedantic, obsessional type of neurotic mother who was full of anxieties and worries about her child had carefully recorded each step in her baby's development, together with snapshots, weight-charts and so on, in neatly bound booklets. She had written down the date of his first teething, when he first smiled, how he first learned to walk or began to speak, and many anecdotes and stories about his behaviour at every stage of his development. Much as the investigator was delighted with this profusion of recorded information, she could not help contrasting the frequently careless fashion in which data about the delinquent child's early years had been lost or forgotten. In the case of large poor families, for example, the mothers' observation of important details of the early years was often hopelessly vague, inaccurate, and unrecorded. This was also true of children whose families had moved about a great deal or had been broken by domestic discord or frequent separations; or of children who had spent some years of their life in institutions. In such cases the data sought for in an investigation of this kind are frequently unobtainable in spite of patient and painstaking inquiry. Typical of the difficulties encountered in research on delinquency are those in the case of Paddy (Case No. 13), where the information needed had perished with the child's mother. In several cases the difficulty proved insuperable.

METHODS OF APPROACH

The procedures used in the project will only be briefly stated here, since I have so presented the results in Part II in such a way that the details of method are implicit. After final selection and matching of the fifty pairs of delinquent and neurotic children, a collection of all the relevant information available about each case was made according to a system outlined in Appendix I (p. 487). From the dossiers collected about each child a case summary was made and all the important factual information for each case was tabulated and transferred to master cards.

After a survey of the theoretical field a list was then compiled of some 300 conditions to be examined and compared as to their incidence in the background and life stories of the children in the respective groups. This method may be compared to sinking shafts into various levels and phases of the children's lives and 'sampling' a wide assortment of the circumstances and experiences which may have influenced them in taking contrasting routes in emotional and social development.

CONDITIONS TO BE INVESTIGATED

In this project emphasis was placed primarily, though not entirely, on the aetiology of delinquent disorders. The chief research procedures were therefore designed to test the validity of certain hypotheses about delinquent character formation and delinquent behaviour. Some items of interest for neurotic development were also included, but a fuller elucidation of causative factors in neurotic behaviour would require much further study.

It was decided to divide the conditions to be compared in these two matched groups of children into three main sections as follows:

I. Those conditions which had led to the child's breakdown in adjustment to community life, i.e. his symptoms, behaviour, and emotional conditions on referral to the clinic.

II. Those conditions which characterized the child's home and family background and related to his social setting.

III. Those conditions thought to have played a possibly significant role in the child's development and personal history.

A summary of the results of the research into these three large areas of observation is presented in Part II under these chapter headings—Chapter III: 'The Child at Large'; Chapter IV: 'The Child at Home'; and Chapter V: 'The Child Himself'. The considerations that led to the decision to divide up the survey of material in this way are given briefly below.

I. *Symptoms, behaviour, and emotional conditions.* This was arrived at

c

by an empirical grouping together and examination of the symptoms, emotional characteristics, and behavioural record for which each child was referred to the child guidance clinic, plus certain observations made on the child while he was examined in the clinic. The intention was to provide data about the child's emotional condition as revealed through the picture he presented to the observer that would serve as a supplement to the factual data examined later. It was also aimed to draw a fairly sharp distinction between disturbances characteristic of the delinquent child and those characteristic of the neurotic child as revealed in the child's general behaviour. An attempt was made to find three groups of emotional characteristics or symptoms that would include, respectively: (1) all behaviour commonly thought to be characteristic of delinquents; (2) all behaviour thought to be characteristically neurotic; (3) a miscellaneous group of other behavioural characteristics not regarded, in common practice, as either typically delinquent or typically neurotic. A certain degree of overlap was clearly inevitable, but this was minimized by the care taken during the selection of cases to omit as far as possible all obviously borderline cases (see p. 45). It was expected to find that the group of delinquent characteristics would appear very frequently in the delinquent group and less frequently in the neurotic group; and that the group of neurotic characteristics would occur very frequently in the neurotic group and less frequently among the delinquent children. Should these assumptions be borne out by the project it would confirm the assumption underlying the decision to select two pathological groups: i.e. that the delinquent and the neurotic form more or less distinct groups and can be distinguished on behavioural and possibly also on aetiological grounds.

In grouping items into behavioural sub-sections (1) and (2) we followed common psychiatric, social, and legal practice in regard to delinquent and neurotic behaviour, irrespective of the expectations of Freudian diagnostic theory. Sub-section (3) included a remaining miscellaneous or 'neutral' group of difficult traits, symptoms, habits, and behaviour for which children had been referred to the clinic. This large loose group consisted of characteristics that do not fall readily into the commonly accepted

54

behavioural descriptions of delinquency or neurosis, or which, though often observed in such children, have not been given a place in the usual diagnostic systems. We considered this miscellaneous group to be of theoretical interest both for the aetiology and treatment of delinquent and neurotic conditions, since it contains characteristics which are treated with varying importance by different theorists, and which we hoped to define in a more exact way.

Two examples from the miscellaneous conditions examined under this sub-section may serve to illustrate this point. First, the child's adjustment at school. It is commonly known that the delinquent tends to be backward in school and that dullness of intellect may contribute indirectly to delinquency. In this project, however, the level of intelligence for both groups was the same. Comparison could therefore be made between the teacher's estimate of the degree of educational backwardness and the educational psychologist's assessment after his diagnostic examination. It was also possible to compare the children in each group who were not generally retarded in school work, but who had undue difficulty in mastering a special subject in the school curriculum; for instance, a boy who was inhibited in all subjects requiring the expression of aggression, or who could not succeed in geography because he could not remember the shape of maps; or a girl who could not compete in subjects such as biology or mathematics or in other fields which she had come to regard as strictly masculine territory. Psycho-analytic theory explains such retardation in a special subject by saying that it arises from unconscious conflicts which have become focused on a particular form of learning. If this explanation is valid, one might expect to find specific learning inhibitions more frequently in the neurotic than in the delinquent children, whereas general educational retardation might be expected to occur in children in either group.

A second example from the miscellaneous section is of particular interest in comparing delinquent and neurotic children, who, from an early age or over a considerable period, imitate the behaviour of the opposite sex. I was struck by the number of times the description of behaviour for which the child was brought to the clinic included complaints of girlish behaviour in boys, or tomboyish, masculine behaviour in girls. The latter type of case was frequently summed up in the remark: 'The trouble is she *ought* to have been a boy.' Freud (1905) showed that some disturbance in the individual's ability to accept his own biological sexual role, or some confusion in the normal identification with his own sex, can be found at the root of many neurotic conditions, and especially in those common forms involving the repression of unconscious homosexual tendencies. By comparing the numbers of children in the two groups who imitated the interests and general behaviour of the opposite sex, it was hoped to find another opportunity of testing the validity of the Freudian theory of the sexual aetiology of the neuroses. Benedict (1939) and Mead (1949) have also shown the vital part played by the child's imitation of or identification with the parent of its own sex in problems connected with proper adjustment to masculinity or femininity. They have shown that sexual inversion among primitives arises only in cultures that regard certain activities as specifically feminine or masculine, and occurs to a lesser extent in those that do not emphasize this sexual distinction.

The wide range of problems that fell into sub-section (3), the miscellaneous section, revealed that almost every aspect or level of the child's life presents difficulties of some kind or other in delinquent or neurotic children. It was therefore decided to break the group up into a number of sub-divisions, and these are described in further detail in Chapter IV.

II. *Home and family background.* This was divided into two main groups: (1) social and environmental conditions; (2) family background. As will become evident, this section owes much, on the one hand, to classical pioneering studies in the psycho-sociology of delinquency such as those of Healy, Healy and Bronner, Burt, Shaw, and Mannheim and, on the other, to the psycho-analytic studies of Aichhorn, Anna Freud, Friedlander, Glover, and Bowlby.

III. *The child's development and personal history.* This set of conditions was concerned with the child's personal history and with some of his developmental and educational experiences. It included the child's health and physical condition, a wide range of items from his earlier history and upbringing, and an examination of his present interests and achievements.

FORMULATION OF HYPOTHESES

At this stage of the work these three research areas were scrutinized and expectations formulated with regard to certain hypotheses about delinquent and neurotic children. To avoid repetition here and constant cross-reference, these hypotheses are set out in the following three chapters in such a way that they may be immediately compared with our findings on the conditions to which each refers.

STATISTICAL PROCEDURES

One of the main objects of my research was to test statistically certain hypotheses about delinquent and neurotic development. A number of statistical procedures are available for assessing the precise significance to be attached to the discrepancies found between actual observation or fact, and the consequences which are deduced to follow from an hypothesis. The first of the modern tests of significance was suggested by Karl Pearson in 1900[1] and is known as X^2 (Chi-square). This test provides an objective assessment of the agreement between fact and theoretical expectation, where the comparison is based upon the counting of instances belonging to certain categories or classes, as distinct from comparison based upon measurement.

My aim was to establish differences between observed and expected distributions of data, i.e. to make a rigorous comparison between the numbers actually observed to fall into any one category and the numbers expected on the basis of an hypothesis. In other words, I wanted to test whether the observed distribution of characteristics in the sample (i.e. the set of observations) was such that it could reasonably be granted to be drawn from a parent population such as was implied in the given hypothesis.

As an index of the relation between the observed frequencies and those expected on the basis of a given hypothesis, I decided to use the statistic X^2 for which the distribution was known, thus

[1] *Philosophical Magazine*, Vol. 50, pp. 157–75.

permitting determination of associated probabilities. Pearson's X^2 distribution was used, together with Fisher-Yates' correction for small samples (Fisher, 1941; see also Appendix 1). The chief advantage of the X^2 test is that it provides a precise measure of the probability that observed and expected occurrences differ significantly. Although data characterized in terms of qualitative differences do not permit the calculation of a correlation co-efficient by the ordinary product-moment formula or by rank methods, an index of the degree of association between a set of scores and a two-category classification such as is given in the present data may be obtained by arranging the data in a 2 × 2-fold table (both variables being dichotomous) and calculating a modified form of the product-moment coefficient, namely, tetrachoric r. The advantage of tetrachoric r is that it allows the calculation of the correlation between two characters of attributes, neither of which is directly measurable, but both of which are capable of being grouped into at least two categories. For example in finding the correlation between delinquency and absence of fathers, the children might be classified on the one hand into those who are delinquent and those who are not, and on the other hand into those whose fathers are absent and those whose fathers are present. For practical purposes it was necessary to make an assumption, when examining various conditions in this special group of delinquents, that neurotics could be treated as non-delinquents. This meant that, as far as delinquency was concerned, the neurotics could be regarded as representative of the general clinic population of maladjusted children from which both samples were drawn. It might be assumed that the groups were evenly distributed in this population. While keeping the arbitrary nature of this assumption in mind, I thought it worth while to include in the results a tetrachoric correlation, which was calculated in each case except where the numbers were very small.

Any attempt to compare the results obtained from the present groups of delinquent and neurotic children with those obtaining in the general population would, in the absence of a 'normal' control group, be premature. Moreover, since a large group is desirable when probability relations are under consideration, the results obtained from the small groups in the present study can carry no very great conviction by themselves. Their value lies rather in establishing preliminary findings that may be checked by more refined methods in larger-scale investigations as our knowledge increases.

In any reasoning from the general principles of probability, great difficulties arise in trying to estimate the 'true' percentage of an hypothetical total population. No exact means, fine enough for the requirements of accurate research, are available for testing the normality of distributions such as we found in our project. For example, among other differences suspected and unsuspected, the sample of delinquent children drawn from the selected clinics was shown to differ in an important respect, namely the social level of the parents, from that reported in the majority of studies of delinquents in other parts of the United Kingdom. The distribution of delinquents, according to the present careful definition of delinquency, is not known either for this county or for any other area, and any estimate is inevitably unreliable. Standards of psychological examination at present in use in child guidance clinics and in the many other organizations dealing with the maladjusted child, vary too much for their existing statistical data to be regarded as comparable. It is to be hoped that with more uniform standards for psychological and psychiatric examinations, more reliable data of this sort may gradually become available. All that can be claimed from the data in this study and the methods used to analyse it, is that in the samples of children actually compared the division into delinquent and non-delinquent did not arise by chance, but is in some way related to the cross-division obtained on the various conditions enumerated. It does not necessarily follow that there would be a similar relation between delinquency and non-delinquency, i.e. neuroticism, in other samples, nor in the general population.

To sum up, the use of the chi-square test in the present investigation was straightforward and the problem a typical one. We tested whether the frequency of occurrence of facts reported in the life histories of the delinquent and neurotic children differed significantly from the frequency of occurrence of the same facts deducible from a Null hypothesis (Fisher, 1941). However, when relative association has been tested by chi-square, the presence of positive associations revealed, and the degree of association calculated as a correlation coefficient, the fact of correlation is not claimed to 'prove' that the condition was an effective cause. In practice, it was possible rather to make statements in terms of good approximations and maximum likelihood than to draw precise conclusions or 'proof' about the operation of alleged causal factors. The methods selected allow only for a statement of more or less strong indication that the hypothesis accounts for, or fails to account for, the whole of the facts.

PART TWO

PRESENTATION OF RESULTS

CHAPTER III

The child at large: a behavioural picture

This chapter describes the results of our research into the symptoms and emotional conditions found in the delinquent and neurotic children on referral to the clinics. It gives, as it were, a dual picture of the two contrasting groups: (a) as seen by the community which reacts to their 'nuisance-value' (i.e. their outwardly observed behaviour), and (b) as seen in the emotional sufferings and psychological symptoms of the disturbed persons (i.e. their inner difficulties as observed in clinical case history records).

The first group of results in this section concern characteristics of delinquent behaviour, i.e. the many kinds of aggressive and antisocial conduct inherent in everyday legal and psychiatric descriptions of delinquency. The tables of results show the frequency with which each condition occurred in the two groups, and the totals, unless otherwise indicated, represent the number out of a possible fifty cases. Where the total for various reasons is less than fifty this has been indicated.

GROUP I. CHARACTERISTICS OF DELINQUENT BEHAVIOUR

1. *Stealing, pilfering, forgery, and embezzlement.* Cases were included where stealing had been repeated or carried on for some period of time; where it was recognized by the child's family as a problem; and, as in the majority of cases, where the problem had failed to respond to ordinary methods of correction.

2. *Lying.* Telling fibs, inventing 'stories', or denying facts to gain material advantage, to get out of trouble, or to get another child into trouble, are referred to here, rather than 'imaginative lying' or 'romancing', which is included in the later miscellaneous section.

3. *Truanting.* Truanting was counted as one of the child's problems only when it was a well-established habit or a frequent occurrence in response to certain situations.

4. *Wandering, running away from home or school, staying out late at night.* This section included all cases of wandering, repeatedly staying out late at night, or running away without adequate reason.

5. *Aggressive or destructive behaviour.* Under this heading was included aggressive or destructive behaviour of an extreme type such as housebreaking, malicious damage, much fighting, marked aggressiveness towards other children, and destruction of other people's or the child's own property. Extreme general destructiveness dating from very early childhood was also included, e.g. Case No. 20, Ian.

6. *Quarrelsomeness; tormenting, provocative behaviour.* This section included quarrelsome, mischievous, trouble-making, or ugly-tempered behaviour that could be regarded as typical of the child in his attitude towards people. Such quarrelsome behaviour is open and undisguised and frequently its object is to provoke other people to respond in a certain way. Quarrelsome and ill-tempered behaviour is typical also of certain types of neurotic condition, but there it is expressed in much more hidden, subtle, or complicated ways. The type of habitually tormenting, provocative behaviour, with violent sado-masochistic relationships, or undisguised callous and sadistic behaviour that is found in many delinquent children, can usually be recognized as distinct from the anxiety-ridden, compulsive aggressiveness of certain neurotic children.

7. *Extreme disobedience and defiance.* Disobedience to and defiance of parents, whether caused by the child's intractability to discipline or provoked by weak or misguided handling by the parents, constitute some of the most frequent reasons for regarding the child as 'difficult'. In this category were placed children whose disobedience and defiance towards those in authority had become troublesome and habitual, but had not yet taken the form of flagrant rebellion described in the following section.

8. *Unmanageable or 'beyond control'.* These were children in whom rebellion against authority was habitual, extreme, and violent, e.g. a child described by a headmaster who had had thirty years' experience with difficult boys as 'beyond my control' (Case No. 17, Monty); or a child described by an equally experienced probation officer as 'the most difficult child I have ever had to deal with' (Case No. 20, Ian). Some of the worst juvenile court cases were included here.

9. *Openly hostile to parents and teachers, or 'up against authority'.* Opposition to authority is typically the starting-point for much delinquent behaviour, and may lead to flouting the codes of social and moral behaviour that the adults in authority represent. Included in this group were children who were hostile, defiant, and provocative towards all authority—parents, teachers, probation officers, and representatives of the law. Also included were those whose rebellion was specifically against authority rather than against social standards only; those who showed their rebellion by being passive, spiteful, and sly; and those who were openly defiant.

10. *Cruelty to animals or younger children.* Cruelty is commonly recognized as a passing phase in childhood that, under educational pressure, is disguised or sublimated into more acceptable behaviour as the child progresses beyond the early phases of his emotional development. Here the children had shown unrestrained and quite outspoken cruelty far beyond the usual age. One child, for example, took sadistic pleasure in torturing cats or birds (Case No. 16, Jonathan); another organized a gang for the purpose of whipping other boys (Case No. 20, Ian). Some were so cruel to younger siblings that they endangered their safety (Case No. 41, Maureen). Cruelty in a more subtly disguised and less easily apprehended form is commonly observed at an early stage in the development of certain neurotic conditions, particularly in obsessional neurosis. This, however, is partially repressed and later becomes closely associated with guilt and anxiety. The cases included here refer only to gross and outspoken cruelty that is in no way disguised, and the motives for which are usually conscious, i.e. the desire to hurt or to inflict pain.

65

11. *Incorrigible, impervious to punishment, does not respond to ordinary discipline.* These consisted of juvenile recidivists and children to whom the ordinary methods of correction in home, school, the juvenile courts, or elsewhere had been patiently and persistently applied without altering the child's behaviour. Difficulties in the treatment and re-education of this type of delinquent are known to be very great because of their emotional hardening and repeated failure to adapt to social standards. Ordinary methods of character education are not likely to succeed since the child has failed to progress beyond a certain level of emotional development, and the basis for moral and social education has therefore not yet been formed. Methods, such as those of Aichhorn and Slavson, that can be expected to succeed in cases of this kind are slowly being developed, but it is of interest to note what proportion of delinquent children fall into this 'incorrigible' category.

12. *Member of tough or aggressive gang.* All these were children who organized or belonged to an aggressive gang. A juvenile court conviction for delinquent behaviour as a cooperative member of a gang was also included here.

13. *Verbal aggressiveness.* Under this heading were included all children whose cheeky, insolent, and rude behaviour, or whose swearing and use of bad language and obscenities, were sufficiently persistent to be complained of by parents or teachers. Aggressiveness on the verbal level is more highly controlled than gross cruelty or physical aggression, and is therefore likely to be found to a considerable extent in some neurotic disturbances. On the whole, however, open verbal aggressiveness is thought to be more characteristic of the delinquent.

HYPOTHESIS: Characteristics of Delinquent Behaviour
We should expect to find that each of the above types of delinquent behaviour occurs more frequently among delinquent than among neurotic children. (Confirmed.)

The results in *Table 5*, Appendix 1, show that there is in each case a significant difference between delinquent and neurotic children in the numbers of cases showing these types of delinquent behaviour. We may conclude that our selection of the characteristics of delinquent behaviour was made on a valid basis, and that the behaviour described can be regarded as characteristic of delinquent children. There is a high positive correlation between delinquency and each of the observed behavioural characteristics in this table.

Examples of Delinquent Behaviour

1. *Stealing, pilfering, forgery, and embezzlement.* Thefts occurred in a number of interesting ways. There were cases of stealing from the mother, stealing in order to spend money upon other children (i.e. riding in a taxi); stealing by collecting money under false pretences in the street (e.g. for a bogus 'Spitfire Fund'); stealing flowers from other people's gardens, stealing and spending sweet coupons not belonging to the child, stealing from the cloakrooms or from other children's coat-pockets at school, stealing from a bookstall, stealing from neighbours' houses; stealing such items as a watch, fountain pen, pencil, etc., from a brother or boy cousin; stealing lipstick, face-powder or make-up from women and girls; stealing from the mother such small objects as a cochineal bottle (at first thought to be red ink), or bottles containing medicine or inhalation (thought to be poison or some other dangerous substance); stealing by not returning change after shopping expeditions; stealing food in an unusual way (e.g. leaving always one part behind, one lump of sugar, one currant, or a tiny portion of cheese after the child had eaten the rest); stealing by 'borrowing' such items as bicycles or tricycles from another child; obtaining money under false pretences (e.g. from the mother on the pretence of buying school savings stamps, or from the neighbours or shopkeepers in pretence of borrowing a shilling for the mother 'for the gas'); stealing trinkets from Woolworth's; stealing from the father (e.g. many cases of stealing the father's watch, the father's jack-knife or fountain pen); stealing the baby's food; stealing sweets; stealing and hiding another child's ring or cap or scarf; having 'a mania for pens'; stealing fruit from fruit barrows; taking jewellery (e.g. necklaces, bracelets, hair slides) from the mother or grandmother; stealing money

67

which is left lying about in the house or near the house (e.g. the milk money, money left for the baker or the insurance money); stealing and tearing up a £1 note; stealing from mother's or sisters' post office savings boxes; stealing unused railway tickets from the booking office at the railway station; stealing a supply of Christmas sweets father had hidden away; stealing mother's cigarette lighter; stealing up to £10 in notes and half-crowns from the grandmother in order to buy books and toys or to go to the pictures; begging money with 'hard-luck' stories; stealing money from school fares or school lunch money; stealing over a long period before and after a time when a child was encouraged to thieve in a concentration camp; breaking a shop window in order to steal a Red Indian suit; stealing over a long period since the age of four or six years such things as eggs from neighbouring farms; breaking into ex-commando's stores and taking hand-grenades; stealing several bicycles in one day; stealing, with the obvious intention of being found out, small items from home or school; stealing a razor and torch and trying to sell them; stealing from an orchard; stealing five pounds' worth of paraffin for a bonfire; embezzling the sum of £50 over a period of months from his employer; forging a cheque in his mother's name and trying to cash it; stealing money from home to buy a pair of skates immediately after the mother had bought him a pair which he considered not good enough; house-breaking and rifling a gas-meter; a long history of stealing in the home (e.g. Case No. 15, Donald. 'Donald has always stolen'); stealing from the mother a wristwatch and throwing it away.

Only three cases of stealing were found amongst the neurotic children and these were: persistent stealing of food from the larder in a home where this was strictly forbidden (Case No. 85: Jean); pilfering paper, string or other oddments left lying about and 'finding' things at school (Case No. 54, Jackie); petty pilfering at school (Case No. 71, Gregory).

2. *Lying.* Lying occurred very commonly in the delinquent children, and its motives were varied. Examples were: lying in order to deny misdeeds and to get out of trouble; deceiving the mother in order to gain the child's own ends; lying in order to get

another child into trouble; pointless and impulsive lying; story-telling, boasting and self-aggrandisement; lying in order to maintain a pose (impostor type); lying for purposes of alibi; lying plausibly with pleasure in deceiving another person; a bare-faced and defiant lie to achieve the child's own ends; lying in order to maintain former lies; lying in order to maintain a fantasy; prevarication; and lying in order to be found out.

The four cases of lying observed amongst the neurotic children were lying to avoid getting into trouble or lying to support fantasied exploits (Case No. 54, Jackie); lying to avoid getting into trouble for meddling with others at school (Case No. 71, Gregory); 'bouts' of lying and fantasying to get other boys into trouble (Case No. 63, Charles); and lying to deceive a hated stepmother (Case No. 98, Ruth).

3. *Truancy.* Truanting occurred among the delinquent children in many forms. Examples were: solitary truanting; truanting in couples or groups; a child who incited other children to go with him; secret truanting over a long period; isolated episodes of truanting; truanting in order to go to the pictures, or to spend a day upon the beach; truanting to avoid facing up to trouble at school; truanting with the purpose of running away from school; truanting in order to go shoplifting; truanting to join undesirable friends; irresponsible and impulsive truanting; truanting in imitation of an admired older boy and father; and truanting with a definite object (to 'check up' on the mother who deceived her).

Truanting occurred in only three cases amongst the neurotic children. One case (Case No. 57, Bertie) who hated school and refused to attend, had been very upset when forced against all his pleadings to return, and later began to truant.Truanting occurred, together with episodes of 'wandering', in one child (Case No. 55, Billie), and another girl truanted to avoid the consequences when the untruth of her 'romances' was discovered at school (Case No. 91, Patricia).

4. *Wandering and running away.* Among delinquent children, wandering and running away usually occurred in a direct and unmistakable form. Examples were: running away from school

or from home; running away after punishment and trouble at home; running away from a home where a child feels rejected; staying out late at night with other boys; staying out with mischievous intent; staying out late with men or 'exposed to moral danger'; sleeping out under hedges, in air raid shelters or in a telephone box; compulsive wandering (wanderlust); running away from home in order to take a job or to try to join one of the Services; repeatedly running away from home to avoid the cruelty of the father; wandering into other children's homes which were happier and more attractive than her own; absconding from a remand home; running away from home to avoid expected punishment from foster-parents; repeatedly running away from boarding school; and cases of aimless wandering.

Among the neurotic children, wandering and staying out occurred only in three boys, and in less definite forms, as when associated with a symptom (Case No. 55, Billie); associated with neglect (Case No. 53, Colin); or in the case of a stepchild who often stayed out all night after punishment (Case No. 63, Charles).

5. *Aggressive and destructive behaviour.* Among the delinquent children, extremely aggressive and destructive behaviour involving malicious damage, housebreaking, much fighting, or sadistic behaviour towards other children occurred in about half the cases. Examples included destroying toys; destroying other people's property; violent behaviour towards teachers and others at school; kicking and doing physical damage during temper tantrums; destructive or violent behaviour towards animals or toys; putting destructive chemicals on dolls' faces; stealing with violence; aggression towards the mother amounting to physical attacks; 'brainstorms' at school in which the child does physical damage; and outbreaks of uncontrollable aggressiveness with screaming and rages.

Among the neurotic children, extremely aggressive and destructive behaviour occurred in only four cases. One case involved a phase in a young child of extreme destructiveness towards toys (Case No. 82, Laura); in another, aggressive behaviour at home was associated with hysterical symptoms, threats to kill the mother and temper tantrums (Case No. 90, Dorothy). In the third case, destructive behaviour, spilling and smashing things in a foolish, clumsy way, was associated with a neurotic disturbance involving greediness and feelings of inferiority towards others (Case No. 94, Juliet). In the fourth, wildly aggressive behaviour, including threats to kill in temper tantrums, occurred in a severely neurotic boy (Case No. 60, Irving).

6. *Quarrelsome and tormenting, provocative behaviour.* This occurred in many of the children who were also described as 'beyond control'. Examples are: Case No. 34, Ellen, who is quarrelsome and so spiteful with her brother and with children at school that she is rejected by them and excluded from their games; and Case No. 7, Felix, who is the 'scapegoat' of the district. In the case of No. 35, Maryann, similar behaviour has reached violent extremes of sado-masochism. Other cases, e.g. No. 38, Susan, and No. 17, Monty, show this behaviour to a pronounced degree towards one parent; their provocation, which goes on 'from morning to night', extends to physical attack. Cases such as No. 48, Monica, and No. 12, Carl, are quarrelsome in all their social relationships, following an aggressive family pattern. Quarrelsome and tormenting behaviour also occurred among a number of neurotic children in varying forms, e.g. Cases No. 86, Elspeth; No. 90, Dorothy; No. 85, Jean; and No. 60, Irving.

7. *Extreme disobedience and defiance.* This was of frequent occurrence among boys and girls alike, and was one of the commonest reasons for referring a child to the clinic. All the cases so far discussed might be taken as examples. Others among the delinquent children are: Cases No. 32, Freda; No. 47, Sarah; No. 41, Maureen; No. 20, Ian; and No. 27, Jeremy. Among the neurotic children disobedience and open defiance were very much less frequent, but occurred in pronounced forms in certain types of neurotic condition, e.g. Cases No. 82, Laura; No. 98, Ruth; No. 86, Elspeth; and No. 76, Rollo.

8. *Unmanageable, beyond control.* None of the neurotic children was described as 'beyond control' by parents or teachers, but this was a description very commonly given to the worst types of

delinquent cases. Examples were Cases No. 34, Ellen; No. 35, Maryann; No. 47, Sarah; No. 3, Derek; and No. 17, Monty.

9. *Hostile to parents and teachers, 'up against authority'*. Examples of cases showing special hostility to parents or teachers, or children who 'carry a chip on the shoulder' and are ready to attack all adults who represent authority, were the following: Cases No. 38, Susan; No. 48, Monica; No. 35, Maryann; and No. 4, Reginald among the delinquents. Certain types of neurotic children, e.g. Cases No. 76, Rollo, and No. 86, Elspeth, also showed this attitude to a marked degree.

10. *Gross or open cruelty to animals or younger children*. Cruelty among delinquent children was found in several cases to be associated with sadistic behaviour, that is to say pleasure in hurting or tormenting others or in being cruel to animals, e.g. Cases No. 20, Ian, and No. 34, Ellen. In one child this appears to have been an isolated and temporary phase of 'torturing birds' (Case No. 16, Jonathan), but in others it was a regular form of behaviour towards other children, for which these children were notorious, e.g. Cases No. 35, Maryann; No. 44, Doreen; and No. 3, Derek.

11. *Incorrigible, impervious to punishment, does not respond to ordinary discipline*. None of the neurotic children was described as incorrigible or impervious to punishment, and all were more or less responsive to ordinary discipline. Examples of the delinquent children who were described as 'incorrigible' and failed to respond to patient and continued application of normal methods of discipline were Cases No. 34, Ellen; No. 35, Maryann; No. 5, Thomas; and No. 12, Carl.

12. *A member of a tough or aggressive gang*. Delinquent examples of this were Cases No. 3, Derek; No. 28, Steven; and No. 20, Ian. No neurotic children were found to have been members of an aggressive gang. (This finding, like several others in this group, is probably a result of the exclusion, as far as possible, of cases showing both delinquent and neurotic tendencies.)

13. *Verbal aggressiveness: cheeky, insolent, rude; swearing and bad language.* Of the eighteen cases in this section twelve were from the group of twenty girls. Their use of bad language, both towards adults and towards each other, ranged from cheekiness, rudeness, slandering, shouting, and insolence to outbursts of violent swearing and 'slanging matches'. These compare with types Slavson has described as 'oral aggressives', whom he found very resistant to group treatment. Examples were Cases No. 48, Monica; No. 44, Doreen; No. 47, Sarah; and No. 35, Maryann. Examples from the delinquent boys were Cases No. 15, Donald, and No. 6, Ernest.

GROUP 2. CHARACTERISTICS OF NEUROTIC BEHAVIOUR

A number of characteristics commonly regarded as typical of neurotic disturbances were grouped under the following headings, and their incidence in the two groups is compared in *Table* 6, Appendix 1. These included neurotic fear and anxiety, passive and submissive behaviour, depression and depressive states, inhibited and subdued behaviour, and hysterical and obsessional traits.

1. *Fears and phobias.* Neurotic fears may be attached to an infinite number of external objects and are usually clearly distinguishable from normal fears, not so much by their content as by their persistence in spite of all 'reasonable' attempts at control. Cases were included here of children who showed, among the problems for which they were referred to the clinic, irrational and persistent fears with which the parents had not been able to deal as they had with objective fears, i.e. fear of real danger, air-raids, etc. Neurotic fears may be prolonged or intensified by the fact that they are also felt by a parent or another sibling, and they may or may not have developed into a true phobia. Attention was paid less to the attachment of a fear to a specified object or content than to the general fearfulness observed in the child's nature. Children were included here who may be described

73

merely as 'extremely fearful' or 'full of fears', or 'afraid of his own shadow'.

2. *Over-anxious behaviour.* Under this heading were included all cases of children who were described as being typically 'over-tense', 'worries a lot', 'easily frightened', 'looks for something to worry about'. These are types of behaviour that, when part of the child's habitual response and not a response to recent individual experiences, indicate the presence of deeper anxieties. Other cases of overt anxiety, 'free-floating anxiety', anxiety states, and so on were also represented here (if not included under the heading of 'Fears and phobias').

3. *'Nervous and highly strung'.* Under this heading were included all children described by family or teachers as 'nervous', 'highly strung', 'over-sensitive', etc. Such behaviour was indicative of marked inability to bear anxiety.

4. *Tearful, cries easily, easily upset.* An unusual amount of crying often indicates a latent state of tension or anxiety, e.g. the child seems to be always depressed and ready for bad luck, failure, or general misery. Included here were all children who were quickly upset and cried easily and inconsolably without adequate cause and at unsuitable times, such as in the street or in school.

5. *Pavor nocturnis, frequent nightmares, or anxiety dreams.* These cases all suffered from some kind of night terror at the time of the research. (They were distinguished from cases who showed sleep disturbance only during early development. The latter were included in a later set of conditions under the heading 'Difficulties in early habit-training'. They were also distinguished from other forms of sleep disturbance included under the more comprehensive heading 'Neurotic disorders of organ function'.)

6. *Babyish, dependent behaviour.* Under this heading were included all kinds of immature behaviour resulting from fearfulness, passivity, inhibition, and other causes. Examples are: inability to separate from mother, demonstrations of helplessness, extreme dependence and babyishness, especially in personal matters, beyond the age at which this can be regarded as normal.

7. *Watches other children, unable to stand up for himself.* These were all children whose fearfulness, timidity, passivity, or inability to compete with others did not allow them to hold their own with other children. Standing and watching other children play, not joining in games, and never defending themselves in a just cause are typical of their behaviour.

8. *Passive, submissive, no initiative or ambition.* Passivity is here used in the sense given by the Oxford Dictionary, meaning 'being acted upon, suffering action, offering no opposition, submissive'. These children took up a passive attitude towards the world in that they avoided active experience, took no responsibility, never started a new activity, and showed no ambition. Such children showed combined helplessness, passive dependence, and refusal of action, as if they did not want to 'start anything' that they might not be able to control, or as if inwardly assured of failure and of the hopelessness of any attempt at an active type of mastery. The motivation behind passivity may be as complicated and multiple as the motivation of any neurotic condition, but the manifestations of this attitude are not difficult to identify. Frequently this very passivity is complained of by parents or persons in charge of the child, who feel it to be either a self-protective or an inhibited-aggressive reaction on the child's part. Such neurotic passivity is to be expected more in boys than in girls, since passivity is compatible to some extent with the girl's feminine aims and accepted feminine role. (A neurotic girl may, of course, tend to express a similar conflict in another way.)

9. *Subdued and inhibited behaviour.* Mild forms of over-subdued and inhibited behaviour are fairly common in normal children in certain phases of their development, but these may reach extreme degrees in the neurotic child. These children were all over-quiet, over-serious, over-slow, and subdued; some were unable to speak up for themselves or spoke only in whispers, or were otherwise socially inhibited.

10. *Cannot express emotion or real feelings, never cries or shows anger.* Neurotic inhibition may take many forms, but often what is inhibited is either action or emotion, particularly aggressive

75

action or aggressive emotions. In many cases this inhibition spreads to the whole of one function, so that locomotion is inhibited (some paralyses) or sight is inhibited (hysterical blindness) or the child is afraid of all emotion or of anything that arouses it (denial of feelings). In these children inhibition of aggression takes the extreme form of their always disguising their real feelings, never expressing emotion freely, and in particular never crying or showing anger.

11. *Timid, hesitant, cautious behaviour.* This is usually associated with undue fearfulness and lack of confidence and frequently to be found in people whose underlying conflicts prevent them from making up their minds or committing themselves. All children who habitually suffered from timidity, hesitancy, indecision, and undue cautiousness in everyday matters were classed in this section.

12. *Awkward, ill-at-ease, clumsy, self-conscious behaviour.* This section included children who were extremely ill-at-ease, clumsy, or self-conscious, always dropping, breaking, or losing things, having many small accidents, or being 'accident-prone'.

13. *Feels inferior, gives up easily, pessimistic, easily discouraged.* In this section were placed all children who were described as lacking in self-confidence or optimism about the outcome of their undertakings. They were deficient, for neurotic reasons, in feelings of self-regard or in 'narcissistic supplies' (Fenichel, 1945). Typically the child feels inferior, gives up easily, feels that he cannot do things, that things always go wrong with him; and he is pessimistic, easily discouraged, intimidated, or habitually adopts a defeatist attitude towards life.

14. *Depression more pronounced than in section 13 and including all extreme forms of depressive behaviour.* These occur in every neurosis, at least in the form of neurotic inferiority feelings, and often in more exaggerated forms. In such cases one expects to find a core of narcissistic injury, conflicts centred on the maintenance of self-esteem, or failures in self-regard. Depressive states are often associated with refusal of food, extreme states of fatigue,

remorse, mourning, grief, extreme regressive behaviour, danger of suicide, suicidal thoughts, excessive greed, monotonous complaining, or exaggerated and continual praying. In a child depression is commonly expressed by accusations towards the parents that they do not love him, or by reiterating 'Nobody loves me', 'I am no good', or 'I hate myself'. Neurotic depressions are usually related to a high degree of ambivalence and hostility towards other persons, or to unconscious guilt conflicts within the sufferer himself.

15. *Fears of dying, preoccupation with thoughts of death or suicide.* Under this heading were placed all cases of children who, whether habitually or in special states of depression, were preoccupied with thoughts of death or with fears of dying, and children who threatened suicide.

16. *Obsessional traits and symptoms.* Under this heading were included all symptoms of any obsessional neurosis, e.g. obsessional rituals, doubts, compulsions, or avoidances; obsessive thinking; counting obsessions; touching or washing manias; repetitions; doing and undoing certain acts; or certain compulsive penance symptoms. These conditions are typical of a well-established neurotic condition of the obsessional type, and it is to be expected that they will occur in a fully developed form only rarely in child cases.

17. *Obsessional reaction-formations and character traits.* This section included all character traits or reaction-formations typical of the alteration in character that occurs in obsessional or compulsive neurosis. Reaction-formations become deeply embedded in every compulsive neurotic's personality in his fight against unconscious hostility, and they may assume rigid forms, for example over-tidiness, over-conscientiousness, over-cleanliness and exaggerated worries about dirt, obstinacy, exaggerated stubbornness, meanness or miserliness, or exaggerated modesty. Because such traits are found in the early stages of obsessional neurosis, we expected to find a larger number of child cases in this than in section 16.

18. *Hysterical traits and symptoms.* This category included all cases of hysterical traits and symptoms that had not been included in any of the foregoing sections, e.g. fears and phobias. For instance, symptoms of an hysterical neurosis, such as hysterical pains; hysterical dream-states or disturbances of consciousness; hysterical disturbances of special senses or of sensation; hysterical hallucination; hysterical motor disturbances; hysterical emotional spells; and exaggeratedly histrionic behaviour. We did not expect that these would occur very frequently in child cases.

HYPOTHESIS: Characteristics of Neurotic Behaviour
We should expect to find that each of the foregoing types of behaviour occurs frequently in neurotic children, but relatively rarely in delinquents. (Confirmed, with the exception of sections 14, 16, and 18.)

In *Table 6,* Appendix 1, correlations are shown between the neurotic cases and the symptoms observed. These results show that there is a significant difference between the delinquent and neurotic children in each of the foregoing sections, except in three groups of symptoms, namely:

14. Depression
16. Obsessional symptoms
18. Hysterical symptoms.

In each of these sections the numbers in both groups are relatively small, and the results confirm the expectation that fully developed symptoms of adult neurosis are not very frequently found in child cases. The number of delinquent children who show hysterical traits is lower than might have been expected since some types of delinquency strikingly resemble certain types of hysterical or histrionic behaviour. Although genuine depression in very young children has been described,[1] it is doubtful whether fully developed depressive states are frequently seen in child guidance clinics. Mild degrees of unhappiness and sad behaviour seem to be more characteristic of the neurotic group.

Rosenheim (1942) described one type of delinquent child—a

[1] E.g. by Spitz (1946b, and in the film *Grief in Childhood*) *et alia.*

78

rejected child—who showed defiant and disobedient behaviour in an attempt to escape from deep torment of a depressed, suicidal type by gratifying every impulse. One child defended this type of behaviour, regardless of the opinions of those about her, by saying it helped her to forget unbearable troubles. Such delinquency in order to ward off periodic depressions has been described as involving the use of special mechanisms similar to those of manic defence.[1] Similar conclusions were reached by Ferenczi (1929). In cases where delinquency is used as a defence against inner depression, it is difficult to discover the hidden depression by the mere external observation and record of behaviour and to make comparisons within the scope of our project.

Examples of Neurotic Behaviour
Neurotic disorders assume such highly individual and complex forms that any attempt to isolate details of behaviour apart from the context of each child's total personality disturbance yields only a spurious and deceptive clarity. It will be of greater value to indicate typical examples of cases that fall into each of the main pictures of neurotic disturbances, as follows:

Obsessional neurosis. Cases No. 76, Rollo, and No. 79, Pierre (well developed.)

Phobias. Cases No. 52, Geoffrey, and No. 51, Maurice.

Hysterical conditions. Cases No. 87, Penelope, and No. 88, Daphne.

Anxiety state. Case No. 77, Rupert.

Anxiety hysteria. Case No. 83, Gertrude.

Neurotic character disturbance. Cases No. 89, Janice, and No. 86, Elspeth.

Primary behaviour disorder with neurotic tendencies. Cases No. 59, Clifford, and No. 90, Dorothy.

It may be concluded that, with the exception of sections 14, 16, and 18, each of the foregoing types of behaviour tends to occur more frequently in neurotic than in delinquent children. We may therefore assume that we chose characteristics of neuro-

[1] By Dr. Augusta Bonnard, Director, East London Child Guidance Clinic (private communication, 1951).

tic behaviour on a valid basis, and that the behaviour described can be regarded as characteristic of neurotic children. There is a high correlation between neuroticism and most of the behavioural characteristics described above, and in all cases the correlation is positive.

(The late Professor J. C. Flugel suggested that we should compare the various types of neurotic difficulties, such as hysteria, phobia, obsessions, etc., with a number of the conditions examined, such as the type of earlier difficulties shown, the kind of discipline experienced, early habit-training or discipline difficulties, psycho-sexual behaviour, etc., but the number of cases when sub-divided into the respective neurotic categories was too small to yield reliable results. This might be possible, however, in a parallel study into the conditions affecting neurotic development.)

GROUP 3. OTHER BEHAVIOURAL CHARACTERISTICS

This group consists of the miscellaneous 'pool' of emotional and behavioural characteristics that are not regarded in common psychiatric practice as typically either delinquent or neurotic. We therefore expected them to occur with the same frequency in both groups. Comparison between the two groups of children on these 'neutral' items has shown some characteristics to be interesting for theoretical reasons, while others are less important. In particular, certain items that are given special significance in psycho-analytic theory for the development of the neuroses or delinquency, but that are not always regarded as significant in general psychiatry or psychology, were arranged in groupings corresponding to certain theoretical expectations and their incidence was examined.

This miscellaneous set of conditions was grouped into nine sub-sections each containing a cluster of related symptoms or emotional and behavioural conditions that had been used to characterize various children on referral.

SOCIAL RELATIONS

We were interested to observe how many delinquent and how many neurotic children showed difficulties in their relations with other children, were unable to make normal social relationships, or showed fear and inhibition in the sphere of social feelings (i.e. in the forces within individuals that favour and maintain group formation and group relatedness.)

1. *Well-behaved, good, and biddable.* We included this section to provide contrast for the characteristics of disobedience, defiance, or being 'beyond control' that were observed among delinquents. Educational psychologists frequently observe that the 'over-good' child, who may withdraw himself and become inhibited in school, is often overlooked by the teacher. Though the teacher may not see him as a problem, he is likely to be more deeply disturbed than the child who makes his difficulties felt. Busy teachers may well fail to pick out withdrawal and depression symptoms associated with grave personality disturbance. In this section were included children who were described as extremely good, well-behaved, and tractable.

2. *Uncooperative and unhelpful in the house.* These were children who failed to cooperate in the normal family tasks, who obstructed family living to such an extent that they were described as 'impossible to live with', or who were in other ways at odds with family living and family responsibility.

3. *No friends, unsociable, does not mix, does not get along with other children.* Children may often fail to get along with other children because of their own difficulties, because of a disturbed relationship with other children, or in some cases because the parents refuse to allow the child to mix with other children in the normal way. All such cases were counted here.

4. *Exhibitionist behaviour.* Two types of exhibitionist behaviour are commonly met with: (a) boastfulness, showing-off, and playing up for pity and attention. Under this heading were placed those children who were actively exhibitionist, dramatized themselves, were histrionically gifted in some way, or were openly

81

braggarts and boasters; (b) playing the fool or clowning before others. These children 'exhibited their defect' or deficiency, i.e. they pretended to be daft or to be a clown; made grimaces or danced about asking stupid questions, inviting laughter and ridicule.

5. *Envy, jealousy, and searching other people's belongings.* Under this heading were included children in whom envy, whether of others' belongings, personal success, or attributes, was pronounced. Jealousy may assume many forms, and isolated incidents (not amounting to theft) have arisen in several schools where one child searches through the belongings of other children or of siblings without being able to give a reasonable explanation for his behaviour. What is sought is probably something less tangible than material goods, and the child envies another for something that he feels to be lacking in himself.

6. *'Easily led', following dominating child.* Under this heading were placed all cases of children who were submissive towards a more dominant child and were easily persuaded to follow the latter's bidding.

7. *Prefers the companionship of younger children.* This included children who preferred the company of smaller ones and either watched or joined in their play as one of them.

8. *Chooses bad companions.*

9. *Gets bullied, victimized.* These children were all bullied, teased, called names, or victimized by others, or feared other children.

10. *Bullies, victimizes other children.* These children were the opposites and partners of those in section 9.

11. *Dislikes meeting people.* Those children who avoided meeting others, refused to speak to strangers or to make new friendships.

12. *Solitary, seclusive, lacks relationships with other children.* Solitariness and seclusiveness were counted when these were thought to be attributes of the child himself rather than due to lack of

opportunities in the environment. The child who lacked relationship with other children, who felt that he was destined to be a 'lone wolf' or that he was somehow different from other children, was included here.

13. *Crushes, many intense friendships or enmities.* This section included those whose friendships or hostilities took unusually intense forms, e.g. children who had 'crushes' on other children or adults, or who had hated and 'deadly' enemies.

14. *Difficult behaviour towards siblings or other children.* This included all types of aggressive, difficult, spiteful, and jealous behaviour towards the child's contemporaries, whether siblings or other children.

15. *Shy, blushes easily, withdrawn, reserved, or retiring.* Blushing and shyness are well-known symptoms of social inhibition and are often the outcome of underlying inhibitions of exhibitionism. They are usually associated with retiring, reserved, or very withdrawn behaviour.

HYPOTHESES: Social Relationships

1. We should expect to find that a greater number of neurotic than of delinquent children were described as well-behaved, good, and biddable. (Confirmed.)

2. We should expect to find that a greater number of delinquent than of neurotic children showed exhibitionist behaviour of the boastful, showing-off type. (Confirmed.)

3. We should expect to find no significant difference in the children of both groups showing the second type of exhibitionist behaviour, i.e. 'exhibiting the defect'. (Confirmed.)

4. We should expect to find no significant difference between delinquent and neurotic children with respect to the other items in this section. (Confirmed, with the exception of item 5.)

The results in *Table 7*, Appendix 1, show a significant difference between delinquent and neurotic children in three of the foregoing sections, namely Nos. 1, 4(a), and 5. In all other cases the difference between the two groups is not significant. This indicates a tendency for neurotic children to be well-behaved, good, and easily managed, in contrast to delinquent children, who tend to be unmanageable. The delinquents tend to be more openly exhibitionist than the neurotics, with a good deal of boasting, showing off and playing up for pity and attention. There was no significant difference between the numbers of children in the two groups who play the fool and clown by 'exhibiting the defect' before others. Neurotic children tend to show jealousy, envy, and covetous behaviour more frequently than delinquent children.

Disturbed social relations occur in a small percentage of cases in both groups. The percentages are highest in both groups, however, for children who are unsociable, who do not mix or get on with other children, who are boastful and show off, who show difficult behaviour towards siblings or other children, who are bullied and victimized by others, who are envious of other children, and who prefer to play with children younger than themselves.

It may be concluded that both neurotic and delinquent children tend to have considerable difficulties in social relations with their fellows.

SCHOOL DIFFICULTIES

16. *Retardation in school subjects.* We examined children whose attainment in school subjects fell below the level of their intellectual capacity. This was usually assessed by the educational psychologist, or in some cases by the child's teacher, or by these two in consultation.

17. *Learning difficulties in special subjects.* Cases were included here where the child showed a specific and isolated difficulty in one subject or group of subjects, e.g. in geography, biology, or reading. These are cases where the difficulty is not related in any apparent way to the child's level of achievement in other subjects, which he is usually able to master.

18. *Cannot concentrate, inattentive, easily distracted, preoccupied, has poor memory.*

19. *Intense dislike of school or teachers, refusal to go to school.*

20. *Does not fit in with school routine.* Under this heading were included all children who were not amenable to discipline, who disobeyed the school rules, and did not adapt their behaviour to ordinary school routine.

21. *Difficult and unsettled behaviour in school.*

HYPOTHESES: School Difficulties.

1. We should expect to find that a greater number of neurotic than of delinquent children show learning difficulties in special subjects in school. (Confirmed.)

2. In all other cases we should expect to find that both delinquent and neurotic children experience school difficulties of the types described here, and that there is no significant difference between them. (Confirmed.)

The results in *Table 8*, Appendix 1, indicate that there is a significant difference between delinquent and neurotic children with regard to difficulties with special subjects in school. The numbers are rather small, but they indicate that neurotic children tend to have more difficulties in special subjects than delinquent children. On all other items in this section the difference between delinquent and neurotic children is insignificant. A high percentage of the children in both groups had difficulties in school, especially general retardation, poor concentration, and difficult and unsettled behaviour.

DAY-DREAMING AND FANTASY

Day-dreaming and fantasying are commonly observed at various periods in the development of normal children. Sometimes they afford a retreat into a fantasy world from attempts at mastery of the external world; sometimes they are the refuge for wishes that cannot be fulfilled, as for example in the invention of imaginary companions. Unconscious fantasy, or more correctly, the impulsive 'acting out' of fantasies, is well known to underlie the irrational aspects of many kinds of delinquent or criminal

D

conduct, e.g. in children's lies and falsifications (Stanley Hall, 1890); in homosexuality and other perversions (Freud, 1905, 1919); in character disorders like the 'criminals from a sense of guilt' (Freud, 1915d); in pathological lying, accusation, and swindling (Healy, 1915b); in certain types of sex delinquency such as fetishistic stealing, exhibitionism, voyeurism, sadism, and masochism (Healy, 1917); or in certain actions of 'impulse-ridden characters' (Reich, 1925). Detailed psychiatric studies of various types of neurotic delinquency have confirmed the role of unconscious fantasies in the determination of criminal tendencies. Some examples of studies on child cases are those of Frosch and Bromberg (1939) on sex offenders; Yarnell (1940) on children showing fire-setting tendencies; Lowrey (1941) on certain older runaways and adult nomads; Rosenheim (1942) on the antisocial and 'persecuted' behaviour of the rejected child; Slavson (1943a and b) on the psychological bases of the many kinds of aggression commonly met with in the re-education of delinquents; and Andriola (1946) on the escape-fantasies of truants. In pathological or imaginative lying it has been suggested by several writers (including Helene Deutsch, 1947) that a pretence of reality is shared by means of the supposed lie with others who are persuaded to believe in the liar's substitutive fantasy. If others also believe that the absurd, fantastic, or unreal things are true, then the liar himself can more easily believe in their reality.

In view of the increasing numbers of such studies, it would be interesting to compare the outwardly observed day-dreaming and fantasy behaviour in the groups of neurotic and delinquent children, on the hypothesis that escapist behaviour is common to both. An examination will be made of the incidence of 'romancing' or pseudologia fantastica, as well as of day-dreaming, fantasy life, and imaginary companions.

22. *Fantasies, over-vivid imagination, day-dreams.* Under this heading were included children with strong fantasy life and day-dreams, revealed by imaginative story-telling, 'living in a world of their own', preoccupation with day-dreams, or having 'magic' thoughts. This behaviour was so outstanding in these children as to be regarded as a problem by parents and teachers.

23. *Having fantasy companions.*

24. *Romancing.* Under this heading were included all cases of imaginative or pathological lying (pseudologia fantastica).

HYPOTHESIS: Day-dreaming and Fantasy
We should expect to find no significant difference between neurotic and delinquent groups in the frequency with which day-dreaming and fantasying occur. (Not confirmed.)

The results in *Table 9*, Appendix 1, show that there is a significant difference between delinquent and neurotic children in section 22, but no significant difference between the two groups in those who have fantasy companions or are prone to romancing. A small proportion of children in both groups was referred to the clinic for symptoms that included romancing. It may be concluded that neurotic children tend to have, or to reveal, a vivid fantasy life more frequently than delinquent children, but romancing is common to a small proportion in each group. There was some reason to suppose that the neurotic child tends to work out his fantasy in more symbolic forms within himself, whereas the delinquent, in his general conflict with his environment, achieves direct expression of his fantasies in action. It was interesting that the numbers in the two latter sections were very small, and these may well have been diminished by the exclusion of the delinquents whose actions were known to be neurotically determined.[1]

DIRTY AND UNTIDY BEHAVIOUR
This heading refers to dirtiness and untidiness to an extent that creates a problem in family life. Certain types of dirtiness and untidiness are common both in very small children and at certain stages in puberty and adolescence. Dirtiness to a greater degree than normal, however, or dirtiness continuing throughout childhood, indicates either a failure in adaptation towards

[1] This result also confirms once more the hypothesis, basic to our project, that there is one large group of delinquents, i.e. the so-called 'antisocial character', that may be distinguished from those whose delinquency arises purely as a neurotic symptom, and that it is of great theoretical and practical importance to distinguish between the two.

normal social habits of cleanliness and tidiness, or in some cases a refusal to give up the infantile irresponsibility and pleasure in dirtiness. We expected this to occur in some types of neurotic children, but to be a more pronounced delinquent characteristic.

25. *Untidy, careless about clothes, toys, or appearance.* This included children who were untidy or careless about their own or others' possessions, and children who were untidy and careless about their own appearance to a degree that created a problem in the family or was complained of by teachers.

26. *Dirty habits.* This section included children who showed all kinds of dirty habits, and children who would not wash or liked being dirty or frequently got very dirty.

27. *Playing with faeces or urine, eating or smearing faeces.* In these children such habits had developed during school age, or had persisted since infancy.

HYPOTHESIS: Dirty and Untidy Behaviour

We should expect to find that the delinquent children showed a greater degree of dirty and untidy behaviour than the neurotic children. (Not confirmed.)

The results in *Table* 10, Appendix 1, show that there is no significant difference between delinquent and neurotic children upon any of the foregoing types of dirty and untidy behaviour. A small proportion of both delinquents and neurotics were found to be untidy and careless in appearance, or to have dirty habits and refuse to wash. Five delinquent children were found to show such crude behaviour as playing with faeces or urine, or smearing or eating faeces. This behaviour was not observed at all in neurotic children. The numbers in each of the foregoing groups, however, are very small, and the results therefore inconclusive.

PERSISTENT HABITS

Goodman and Michaels (1934, 1939) in their studies on the relationship between persistent enuresis and delinquency found that five traits, enuresis, thumb-sucking, nail-biting, speech impediments, and temper tantrums were commonly found in combination, the last four being specifically correlated with enuresis.

Michaels (1938, 1940), in analysing the incidence of enuresis in 100 delinquent cases and 100 sibling controls, found a higher incidence of thumb-sucking, nail-biting, left-handedness, temper tantrums, and poor sleeping habits in delinquents than in their siblings. Greenacre (1944) and Levy (1944) in tracing the course of infantile aggression and the emergence of later general restless behaviour, observed the reactions of infants to movement-restraint. Greenacre found that prolonged early restraint tended to increase the sado-masochistic elements in character, and to exaggerate the child's over-activity and 'difficult' behaviour. In some cases movement-restraint produced over-activity and restlessness similar to that commonly observable in tiqueurs. Levy (1944) collected observations upon tics, stereotyped movements, and hyper-activity in dogs, chickens, hens, horses, and animals in captivity in the Zoo, and found a close relation of these movements to states of tension. He also observed the emotional response of children whose movements were restrained in various ways: for example, in the playpen, on the beach, who were locked in rooms, prevented from crawling, necessarily immobilized in plaster-casts, or subjected to common forms of restraint and prevented from sucking their thumbs. This hyper-activity resulted in certain psychological characteristics between the ages of three and five years such as mood habits, confusion, impulsive irritability, and wildly destructive behaviour. Levy concludes that restraint of movement tends to produce psychic tics, compulsive accessory movements, and generally heightened aggressiveness.

Under the heading of 'persistent habits' we made a study of the numerous bodily habits (usually referred to as 'nervous habits') that involve picking, pulling, sucking, jerking, twisting, or manipulation of certain parts of the body, habits of movement and gait, and so on. These were conditions about which complaints had been made on referring the child to the clinic and which parents had been unable to eradicate. They were arranged in four groups, as follows:

DELINQUENT AND NEUROTIC CHILDREN

28. *Tics, twitchings, grimacing, habits of movement and gait.*

29. *Sucking thumb, fingers, lips, or lapels, sleeves, handkerchiefs, or any other type of sucking activity.*

30. *Nail-biting.*

31. *Other bodily habits.* These included picking the teeth or nose, picking at skin or clothes, dribbling, wriggling, sniffing, grunting, chewing, smelling, blinking, shrugging, biting the lips, or having a persistent nervous cough.

HYPOTHESIS: Persistent Habits
We should expect to find no significant difference between delinquents and neurotics in any of the foregoing habits. (Confirmed.)

The results in *Table* 11, Appendix 1, show that there was no significant difference between delinquent and neurotic children with respect to any of the items in this section.

SEXUAL BEHAVIOUR
The psychodynamic problems of the crude sex offender were analysed by Freud (1905), who provided the first scientific basis for an understanding of his behaviour. Juvenile sex offenders were described by Healy (1915a, 1917) as forming a high percentage of the most difficult juvenile cases. Healy found that most of his sex delinquents (voyeurs, exhibitionists, cases of fetishistic stealing, etc.) when submitted to a form of 'mental analysis' (i.e. the exploration, on the conscious plane, of fantasies, recurrent worries, images, or ideas) repeatedly reverted to sex curiosity and sex items. They also revealed a half-knowledge of illicit sex behaviour on the part of their parents, and knowledge of adult sex behaviour observed elsewhere. Healy and Bronner (1929) extended their investigations to include certain behaviour disorders such as predatory sexual offences and other antisocial peculiarities of behaviour which had not been severe enough to come before the courts, and demonstrated what can be accomplished for many such delinquents by probation or foster-care, when the home environment is unsuitable.

The problem of the sex offender and of juvenile aberrant sexual behaviour received relatively little systematic attention in the objective studies of the 'twenties and 'thirties, except in certain types described by Burt (1925). Stekel (1925) found disturbances in psycho-sexual development and various disturbances in early instinctual and emotional behaviour in certain kinds of criminal behaviour, such as kleptomania and pyromania. He repeatedly found, in the case histories of such offenders, experiences in early life that provided the stimulus for perverse sexual satisfactions, symbolized or directly obtained in specific violent antisocial actions. Henderson (1939), in his textbook on psychopathic states, classified certain types of sex variants and suicidal cases as psychopathic states, whereas most dynamically orientated psychiatrists, including Healy and Karpman, view these as neurotic disorders '. . . for they can be treated and cured as neuroses' (Karpman, 1948a), and 'the structural organization of the personality in these cases is essentially that of the neuroses'.

Abnormalities or retardation in psycho-sexual development were reported by Mowrer and Mowrer (1938) in studies of the aetiology and treatment of enuresis in delinquent and other juvenile cases; by Menaker (1939) in a study of stealing as a neurotic symptom in boys; by Yarnell (1940) in a study of juvenile fire-setters; and by Karpman (1939, 1941, 1947, 1948a) in his various studies of psychopathic personalities. Shaskan (1939) examined 100 cases of adult and adolescent male offenders who were committed for various sex crimes. Psychosis, mental deficiency, perversions, and alcoholism were found to be common in these offenders. Evidence of sexual, marital, and other maladjustment was found in nearly all the cases.

Frosch and Bromberg (1939) in a psychiatric study of 709 sex offenders suggested that Shaskan exaggerated the influence of alcohol. No cases of psychosis were found in this group and mental defect played only a minor role. The authors re-emphasized the role of social and psychological factors, and noted a high rate of strong religious affiliation among sex offenders. They also found indications of strong sexual fantasies and excessive, over-compensatory reaction-formations in the form of moral preachments and harpings, projection, denials, and rationalization. The offenders with minors frequently denigrated their child victims' personalities, and saw them as aggressive and offensive persons who forced them into the act, e.g. (Frosch and Bromberg, 1939) 'they ... (little girls) ... are worse to the public than any criminal. They are cunning, devilish, tricky. You can't help blushing when you are in their presence'. Frosch and Bromberg assert that no drastic solutions for dealing with offenders can replace the need for painstaking re-education and psychotherapy of the individual offender and a wider education of the public.

Waggoner and Boyd (1941) studied twenty-five cases of juvenile aberrant sexual behaviour, where perverse sexual practices were not circumstantial or casual but 'unnatural' in the sense that they were the child's regular and preferred pattern of behaviour. The perverted sexual behaviour in each case was inextricably connected with the general personality and delinquency pattern of the offender and other misdemeanours were frequently observed to originate in the same causes. Investigation showed that the perverse sexual practices had begun at six to ten years of age, and that the child's sexual interest had been awakened by other individuals, but the practice continued because it fitted in with the child's personality problems. In school the children were found to be either docile and models of good behaviour, or characterized by restless, impulsive behaviour and overt sex acts. Waggoner and Boyd also found that the majority of the cases studied were deeply interested in church and religion, but this failed to produce a practical sexual morality. In this study only cases of overt sexual offences were studied, and no special attempt was made to observe the development of children who prefer to imitate and identify with the interest, activities and behaviour of the opposite sex.

Bender and Paster (1941) studied the factors determining homosexuality in twenty-three boys who showed marked homosexual tendencies. The authors accepted the formulations of Freud, Alexander, and Ferenczi on the psychological determinants of homosexuality, and evaluated the early environment of their cases to determine the points at which these patterns of behaviour were adopted. It became evident that this was not due to basic physical 'femininity' in boys and 'masculinity' in girls.

The factors that determined the development in these children of psycho-sexual trends contrary to their constitutional pattern were multiple and arose from faulty family relationships (Bender and Paster, 1941, p. 741). 'Most of the parents were found to be emotionally unstable with evidence of strife between mother and father. The parents of the same sex were either grossly abusive, played a negative role, or were altogether absent in approximately 90 per cent of the cases. Conversely, the parents of the opposite sex were either more dominant, or over-solicitous, and a certain amount of seduction by the latter was evident in some of the cases. Where rejection was not apparent the parent or parent-substitute of the same sex displayed homosexual tendencies and openly influenced the child. The children thus tended to identify themselves with the parent or parent-substitute who stood out before them as a source of strength, affection and security.' In many cases of boys, an additional factor influencing the adoption of a feminine role was the more favourable position of their sisters in the family group, or the feminine role of the mother was frequently exaggerated by over-solicitous aunts or grandmothers. All cases were characterized by feelings of inadequacy and were preoccupied with problems of femininity and masculinity. Tension, restlessness, and bewilderment reflected their underlying emotional disharmony and inability to adjust their inner lives to socially acceptable standards of behaviour for their sex.

Wortis (1939) made a further contribution to understanding the problem of sex offences and sex offenders, by examining certain sex taboos and customs which operate in our society but not in others, and the relativity of cultural standards with regard to sex offenders and the law. He regards sex offenders as individuals whose behaviour runs counter to contemporary sexual taboos in a given community. Wortis submits evidence that the majority of revolting sex crimes are committed by persons who are not legally insane, and he lays a store of blame on a society which (Wortis, 1939, p. 563) 'provides inadequately for the inculcation of normal sex habits in its individual members', and often 'deliberately undertakes to obscure and befuddle the problem for the young, or frequently denies opportunities for the practice of normal sexuality in maturity'. Benedict (1939) and other

93

anthropologists prefer to place sexual offences within their relevant cultural context. Certain cultural arrangements make homosexual temptations meaningless and their practice unsatisfactory, and a 'free access to an honourable and satisfactory sex life' can make certain perversions appear ridiculous (Benedict, 1939, pp. 571–3ff). Benedict agrees with Wortis that sex perversions are usually indulged in where the environment denies the individual a better way. She thinks that criminality, like neurosis, also provides for the delinquent *faute de mieux* a way of life which he can handle but which is, at base, 'rooted in deprivations'. Benedict presents evidence that sex offences are rare in primitive societies and that sex perversions originate in relation to the tribal distinction between the role of man and that of woman. Among Plains Indians of North America a boy who baulks at deeds of daring required on the warpath, which alone prove his manhood, may take the role of woman by becoming a *berdache*. He might nevertheless be respected as the 'best wife' in that he outshone women at their own occupations, was strong, industrious and could provide game for the larder which women could not do. The *berdaches* were seldom distinguished physiologically from other men, nor were their characteristics evident from early childhood. Benedict claims that 'the aetiology of homosexuality . . . in this and other cultures although it may be physiological in certain persons is overwhelmingly social . . . homosexuality correlates with the allotment of contrasted roles to men and women'. Tribes where men and women are not culturally differentiated, e.g. where a woman may hunt, go on a warpath, or divorce her spouse as can the men, have no *berdaches*. Benedict offers the corollary that the control of sex offences on a community-wide scale can be not merely medical but also social. 'Deprivations, humiliations, discriminations against minority groups, all take their toll in that a certain proportion of people will take up a-social or unorthodox ways of life *faute de mieux*'.

Mead (1931, 1935, 1949) has strikingly shown how a blanket conception of what is masculine and what is feminine is involved in a child's identification with its father or mother, and how often this is basic in problems having to do with a male's or female's proper adjustment to masculinity and femininity. Freud (1905) has shown the basic emotional factors involved in homosexuality to be avoidance, fear and hatred of the opposite sex. Kardiner and Linton (1939) have shown how completely the functions of men and women in certain polyandrous and polygamous societies run counter to our Western customs.

An interesting corroboration of psycho-analytic studies of the relation of sexual disturbance to neurotic conditions has been made in the study of animal neuroses by Horsley Gantt and his collaborators (1944), who published the result of the first twelve years of their researches into the study of nervous imbalance and the development of artificially produced nervous disturbance in dogs. Using an objective approach of the type pioneered by Pavlov, Horsley Gantt was able to produce and study patterns of dysfunction in the nervous system related to characteristic anxiety states. Disturbances of behaviour such as eating disturbances, refusal to eat, and excretory and sexual disturbances were artificially produced by this method. Sexual difficulties were manifested in 88 per cent of the dogs' anxiety attacks. A marked inhibitory effect upon anxiety reactions was produced by strong sexual stimulation and a striking improvement in the behaviour of neurotic dogs followed after reunion and companionship with the female dogs in the paddock. From many similar observations Horsley Gantt concluded (1944, p. 186) 'The widespread connections of the sexual function, its intensity and predominant influence, are facts which cannot be doubted . . . in the general explanation of all nervous disturbances.' He also submitted his findings to a social anthropologist (Leighton), a psycho-analyst (Saul), and a physiologist (Ischlondsky) who offered interesting mutually consonant explanations of his findings.

Under the general heading of 'Sexual Behaviour' an examination was made of the main types of sexual behaviour which had been regarded as constituting a problem in some of the delinquent and neurotic children in this study.

32. *Exaggerated masturbation.* This included cases of children beyond the age of five or six who masturbated in public, who masturbated openly in school, and all other cases of compulsive masturbating.

33. *Precocious sex games, sexual notes, offences, etc.* This section included behaviour of the type usually referred to the juvenile courts as 'sexual offences', such offences being commonly regarded as sufficient reason by themselves for referring a child to the juvenile court (i.e. without further delinquent behaviour). This behaviour usually relates to exaggerated sexual curiosity, various methods of making sexual investigations, exhibiting and 'peeping'. According to psycho-analytic theory, a certain degree of sexual curiosity and more or less secret investigation might be expected to occur in delinquent, neurotic, and normal children's behaviour alike at certain age levels. However, the apprehension of the child usually indicates that, since he has been unable to hide his curiosity or investigations, or since they have taken undesirable forms, the problem has become an acute and severe one for him. Juvenile court officials who show an increased readiness to refer all cases of sex offenders for psychological examination, have begun to recognize that this behaviour may form part of the neurotic as well as of the delinquent picture.

34. *Imitation of the opposite sex.* (a) Girlish behaviour, interests, and activities in boys. (b) Boyish behaviour, interests, and activities in girls.

We next examined imitation of the behaviour of the opposite sex in an attempt to test one aspect of the Freudian theory of the sexual aetiology of the neuroses. Freud (1905) traced the origin of homosexuality to unconscious fear and hatred of the opposite sex, allied with a reluctance on the part of the individual to accept his or her biological sexual role. He succinctly described the neurosis as 'the negative of the perversion', and many neuroses were found to involve, among other things, a problem of unconscious sexual inversion (the so-called 'negative Oedipus complex'). This was usually based upon early dissatisfactions with the individual's own sex and an attempt, in fantasy or in reality, to take over or to imitate the role of the opposite sex in relation to the parent of the same sex, whom the child had taken as his Oedipal love-object. Where the Oedipus complex was not worked through in the normal way, these aim-inhibited strivings were thought to lead either to neurosis, to homosexuality in later life, to confused sexual identification patterns in the character, or to some configuration of these in combination. The resultant character disturbances might be as manifold in form as the infantile experiences themselves.

We thought it of especial interest, since childhood neurotic conditions are thought typically to represent earlier stages in the development of adult neuroses, to see whether any tendency towards confusion with regard to the male or female role, or reluctance to identify with the parent of the same sex and to accept the standards and behaviour which are normal for the child's own sex, could be observed in the behaviour of the neurotic children. We examined the data and included cases which showed this tendency to a marked degree. Typical examples are (a) a girl (Case No. 100, Frances) who '. . . is interested only in farm work, hammering, sharing in breeding pigs; works outdoors with her father, plans to be a farmer, does not like sewing, femininity, glamour, or housework, and likes to dress as a boy'; (b) a boy (Case No. 72, Alexander) who '. . . makes doilys, lampshades, draws patterns, prefers to stay with mother or play with girls, likes to cook, has feminine hobbies'.

HYPOTHESES: Sexual Behaviour

1. We should expect to find that neurotic children show a tendency towards imitation of the behaviour, interests, and activities of the opposite sex and that delinquents do not. (Confirmed.)

2. We should expect to find no significant difference between delinquent and neurotic children in other items of sexual behaviour. (Confirmed.)

The results in *Table* 12, Appendix 1, show that there is a highly significant difference between delinquent and neurotic children in the imitation of the behaviour, interests, and activities of the opposite sex. This occurred much more frequently in the neurotic children than in the delinquents. No significant difference was found in the incidence of exaggerated masturbation or precocious sex games and offences. They occurred to a minor extent in both delinquent and neurotic children. There is a small correlation between delinquency and sex offences but the numbers on which this is based are very small.

'DIFFICULT' BEHAVIOUR AND EMOTIONAL CHARACTERISTICS

There remained a varied assortment of behaviour traits and emotional attitudes, couched in the descriptive language of parents, teachers and others who had found the children 'difficult' to cope with for a number of reasons. For ease of reference, rather than because they fitted into any complete or mutually exclusive groups or patterns of behaviour, these have been arranged in four sub-sections, as follows:

(a) 'Tough-Guy' Attitudes

A number of writers have referred to the tough, 'don't care', emotionally hardened attitude observed in many delinquents. Healy (1917) referred to these as 'rough' rather than 'sensitive' characters, and in some cases he found a coupling of hyper-sensitiveness on the one hand with extreme callousness on the other. Makarenko (1935) found many characters of this type among the violent delinquents in the Gorki colony. Aichhorn (1925) described similar types among the aggressive delinquents for whom he evolved a special technique, the 'moment of surprise',[1] to re-awaken a once-existent positive emotional tie, and he manipulated this for the establishment of a certain type of transference without which he considered genuine re-education and character change to be impossible. Michaels and Goodman (1939) have referred to the 'impenetrable armour' with which such children surround themselves, and which frequently proves impervious to ordinary therapeutic approaches. Bowlby (1944) has described a similar character structure in his 'affectionless thieves' who were characterized from infancy by a remarkable lack of affection or warmth of feeling for anyone. Schmidl (1947) found on the basis of Rorschach experience with juvenile delinquents certain types of characteristically evasive responses significant of '. . . a deep-rooted tendency to be secretive, not to reveal anything, whatever the situation may be. . . .' (ibid., p. 157).

---

[1] See also Biddle (1933).

Under the general heading of 'tough-guy' attitudes the follow-ing constantly recurring types of behaviour were examined in the delinquent and neurotic groups:

35. *'Don't care' attitude, bravado, acts 'tough-guy', pretends unconcern.*

36. *Affectionless, callous, hard, shows no affectionate feelings.*

37. *Uncommunicative, evasive, denies difficulties.*

HYPOTHESIS: 'Tough-guy' Attitudes
We should expect to find that 'tough' behaviour and character occur more frequently in delinquent than in neurotic children. (Confirmed.)

The results in *Table* 13, Appendix 1, show that there is here a significant difference between delinquent and neurotic children, and that 'tough-guy' attitudes are characteristic of the delinquent rather than of the neurotic children.

(b) The 'Antisocial Grudge'
Healy (1915a, 1917) first drew attention to the number of cases in which bitterness and dissatisfaction were among the most typical characteristics of the delinquents' mental make-up. He noted (Healy, 1915a, p. 34) '. . . the chronic attitude of the offender re-presenting himself to be as one like Ishmael, whose hand shall be against every man and every man's hand against him'. He des-cribes (ibid., p. 376) what he calls 'the remarkable phenomenon of the antisocial grudge' and notes '. . . its extensive appearance at a very early age in the development of antisocial feeling'. Many writers since Healy have noted in passing the same or similar characteristics in young offenders. Karpman (1939, 1948a) has noted the extent of this grudge in psychopathic personalities, and he feels it to be a reaction at the deepest level to frustrated and unrequited love in the earliest years accentuated by a 'vicious' environment that stimulated aggression without providing satis-factory repressive and sublimating influences. The delinquent's bitterness he holds to be typically related to early psychic trau-mata, to early deprivation of love, and lack of normal emotional security within a family unit. Karpman feels that such an attitude

is based on psychopathic egotism and selfishness which cannot be modified by ordinary educational procedures. Such a child lives entirely for himself, using others only for what he can get out of them or for 'what the world owes him'. As against other types of delinquency, no environment, however considerate, will help him, in Karpman's opinion, since no ordinary environment can provide the catering and ministering to his wishes that he craves and demands. A cure, in such cases, can only be achieved when a change in the 'grudge-attitude' has been effected by psychological treatment and a more satisfactory environment provided.

Bartemeier (1930), Levy (1932b), and Tiebout and Kirkpatrick (1932) severally found in delinquents aggressiveness, bitterness and resentment that for a number of reasons had been heightened by experiences in infancy. Topping (1941, 1943) also described a similar group of aggressive, resentful boys, in whom she found a complete lack of humour, lack of insight, a 'capacity for deadly attack', and what she described as 'warped' or 'scarred' personalities. Rosenheim (1942) found a similar attitude in the rejected child who, unloved from childhood, maintains an attitude of complete justification for antisocial behaviour at all times. He never confesses his thefts; indignantly complains of the injustice of the accusation of stealing; feels persecuted and hated by everyone; in some places even appears to simulate hostility in order to keep people at a distance, and by deliberately unfriendly means provokes punishment. Reich (1925), Aichhorn (1925), Stekel (1929), Friedlander (1947), and other writers on the problem of sadism and masochism have thrown considerable light on the origin and morbid forms of such quarrelsome, narcissistic, sado-masochistic attitudes to authority. Friedlander in particular has described in detail how the typical 'grudge against society' attitude met with in so many offenders develops out of the sado-masochistic type of object relationship.

In the present section, under the general heading 'the antisocial grudge' (adopting Healy's useful term), the following character traits were compared in the groups of delinquent and neurotic children:

38. *Whining, complaining, self-pitying behaviour.*

39. *Blames and accuses others, is resentful and bitter, bears a grudge, nurses his grievances.*

40. *Martyr attitude, sullen and sulky, thinks others are against him.*

41. *Revengeful, spiteful, tell-tale, gossiping.*

42. *A ringleader for trouble, mischievous, incites others, is blamed, scapegoated.*

HYPOTHESIS: the 'Antisocial Grudge'
We should expect to find that bitter, grudging attitudes occur more frequently in delinquent than in neurotic children. (Not confirmed, except for items 41 and 42.)

Table 14, Appendix 1, shows a significant difference between delinquent and neurotic children only in items 41 and 42. This indicates that delinquent children show revengeful, spiteful, tell-tale, gossiping behaviour, that they are mischievous ringleaders, and that they get blamed and scapegoated for misconduct more often than neurotics. It is the more aggressive, actively vengeful types of 'grudge-behaviour' that are characteristic of the delinquents. The more passive, sulky, 'smouldering' grudge-attitudes were found in a small proportion of both the delinquent and the neurotic children. No significant difference was found between the numbers in each group who are whining, complaining, self-pitying; blame and accuse others, nurse grievances; adopt a 'martyred' attitude; and think others are always against them.

(c) *Defective Super-ego Development*
Faulty conscience development, or failure of the conscience to direct action in accordance with an established ethical code, have always been recognized in everyday 'common-sense' observations of delinquent behaviour. Such recognition, however, has been implicit rather than explicit, and often confused by the failure of normal people to comprehend the delinquent's deficiency in moral sense. This has led in the past to labelling such children as 'morally defective', with little further interest in the nature of this defect. It is surprising that more intensive study by

the 'objective' method of delinquency research has not been made of the aetiological and structural aspects of arrested growth and distortion in conscience development. A study of this aspect of delinquency from the psycho-genetic and structural approach might help towards an understanding of the tendency variously described as 'latent delinquency', 'susceptibility to delinquency', or 'antisocial character formation'.

McDougall (1908), in his analysis of volition and the organization of the sentiment of self-regard, traced the growth of self-consciousness and observed several stages in the development of the conscience. He separated the acquirement of an ideal with regard to certain lines of conduct from the development of a sentiment towards it. He distinguished the development of these two, and described which relationship between them will suffice to secure the realization of the ideal. He also assessed the role of reward and punishment, and the stages of development towards varying degrees of independence of the conscience from the authoritative figures upon whom it first depends. Freud (1914, 1917), in his papers on 'narcissism' and on 'mourning and melancholia', laid the groundwork for a psycho-analytic theory of conscience formation. On the basis of this many subsequent studies of far-reaching importance have been made on this topic by psycho-analytic workers. Freud related the 'watching', self-criticizing function of the conscience to the incorporation by the small child of the demands of his parents and educators which he takes over and makes into his own demands and ideals of behaviour. Conscience formation develops through the child's repeated partial identifications with a loved person that usually occur after he has temporarily withdrawn his love following frustration of his instinctual urges. This identification results in the ego changing in order to resemble the loved person; in a sense the child obtains his independence at a price, i.e. he introjects his parents' demands in order to be free of them and of other external controls. In conditions such as mourning and melancholia, the normal course of a gradual detachment of love from the lost loved one, through grief and identification, may miscarry, and under certain pathological conditions the conscience becomes diseased and severe mental illness results.

Miss Anna Freud, in her lectures and teaching, has stressed that in delinquents the development of the conscience, and therefore general social development also, have typically been disturbed. The strength of the conscience is directly dependent upon the strength and number of the child's early love relationships and a weakening of the earliest emotional ties is reflected in a corresponding weakness in the super-ego or conscience. Frequently it is not the loss but the withdrawal of the loved person which leads to a lack of identification. In delinquents the love relationship has been progressively weakened and is not of a kind that will produce identifications and growth of character. Such a child's emotions are shallow and he is quick-changing and primitive in his relationships, expecting satisfaction without giving a return. The resultant conscience formation is therefore weak and incomplete. Separations from the loved person, especially during the period from the sixth to the eighteenth month of age, are thought to be especially likely to lead to a failure in conscience formation since each separation produces a weakening in the next relationship. When this happens several times there is a definite deterioration in the quality of the attachment. Children vary a great deal in their reactions to such experiences, but commonly they either withdraw and become narcissistic, forming weak relationships in general, or they may develop a 'love-hunger' and change their affections frequently, making a quick withdrawal when frustrated, and as quickly adopting new relationships, none of which are very deep or satisfying, or likely to lead to the child making further steps in social development. Miss Freud has stressed that it is not the traumatic reaction to the loss of the mother which leads to this failure in the delinquent; it is the absence of the daily interaction, and the repetition of the pattern of loving-frustration-withdrawal-identification, which would have led him to gradual changes in character, based upon strong and well-knit identifications with the parent and later with others.

Greenacre (1945) maintains that the conscience in the psychopath and in many delinquents is defective, devitalized or degraded in characteristic ways, and she presents an analysis of its faulty structural development. In most cases she has found a heightening of the quantity of original infantile aggression by various means such as infantile illness, discomfort, somatic frustration, restraint, or neglect, all of which combine to form a predisposition to anxiety. This heightened early aggressiveness, in her opinion, combines with certain later elements to form the essential nucleus for the character formation of the psychopath. Greenacre (1948) in a later contribution to the study of the development and structure of the super-ego, divides the growth of the conscience into four stages, in any one of which disturbances may occur with varying severity. She considers that the first primitive roots of conscience lie in the early introjective-projective stage of the first eighteen to twenty-four months of life: the second stage in the years of habit-training, gaining of nursery morality, and the mastering of body urges; the third stage includes the tremendous advances stimulated in the three-to-six-year period with the struggle and renunciation of emotions focused on the parents leading to an independent self-criticizing function. This is allied with an extension of the child's world following physical and intellectual maturity, and an advance in character formation and independence inherent in the child's identification with the parent of the same sex. The final stage (a corollary to the third stage), occurs in the school-age period and adolescence, when many minor changes and reinforcements in the form of the conscience are produced under social and community influences and augmented by supporting parental figures. In this period character traits and ideals become integrated in an acceptable way and the individual conscience fuses more or less successfully with the social conscience of the community and the general cultural pattern.

Greenacre (1945) gives a good description of the influence on, and resultant structural distortion in, the super-ego, resulting from the presence of certain family constellations such as the combination of a vain, frivolous, insincere, flighty or capricious mother with a hypocritical, self-righteous and punitive father. Aichhorn (1925) has also described the influence upon the delinquent's character formation of contradictory patterns of maternal indulgence and stern paternal severity in which the child flies from one parent to the other in his attempts to escape reality and to evade educational demands—and ends, typically, by rebelling against the authority of both. Reich (1925) also traced deficiencies in the strength and content of the conscience to conflicting patterns of severity and indulgence in the parental figures. Healy and Bronner (1929) in their study of the influence of foster-home placement on problem children, also found many case histories where the delinquents' family constellations showed similar contradictory patterns.

Karpman (1948b) offers another version of the theory of conscience disturbance in the psychopath, and stresses the lack of ethics as an original condition seemingly unmodifiable by the environment. Karpman found, in psycho-analytic studies of psychopaths, that in a minority of cases no psychogenic aetiology could be demonstrated with present techniques of investigation. In a number of other cases he found neurotic conditions in which seemingly psychopathic behaviour was an expression of a disturbed conscience, but a disturbance which was both approachable and curable by psycho-therapy. In other cases he maintained that no conscience, disturbed or otherwise, was demonstrable, nor were there any deep or permanent emotional attachments. He reiterates (Karpman, 1948b, p. 490) that 'the particular emotional factors which contribute most to the formation of antisocial reaction are unrequited love, guilt and hostility', and describes various ways in which these emotional reactions may manifest themselves to produce a disturbed or weakened conscience. Greenacre (1945), however, denies the existence of the conscienceless delinquent or psychopath, and stresses early predisposition to anxiety and aggressiveness and the negative narcissistic parent-relationship. Wherever lies the truth with regard to the failure in conscience development observed in psychopaths and in many delinquents, a number of writers including Levy (1934, 1943), Bender (1943), Lowrey (1940b), Goldfarb (1943, 1944, 1945), Greenacre (1945), Karpman (1948a), and Burlingham and Freud (1942, 1943), as well as earlier investigators such as Aichhorn, Healy and Bronner, and the Gluecks, have agreed, with varying degrees of emphasis, that early deprivation and emotional disturbance lie behind the defective super-ego formation of psychopaths and delinquents.

Aichhorn (1925) has given us an account of a special technique he developed for the re-education of 'incorrigible' delinquents whose ego and super-ego formation are grossly disturbed; by manipulating a certain type of transference he reproduced a process which takes place in the rearing of every child, namely that of identification with the parental figure by means of an incorporation of his ideas. He aimed at bringing about, not a removal of symptoms, but a change in the delinquent's character structure. Friedlander (1947) has described the delinquent's failure to develop a reliable, independent ethical code or conscience in terms of failures or disturbances in the normal course of the socialization process. She describes the typical delinquent characteristics of lack of guilt, inability to wait for satisfaction of impulses, untruthfulness, demandingness, lack of regard for consequences, living for pleasure's sake, lack of a sense of regret or remorse or wish to make reparation for wrongdoings, lack of an independent self-criticizing function, lack of normal feeling for others, and unmodified antisocial impulses (such as greed, cruelty, spite, etc.). She offers an explanation for the persistence of these characteristics on the basis of the Freudian theory of personality development. In many of its aspects the conscience of the delinquent is regarded as being undeveloped beyond a certain level which may be observed in young toddlers. The fact that the super-ego is now known to be a complex group of functions, rather than a single entity; the fact that the dynamic roots of the super-ego (using this term with Freud's original meaning) lie in the unconscious mind, in contradistinction to the concept of conscience as used by McDougall and others in referring to consciously observable functions or processes; and the fact that certain aspects of the defective super-ego of delinquents may be found to correspond with arrested stages in the development of the conscience in normal children, emphasize the outstanding need in delinquency research for a greater understanding of the various aetiological, structural, and dynamic aspects of defective super-ego formation.

In the following section a number of behavioural traits and emotional attitudes that were thought to be indicative of certain aspects of defective super-ego formation, and that were found in the two groups of children on referral to the clinic, are grouped under the general heading 'Defective Super-ego Development'. These are character traits which have been described in the writings of various exponents of Freudian theory who have undertaken psychological re-education of chronic delinquents (e.g. Aichhorn, Reich, Alexander, Karpman, Biddle, Hoffer, Friedlander, Glover, Schmideberg, *et al.*).

43. *No sense of guilt or shame, plausible in excuses.*

44. *Does not own up, repent, or make good his misdeeds, shows no remorse or regret.*

45. *Impulsive, wilful, poor control over impulses.*

46. *Shows no concern for the consequences of his behaviour, heedless of advice or warning.*

47. *Cannot bear frustration or thwarting, resents criticism and correction.*

48. *Mistrustful of adults and fearful of authority, cringes and flinches easily.*

49. *Cannot wait, must have immediate satisfaction for his impulses, impatient.*

50. *Greedy, demanding, dissatisfied, insatiable, gluttonous.*

51. *Greedy, demanding, and extravagant attitude towards money and material goods.*

HYPOTHESIS: Defective Super-ego Formation
We should expect to find behaviour indicating defective or distorted super-ego development more frequently in delinquent children than in neurotics. (Confirmed, with the exception of items Nos. 49 and 50.)

The results presented in *Table 15*, Appendix I, indicate a significant difference between delinquent and neurotic children in most cases. Exceptions are items No. 49 and 50 where the X^2 level is not significant but correlations remain positive. It can be said with some degree of certainty that each of the foregoing items tends to be found in delinquent children more frequently than in neurotics, with the exception of items 49 and 50 which are found equally in both groups. With these exceptions it may be concluded that the group of traits tested in the hypothesis about defective super-ego formation offers a valid description of certain aspects of the delinquent character.

OTHER 'DIFFICULT' BEHAVIOUR

The following section contains a miscellaneous group of other behavioural traits and emotional attitudes for which some of the children in the two groups were described as 'difficult' on referral to the clinic.

52. *Temper outbursts:* (a) temper tantrums, screaming attacks, outbursts of rage; (b) bad-tempered, irritable, easily becomes angry and resentful.

53. *Stubborn, obstinate, negative behaviour.*

54. *Unreliable, irresponsible at school or at work, cannot be trusted, cannot keep jobs.*

55. *Restless, discontented, easily impatient and bored, changeable.*

56. *Lacks persistence, does what takes his fancy only, gives up if criticized, incapable of sustained effort.*

57. *Lazy and idle.*

58. *Selfish and inconsiderate for others' feelings for property, cannot share or take turns.*

59. *Moody.*

60. *Unemotional, apathetic, lethargic.*

61. *Absent-minded and forgetful.*

62. *Fidgety, irritating habits.*

63. *Religious doubts and difficulties, worries over 'unforgivable sin' etc.*

64. *Self-punishment, hurting self or getting hurt, provoking punishment.*

65. *Unhappy, seldom smiles, often dejected and miserable.*

66. *Feels unwanted, rejected, and disliked.*

HYPOTHESIS: Other 'Difficult' Behaviour
We should expect to find no significant difference between delinquent and neurotic children on any of the foregoing traits. (Confirmed, with the exception of item 60.)

The results presented in *Table* 16, Appendix 1, indicate that there is no significant difference here between the two groups, with the exception of item 60, which is seen to be more characteristic of neurotics than of delinquents. It may be concluded that *both* neurotic and delinquent children tend to show in varying degrees and in a high proportion of cases temper outbursts, either in the form of temper tantrums, screaming attacks, and rages or of bad-tempered, irritable behaviour, or easily becoming angry and resentful. Both groups include children who are stubborn, obstinate, negative, restless and discontented, easily become impatient and bored, are changeable, selfish, inconsiderate of others' feelings and property, cannot share or take turns, are unreliable, irresponsible at school or at work, unable to be trusted or to keep jobs, moody, absent-minded or forgetful, have fidgety, irritating habits, are lazy and idle, lack persistence, do what takes their fancy only, give up if criticized, and are incapable of sustained effort. Both groups contain children who are unhappy, seldom smile, are often dejected and miserable, punish themselves, get hurt or provoke punishment, feel unwanted, rejected and disliked, or have religious doubts, worries or difficulties.

QUEER HABITS AND 'ODD' BEHAVIOUR
In this section was grouped a miscellany of queer or 'odd' types of behaviour shown by children on referral to the clinic that marked a child as 'queer', 'different from other children', and so on. Four items were included in this section:

65. *Queer habits, 'odd' behaviour, bizarre ideas.*

66. *'Old for his age', unchildlike, does not play like other children.*

67. *Humourless, rarely smiles or laughs, never jokes or plays pranks.*

68. *Morbid interests.*

HYPOTHESIS: Queer Habits and 'Odd' Behaviour
We should not expect to find a significant difference between delinquent and neurotic children on the items in this group. (Confirmed.)

The results presented in *Table* 17, Appendix 1, show that there is no significant difference between delinquent and neurotic children found on any of this group of items, which were, however, observed incidentally and are not relevant to the main lines of our inquiry. Both delinquent and neurotic children showed certain types of queer habits or odd behaviour, but in most cases the numbers in each group were very small. It is interesting to note that nine cases of delinquent children and eleven cases of neurotic children are described as humourless, never really smiling or laughing, and never making jokes or pranks.

NEUROTIC DISORDERS OF ORGAN FUNCTION
Much study has been made of the relation between delinquency and enuresis, and Michaels (1940) has gone so far as to maintain that there should be differentiated a special type of 'persistent-enuretic delinquent'. The evidence for this, however, appears to be inconclusive. Very little research material appears to be available, moreover, about the specific relationship between delinquency and other disturbances of organ function frequently met with in chronic delinquents, such as encopresis, queer feeding habits, poor sleeping habits or nightmares, speech disturbances or gastric upsets. It was interesting to study the incidence of some of the disorders of this type in the delinquent group as well as in the neurotic children.

Several authors have claimed to establish a relationship between delinquency and persistent enuresis. Goodman and Michaels

(1934) studied the incidence and intercorrelation of enuresis and other neuropathic traits in children. Five traits (enuresis, thumb-sucking, nail-biting, speech impediments, and temper tantrums) were found to occur more often in combination than in isolation, and specifically the last four in combination with enuresis which was regarded as a common indicator of this type of symptom complex. The highest percentage of enuresis was found in the rejected or neglected children (including delinquents) and the lowest in over-protected children.

Mowrer and Mowrer (1938) examined the literature on the aetiology and treatment of enuresis, which ranged from exclusive emphasis upon faulty habit-training to suggestions for various automatic and mechanical training arrangements for its cure. Most of the current theories they found to be inconclusive and unsatisfactory. Enuresis is regarded as a continuation, due to inadequate training, of the physiological incontinence of infancy; or it is caused by certain emotional needs not finding appropriate expression during the child's waking hours; or enuresis is seen in boys as a substitutive form of gratification for repressed passive sexuality; or as a regression in response to sibling rivalry or traumatic experiences; or as a symptom of deep-seated fears and anxieties; or as disguised expression of repressed hostility towards the parents; or a masked form of masturbation and often as emission or orgasm-equivalent allied with a high degree of aggression. They reported that Hirsch found a high positive correlation between enuresis and delinquency. Karpman (1948a) mentions other factors in connection with enuresis, such as emotional instability and immaturity, feelings of insecurity and inferiority and hyper-suggestibility, all of which might also be regarded as part of the general picture of a neurosis, and he suggests that enuresis may be merely a concomitant of delinquency where both are part of a special neurotic constellation.

Michaels (1938) analysed the incidence of enuresis and the age of its cessation in 100 delinquent cases and 100 sibling controls. He found a higher incidence and a longer persistence of enuresis (and also a higher incidence of poor sleeping habits, left-handedness, thumb-sucking, nail-biting and temper tantrums) in delinquents than in their siblings. This result strengthened the conception of an intimate relationship between delinquency and enuresis but Michaels, like Karpman, prefers to regard these both as expressions of some common fundamental disorder of the personality, rather than as linked in a cause-effect relationship. Michaels and Goodman (1939) studied 1,000 neuro-psychiatric patients, and found the highest incidence of enuresis to be in delinquents and psychopathic personalities, both of whom were largely male. They regard enuresis as reflecting (Michaels and Goodman, 1939, p. 64) 'malintegration and disharmony' or 'a disturbance in the psycho-biologic integration and maturation with more physiological manifestations. Delinquency represents a disturbance in the culture-personality integration and maturation with more socio-biological manifestations'. Michaels and Goodman suggest that both delinquency and persistent enuresis offer an 'impenetrable armour' to ordinary therapeutic approaches, and that this can be accounted for by a weak ego, deficient inhibitory tendencies, lack of maturation, and a faulty integration of the component levels of personality. A further parallel might be found in that both delinquency and persistent enuresis are rooted in unbridled and unmodified instinctive drives. An explanation going deeper into the instinctual origins of human motivation has been offered by Alexander and Staub (1931) who regard enuresis as a persistent instinctual act, a kind of anachronism or 'psycho-biological infantilism' that has resisted the restrictions of instinctual activity which education would involve. It remains in a primitive form, regulated neither by adjustment to the outside world nor by the establishment of an internal inhibiting agent within the personality.

Goldman and Bergman (1945) carried out Rorschach Tests upon adult persistent enuretics and offered a challenge to Michaels and Goodman's findings. They found a paucity of psychopaths amongst the enuretics studied and a high frequency of psychoneurotic types. They suggest that many of the enuretic children who do not overcome the symptom may develop into psychopaths, but this can only be shown by follow-up studies of a random group of enuretic children, and not by a study of the past history of childhood enuresis among institutionalized cases, such as Michaels and Goodman carried out.

We examined a number of disorders of organ function found in our 100 cases. These results refer to the child's symptoms at the time of referral and not to disturbances occurring during his earlier developmental history. The latter are included in the sections dealing with difficulties in habit-training, sleep disturbances, etc., during the child's early history (see Chapter V). The present section includes:

69. *Feeding disturbances*, e.g. loss of appetite, excessive greed or queer eating habits, anorexia nervosa.

70. *Sleep disturbances*, e.g. all cases of sleep-walking, much sleep-talking, insomnia, very restless sleep or nightmares, or night terrors.

71. *Speech disturbances*, e.g. stammering or stuttering, inhibition of speech, loss of speech, speaking only in whispers, etc.

72. *Disturbances in bladder control*, e.g. diurnal and nocturnal enuresis and frequency of micturition.

73. *Disturbances in bowel control.* Under this heading were included all cases of encopresis, faecal incontinence, and soiling episodes.

74. *Disturbances in the alimentary system*, e.g. disturbances such as gastric upsets, colitis, constipation, diarrhoea, etc.

HYPOTHESIS: Neurotic Disorders of Organ Function
We should expect to find no significant difference between neurotic and delinquent children in the number of cases showing neurotic disorders of organ function. (Confirmed.)

The results presented in *Table* 18, Appendix 1, indicate that there is no significant difference between delinquent and neurotic children on any of the items listed in this section. The item 'speech disturbances' tends to fall near the borderline, and the correlation indicates some tendency for speech disturbances to be associated with neuroticism rather than with delinquency. It is interesting to note that in several cases the numbers for both delinquent and neurotic children are very high in this section. It may be concluded that a large number of both neurotic and delinquent children suffer from feeding disturbances, sleep disturbances, and disturbances of bladder control, and a smaller number of children in each group show speech disturbances, disturbances in bowel control and disturbances in the alimentary system.

LABILITY OF NERVOUS SYSTEM AND ALLERGY

Under this general heading the following symptoms were found to occur and their incidence was examined in both groups:

75. *Headaches and temperatures.*

76. *Sick turns with vomiting, train-sickness, etc.*

77. *Fainting turns.*

78. *Asthma.*

79. *Urticaria.*

HYPOTHESIS: Lability of Nervous System and Allergy

We should expect to find no significant difference between delinquents and neurotics in lability of nervous system and allergy. (Confirmed, with the exception of item 78.)

A significant difference between delinquent and neurotic children was found on one item only—the symptom of asthma—which tended to occur more frequently in the neurotic than in the delinquent children. *Table* 19, Appendix 1, shows that the numbers in all cases were very small, and no general conclusion can be drawn from this section.

CHAPTER IV

The child at home:
his family background and social setting

This chapter presents the results of comparing the delinquent and neurotic children on the conditions observed under the general heading 'Home and Family Background'. The tables, as before, show the frequency with which the observed conditions have been found in each group, and chi-square has been calculated, except in cases where the numbers are very small.

SOCIAL AND ENVIRONMENTAL CONDITIONS

Earlier studies of the sociological and psycho-social background of delinquents emphasized various aspects of their environment. Most of these studies have shown that the delinquent child tends to come from homes in the lower social strata, from working-class homes, from poverty-stricken, slum-type homes, or from demoralized families living in areas of community disorganization (Healy, 1915a; Burt, 1925; Shaw, 1929, 1942; Carr-Saunders, Mannheim and Rhodes, 1942; Mannheim, 1948; Rose, 1949, et alia). However, in later studies Healy found the environmental circumstances of his misdoers most diverse, and '. . . they appeared to come from all classes and conditions of society' (Healy, 1917, p. 313). Gordon (1928) maintained that studies of the environmental conditions of delinquency (housing, opportunities for leisure pursuits, area, health, and so on) can only be regarded as studies of 'secondary influences' and may well be meaningless without postulates concerning underlying psychological factors, since for every one case of juvenile misconduct that has been subjected to any of these influences, there can always be found a dozen law-abiding children living under exactly the same conditions. Gordon also stresses the relativity of various types of social misconduct in different classes and in different cultural patterns.

Aichhorn (1936) was concerned less with the external conditions or circumstances of delinquency than with the psychogenesis of the emotional aspects of the child's life. He makes the useful distinction between cases showing overt delinquent behaviour, which he calls 'manifest delinquency', and cases where a tendency towards misbehaviour exists but has not yet expressed itself— 'latent delinquency'. This tendency may lie dormant until suitable circumstances, e.g. certain traumatic experiences, arise and turn the latent into manifest delinquency. Aichhorn does not dismiss the importance of environmental factors in latent delinquency but considers them of secondary importance as precipitating factors (ibid., p. 41); 'We see now the bearing bad company has on the real problem. To find the causes of delinquency we must not only seek the provocation which made the latent delinquency manifest, but we must also determine what created the state of latent delinquency. . . .'

Carr-Saunders, Mannheim, and Rhodes (1942) reached a similar point of view when they emphasized that a little-understood 'tendency or susceptibility to delinquency' rather than the occurrence of delinquency itself, is the 'proper field for psychological investigations'; that is to say, not how or how often an offender breaks the law, but what psychological characteristics or motives form the precondition for becoming delinquent. Friedlander (1947) in her analysis of 'primary factors' and 'secondary factors' leading to the development of what she has termed 'anti-social character formation' has grasped the same prolem.

Shaw (1929) analysed the geographical distribution of delinquency and the relation of this to certain social and industrial areas of the community. He showed that the proportion of juvenile delinquents varied in different regions of the same city, and concluded that many criminal careers may originate in local areas or in the 'delinquent climate' of boys' gangs. He also found that the closer the area to the centre of the city, to industrial areas, large railway yards, etc., the more marked is the incidence of apprehended delinquency.[1] Psychological interpretation of these results, however, is difficult since similar conclusions might be found, as has been pointed out by Alexander and Healy (1935) and by Karpman (1948a) if one studied the incidence of business or financial transactions, or of typists and factory workers in relation to areas of the city. Studies like that of Shaw's 'Jack-Roller' (1930) although isolating and enumerating the external influences upon a boy's life, do not throw any light on the problem of which of the manifold harmful environmental forces have influenced the child in which way.

Levy (1932b) attempted to coordinate what was known about the influence of 'the delinquency-fostering milieu' and to differentiate neurotic delinquency from that produced by the environment. The delinquent act he describes as a product of an interaction between the individual and society. What determines this act may be chiefly (1) the social environment, (2) the interaction of the child's personality with the personalities of others about him (especially in the family situation), or (3) the mental mechanisms in the patient himself. In every act these stresses may vary or combine, or they may predominate in one of three ways (Levy,

[1] In 1942–5 I took part in a parallel study to that carried out by Shaw in Chicago, which was organized by the late Asst./Prof. H. L. Fowler in an unpublished survey for the Australian Council for Educational Research, of delinquency areas in the metropolitan area of Perth, Western Australia. The findings were strikingly similar in almost all respects to Shaw's. However, when the shift of delinquent population over a period of ten years was later analysed it was found that the *rate* of apprehension in these areas also varied considerably according to different social pressures and local conditions. Much minor delinquency remained unapprehended in the 'better' areas where its consequences were less severe, or were concealed, or dealt with by the parents by other means (such as sending the child to boarding school, or shielding him from the public consequences of his delinquency through reasons of family pride). Also, when a subsidiary study was made of the activities of one juvenile gang, it was discovered that the reported 'incidence' of delinquency varied significantly from one end of a long suburban street (where most of the gang lived) to the other. Reasons for this variation were found by studying the geographical distribution of those who *referred* the juvenile delinquents to the courts. At the 'referring' end of the street were situated (a) a station for the training of police officers, (b) a convent, (c) several churches, and (d) the residences of several retired school teachers. At the 'non-referring' end of the street were the habitations of kindly and lenient Chinese market gardeners who tolerated a great deal of 'raiding' of their gardens by the boys, but distributed swift and direct justice of their own when the boys teased them with taunts and ribaldry, or came near their homes. This finding emphasizes once more the need for studying 'non-court' as well as 'court' cases of delinquency, to which Mannheim (1949) has drawn attention.

ib. p. 197 ff.). 'If a child who steals and truants is found to have learned all his lessons in life from a criminal father and an alcoholic mother in a poverty-stricken home in a delinquent neighbour-hood . . . then one does not need to look far beyond the social causes.' Levy adds that in selecting cases to illustrate delinquency resulting directly from social factors '. . . we play safe as long as we stick to extreme cases. As they approach nearer and nearer to the norm, explanations of behaviour principally of social causation become increasingly untenable.' The term 'social factors' he uses to indicate influences which tend to produce delinquency in a direct way, i.e. 'the child develops delinquency in this environ-ment as naïvely and directly as the use of his mother tongue', and personality and other factors are therefore relatively unimportant considerations. As the environmental pressure towards delin-quency is lessened, however, attention must become focused upon '. . . the development of aggressive, dominating tendencies in the patient and upon such major human relationships as mater-nal over-protection, father hostility and sibling rivalry . . . (which) . . . are markedly influenced if not entirely shaped by his early intra-family relationships'. Levy suggests that the most frequent cause of delinquency is a combination of aggressive trends and a delinquency-fostering milieu. The basic problem he sees as the child's failure to modify his aggression to social needs. Frequently this is exaggerated by an indulgent, over-protective mother who is unable to deny or discipline her offspring, yields to his every whim, and yet refuses to give him any independence. This pre-pares him only for one way of living, gives momentum to aggres-sive forces and magnified infantile behaviour. Levy thinks that when aggressive trends are extreme, delinquency may result even when environmental pressures are slight; his commonest finding in delinquent cases, however, is neither a severe milieu nor severe aggression but combinations of both. By whatever routes the normal modification of primary aggression comes about, it seems that it must be fostered in direct response to social relationships.

Shaw (1938) studied the sociological and mass influences upon the antisocial behaviour of five delinquent brothers. The in-fluences of poverty, broken homes and poor environment were given greater significance than individual motivation. These cases represent an extreme example of what Burt has called 'the vicious home' and Levy 'environmental delinquency', where there is no course open to the child but to follow the delinquent habits of his family which he has learned in the same way as he has learned language. Shaw stressed, and most authors fully agree with him, the need for correction of the environmental factors productive of crime.

Shaw and McKay's *magnum opus* (1942) represented twenty years' analysis of the effect of physico-geographic and socio-economic factors on juvenile delinquency. In each of twenty large American cities the incidence of juvenile delinquency corresponded to the physical structure and organization of the city. Higher delinquency rates were found in the inner zones, lower rates in the outer zones, and these rates declined regularly with progression from innermost to outermost zone. Juvenile delinquency was shown to be concentrated in areas of physical deterioration and neighbourhood disorganization, or in areas adjacent to centres of commerce and heavy industry. Only the legally apprehended delinquents, who were of official concern to the public, were included in this investigation. Delinquency was found to be closely correlated with such separate factors as (1) population change, (2) bad housing, (3) adult crime, (4) poverty, (5) foreign or negro birth, (6) tuberculosis, (7) mental disorders. They conclude that the basic solution of this and other problems of urban life lies in a programme of physical rehabilitation of the slum areas and the development of community organization, since 'delinquency has its roots in the dynamic life of the community'. (Shaw, 1942, p. 441 ff.) A preventive programme should decrease the delinquency rate of that area, because, writes Shaw, '. . . if the delinquent tradition did not exist and the boys were not exposed to it, a preponderance of those who become delinquent in low income areas would find their satisfactions in activities other than delinquency'. Shaw does not indicate how he believes the influences described produce their effect, or how juvenile delinquency other than that apprehended by the law can be disposed of in this manner, i.e. by decreasing the temptations which face the normal youth, rather than by increasing his resilience and strength of character in overcoming them.

Freud, Healy, Karpman, and many others have repeatedly demonstrated that subtle early environmental influences contribute to character formation in a way that leads to weakness in the face of temptation or in the face of selfish instinctual impulses. Healy and Bronner have shown that many factors, especially environmental factors to which delinquency is often attributed, also operate in the lives of non-delinquents. Shaw's studies, although telling us a good deal about the 'delinquent climate', tell us nothing of why one particular boy in a broken home in a disorganized community becomes delinquent and another in the same home does not; nor what are the psycho-genetic factors or specific experiences which go into the making of a delinquent, and which produce delinquency in many children who do *not* experience these environmental pressures. In Mannheim's terminology (1949), Shaw's studies should rightly be regarded not as psychological, but as 'ecological', in the sense of being concerned with the individuals's habits, modes of life, and relations to his surrounding environment.[1]

Carr-Saunders, Mannheim, and Rhodes (1942) undertook a large-scale sociological survey of young offenders in Great Britain which gave statistical verification to findings of earlier writers. For example, the authors show that broken homes produce three to four times as many delinquents as do stable and harmonious homes, and that delinquency is the outcome of an interaction between heredity, or the little understood 'tendency of susceptibility to delinquency', and various unfavourable environmental pressures. The authors limit themselves to strictly sociological and statistical aims and have presented some very valuable information about the environmental and social circumstances of 1,953 delinquents whose records were compared with those of 1,970 non-delinquents used as controls. The report deals with court cases of delinquency only and with boys only and, as the authors point out, information upon subtler psychological issues could not be included. Mannheim's very interesting smaller-scale local study

---

[1] The perspectives of time may show that findings about the inadequate social background of delinquents may have been given undue weight because the majority of statistical studies have been concentrated on juvenile delinquents who are referred to courts.

'Juvenile Delinquency in an English Middletown' (1948) is aimed at giving a comprehensive sociological picture of the setting in which delinquency occurs rather than of the psychological factors leading to delinquent behaviour. It provides (Mannheim, 1949. p. 12) 'useful beginnings in the direction towards a more scientific *ecological* study of the criminological situation existing in different parts of the whole country'. He makes a plea for more active collaboration between criminologists and lawyers on the one hand and psychologists and sociologists on the other in 'regional research' into juvenile delinquency and its treatment. Mannheim stresses that the scope of inquiries should be extended beyond the delinquent court case to those who do not come into court, and also those non-delinquents who are in essential characteristics similar to delinquents. He suggests an inquiry distinguishing between (a) court cases of delinquents, (b) court cases of non-delinquents, (c) non-court cases of delinquents, (d) non-court cases of non-delinquents. This, if related to a background of sociological and ecological studies that treat delinquency as one of many sociological aspects of a locality, would contribute to the filling in of many gaps in our knowledge. Mannheim is of the opinion that the scope of controlled experiment in the study of criminology, although involving risk, has perhaps been underestimated, and he is in agreement with Burt (1949, p. 42) that 'certainly it would be perfectly practicable to take paired groups and subject them to planned experiments in alternative lines of treatment or training', and that 'so far as the study of delinquency is concerned nothing short of a vigorous scientific approach will suffice. All possible roads should be followed by a coalition of specialists in all the relevant fields'.

Greenacre (1945, p. 496 ff.) refers to an adverse sociological environment as holding '... influences which complicate and often supply secondarily reinforcing involvements for the delinquent ... (which) ... are often used as rationalizations and given over prominence in many hospitals and court clinics'. She found that psychopaths seen in private practice frequently came from a relatively secure economic background and were free of such influences. Powdermacker, Leves and Touraine (1937) also described, among three main types of juvenile delinquent whose psychopathology they studied in treatment, a group who were typically the 'spoiled child', frequently a middle-class or 'highbrow' type, who became dissocial as a result of indulgence and indiscriminate and super-abundant love. Other writers like Aichhorn (1925), Biddle (1933), and Banister and Ravden (1944) have also stressed that a certain type of 'problem child' or spoiled, over-indulged delinquent tends to come from stable, middle-class homes. Friedlander (1949b) has stressed that neurotic children tend to come almost evenly from homes of working-class and middle-class levels.

SOCIAL LEVEL OF THE HOME

Because of the difference between rural conditions in this county and the crowded life of large industrial cities, it was thought to be of special interest to compare the social level of the homes from which the groups of our selected delinquents and neurotics came. This was done by slightly adapting Booth's scale (as used by Burt, 1925) to the local conditions, and by distinguishing particularly between 'working-class' and 'middle-class' homes. An index of the social and economic level of the home was given by the occupation of the father and, in some cases, of the mother. Since this study was carried out in an immediate post-war period many fathers had spent recent years in H.M. Forces, and categories were therefore included for various ranks in the armed forces. A new category, 'poor middle-class', had also to be introduced to describe a few homes which under contemporary conditions were impoverished but remained definitely middle-class in standards and cultural level.

The cases in both groups were examined and arranged according to parental occupation in the following scale:

Working-class

1. *Very poor working-class:* irregular earnings; casual, unskilled labour; light work; semi-illiterate labourers; the family has periods on relief; father does not support; or mother works and has grave financial difficulties in supporting herself and her child.

2. *Poor working-class:* small but constant earnings; unskilled but regular labour; employed labourers in steady work.

3. *Comfortable working-class:* regular standard earnings; artisans; small shop-keepers (with assistants); owners of small one- or two-man businesses; regular Navy, Army, or Air Force (without commissioned rank).

Middle-class

1. *Poor middle-class:* Culturally middle-class but impoverished homes; families who have 'come down in the world' but struggle to maintain their former standards (e.g. an elderly eccentric 'old college boy' married to the educated granddaughter of a vicar, now living on a very small income and old age pension).

2. *Comfortable middle-class:* high-class labour; well-paid foremen; best-paid artisans; supervising shop assistants.

3. *Well-to-do middle-class:* lower middle-class shop-keepers; tradesmen; businessmen; small employers; clerks, lower commissioned ranks in the Services.

4. *Professional well-to-do middle-class:* professional men, servant-keeping families, and senior commissioned ranks in the Services.

HYPOTHESIS: Social Level of the Home
We should expect to find that a greater number of delinquent than neurotic children tend to come from working-class homes. (Not Confirmed.)

The results presented in *Table 20*, Appendix 1, show no significant difference between delinquent and neurotic children in the numbers who come from working-class homes. The tetrachoric correlation showed a slight tendency for delinquents to come from working-class homes and neurotics from middle-class homes, but this was not large enough to be significant on the chi-square test, and has been disregarded. (It should be remembered, in interpreting this finding, that intelligence has been controlled in the two groups, and that many of the delinquents were non-court cases.)

GROSS ENVIRONMENTAL DISTURBANCES
Studies of the influence of social conditions on delinquency have

emphasized the significance of gross disturbances, such as over-crowding, unsettled home, frequent moves, 'vicious homes', etc. (Burt, 1925; Levy, 1932b; Healy and Bronner, 1936; Carr-Saunders, *et al.* 1942). Burt (1925) found that 55 per cent of young offenders in London came from homes that were below the poverty line. He found that 26 per cent of his cases came from 'vicious homes', and in looking for causes found that in approximately 32 per cent the chief cause was an environmental one. In most cases, however, a combination of factors was found. 'The typical delinquent (Burt, 1925a, p. 3) . . . is a child with a dull un-educated mind, struggling to control an emotional and impulsive temperament, both housed in a weak, afflicted body, and living with a demoralized family in an impoverished home'.

Lindner (1944) undertook the hypno-analytic treatment of a criminal psychopath and stressed the importance of very early emotional traumata, especially the repeated witnessing of noc-turnal sexual scenes which stimulated the child's fear and aggres-sion and led subsequently to the development of neurotic scopto-philia. Greenacre (1945, 1948), among others, has pointed out that there may be an unrecognized psychological factor in the over-crowded and unsatisfactory sleeping arrangements in the slum homes from which criminals so frequently emerge. Collis and Poole's (1950) description of children's life in a degraded in-dustrial slum gives a picture of early sexual experience and not uncommon sexual assault of children which suggests that this view merits further investigation.

In the present section I propose to examine some of these in-fluences in detail, and to include also such items as periods of hospitalization, air-raid experiences, and evacuation, about the effects of which evidence is not conclusive (Mannheim, 1948). Gross environmental disturbances of all types are likely to weaken family ties and disrupt that family unity which is essential for normal adaptation to social life. For these reasons one might ex-pect to find environmental disturbances occurring typically in the histories of delinquents. This does not necessarily follow, how-ever, since the fact that he has been in hospital, in air-raids or evacuated, gives only a rough indication of the inner meaning of such an event for the child at a particular stage in his development

(Burlingham and Freud, 1942, 1943). Many subtle factors such as the way the child was prepared for his experience, the parents' attitude to it, the child's earlier emotional relationships with his parents, and possibly the parents' own fear or opposition to the event, are important as well as the child's way of dealing with his individual experience.

Friedlander (1947, 1949b) has re-emphasized that delinquent children tend to come from broken homes, but that neurotic children frequently come from stable and secure homes. The results presented by Banister and Ravden (1945) also indicate that the 'nervous' type of problem child tends to come from stable 'accord' homes, and the aggressive and delinquent children from various types of broken homes.

It was decided to examine the number of children in both groups who had experienced the following environmental conditions or influences:

a. *Unsettled homes, frequent moves:* e.g. a family which has never had a settled home; or has had an unsettled home for long periods with frequent moves; or constant changes of home and of family personnel, friends and surroundings.

b. *Overcrowded conditions:* e.g. a home in which conditions have always been, or have been for a long time, overcrowded, such as a large family living in an inadequate house; two families living together in a small flat; a large family sharing a house with relatives or friends; a mother living in rooms with her children for a long period.[1]

c. *Periods spent in foster-homes:* e.g. children who had lived in a foster-home for long or short periods, or children whose lives had been spent entirely in foster-homes.

d. *Absence from home with relatives or friends.* Children who for varying periods had been sent to live with relatives or friends were included here when this meant that the total care of the child

[1] As a rough guide a home is regarded as crowded where there are more than two persons per room. In practice, however, the decision to rate a home as over-crowded rested with the psychiatric social worker who took into account such factors as the size of the rooms, or whether there were gardens, and various difficult conditions in sharing houses.

was taken over by someone other than the parents. A holiday visit where there is no question of the child's remaining away indefinitely was not included. Typical cases are those where the grandmother takes over the child while the mother goes out working following separation from the father; or the child is sent away repeatedly and for long periods during times of family emergency, such as mother's illness, or the arrival of a new baby; or the child is sent away on account of difficult or unmanageable behaviour in the hope that a period with a stricter grandmother or less burdened aunt may discipline him. Evacuation to relatives during the war was not included here but counted under the general heading of 'evacuation'.

e. *Evacuation.* This included all children who were evacuated from home during the war and separated from parents or families, whether this was for a long or short time and regardless of whether the evacuation was to the home of friends or relatives, or to billets with strangers.

f. *Travel abroad:* e.g. children who had spent a part of their lives in foreign countries, or in travelling in India, China, America, or elsewhere. Such experience is likely to place strain upon the ties of family life and to expose the child to numerous unusual environmental experiences such as hotel or shipboard life, living in rooms or temporary quarters, dealing with a foreign language, being cared for by foreign servants.

g. *Hospitalization:* e.g. children who had spent time in hospital for any reason at all, regardless of whether or not the experience was mild or severe, or whether a satisfactory family contact had been maintained. More detailed information than it was possible to obtain here would be necessary to ascertain in every case whether or not the event was a traumatic one for the child, especially when the period spent in hospital occurred many years ago (cf. Spitz, 1945, 1946a; Bowlby, 1951).

h. *Experience of air-raids:* e.g. children who experienced major bombing or air-raid attacks, who underwent shelter life, or were
126

in any way exposed to the dangers, hardships or other effects upon civilian life of air-raids.[1]

i. *'Vicious homes'*: e.g. demoralized homes in which the family standards of conduct are low; or where the child's delinquency is condoned or encouraged, so that his behaviour is no more than a copy of the parents' or older children's behaviour (Burt, 1925; Levy, 1932b).

HYPOTHESIS: Gross Environmental Disturbances
We should expect to find that delinquent children will have experienced more gross environmental disturbances than neurotics. (Hypothesis confirmed for items a to c and not confirmed for items d to i in *Table 21*, Appendix 1.)

Table 21 indicates that the differences between neurotic and delinquent children are significant for unsettled homes and frequent moves, overcrowding, and periods spent in foster-homes. They also show marginal significance for absence with friends and relatives. The results were not significant in the case of evacuation, travel abroad, hospitalization, air-raid experience, or 'vicious homes'. About one-third of the children in *both* groups have spent periods in hospital at various times of their lives, and a smaller proportion of both groups have experienced evacuation, air-raids and travel abroad. The numbers in these latter groups, however, are too small to allow any conclusions to be drawn. There is a positive correlation between delinquency and unsettled homes, overcrowding, and periods spent in foster-homes or absent from home with friends and relatives.

Examples of Gross Environmental Disturbances
Many of the children in both groups have experienced more than one of these environmental disturbances. Nine delinquents have experienced gross and continued environmental disturbances throughout the whole of their lives. Three examples are the following:

[1] Two children among the present delinquent cases had also spent periods in internment camps overseas.

Case No. 35. *Maryann* is the child of an unstable middle-class girl who married a man twenty years older than herself, and went with him to Burma, only to find there that he was an alcoholic and a drug addict. Maryann's parents were divorced shortly after her birth, and as a child she was moved around from place to place and from person to person, living alternately with the father, the mother, the mother's second husband's family, the grandmother, in a rigid children's home, and then in a sequence of eight boarding schools, from all of which with monotonous regularity she was expelled for violent conduct. At present the child lives with her grandmother who has taken her to four child guidance clinics, accepting no advice other than that which supports her own wish to send the child away again. The mother has separated from her second husband and refuses to have Maryann with her on account of her violent behaviour to the new baby.

Case No. 47. *Sarah,* aged fourteen, is a rejected child of an unhappy broken marriage, and her mother has sent her away repeatedly on flimsy excuses since her early school years. She has placed her in a convent, in a mental hospital, in a children's home, and in another religious home. She broke off treatment at the clinic, in spite of the girl's satisfactory progress, when help was not forthcoming for her to send the child away again.

Case No. 21. *Bobbie* is a war-baby born illegitimately while his mother's husband was overseas and the family living under very unsettled home conditions. His mother died when he was two years old, and he then lived with a maternal aunt for three years. Next he returned to live with the husband and his second wife, but this was an unsuccessful marriage and the child was unhappy and delinquent there. He now lives with the husband and the latter's mistress and at the age of eleven is again delinquent, truanting and running away from home repeatedly.

INSTITUTIONAL AND 'DEPRIVED' CHILDREN

There have been a number of studies of the influence of institutional rearing on personality development, and the unfavourable

effects resulting when there is not sufficient provision of opportunity for each child to establish an enduring emotional attachment
to one person from his early years. Spitz (1945, 1946), Burlingham and Freud (1942, 1943), Lowrey (1940), Goldfarb (1943,
1944, 1945, 1947, 1949), and Bowlby (1944, 1951) have severally
demonstrated not only that the old-fashioned type of institutional
rearing (where many small children have to share the love and
attention of inadequate and frequently changing mother-substitutes) tends to produce children with all-round personality
impoverishment, but that the whole process of successful upbringing is much more difficult to achieve in institution-reared
children. As I have previously stressed, an adaptation to social
needs comes about, according to psycho-analytic theory, as a
result of the small child's identifying himself with his love-object,
i.e. the person on whom he depends for his intimate daily care,
and so learning to adopt his or her standards of behaviour.
These processes of identification can take place only in response to
complicated psychological interchanges and on the basis of a long-
term, secure emotional dependence. Since institutional life, as
it has largely been organized in the past, endangers the perman-
ence, the exclusiveness, and the depth of such relationships, our
theoretical expectations must lead us to suppose that failures in
the socialization process such as occur in delinquency will occur
more frequently among institution children than among others.

Lowrey (1940b) investigated the influence of isolation and
'affect hunger' upon children who lived their early years in institutions. He found a high frequency of language defects, slowness
of development of speech, marked general inadequacy, and a
voracious 'appetite for affection' which was almost insatiable.
When removed from the institution to foster-homes they were
'isolated children' who were unable to live in a group or to accept
smoothly a position as centre of attention and affection or to make
friendly social relationships. They became wild, demanding,
aggressive, jealous, and negativistic, and sometimes showed
various regressive and neurotic symptoms. In a number of cases
emotional development was retarded, and markedly sadistic behaviour continued until the age of four years. The emergence of
sadism seemed to be both delayed and therefore excessive, and

at the same time was stimulated in some way by alterations in the environment. Lowrey concludes that infants reared in institutions (ibid, p. 485) '... undergo an isolation type of experience, with resulting personality distortion, characterized by unsocial behaviour, hostility and aggression, inability to understand or to accept limitations and marked insecurity in adapting to the environment...'. Lowrey states his opinion that infants should not be reared in institutions, and society should recognize that experiences such as institutional rearing have ill effects on the formation of personality, and provide accordingly. Children who do not receive the normal amount of love and care necessary to stimulate development tend to develop a recognizable composite picture of personality distortion.

Burlingham and Freud (1942, 1943) presented the fruits of their long experience in the observation of infants and children absented from their families in wartime. Detailed accounts are presented of the influence upon young children of early and sudden separation from their mothers, of sudden weaning consequent in many cases upon this separation, and the child's reactions and ways of getting over these events. Valuable material was collected on the separation of the child from the mother at the stage of his intense and dependent relationship in the first years. The small child's overwhelming grief, and the development of many disturbing symptoms during his evacuation, were explained by the nature of his experience of this separation at varying ages, and it was not always possible to overcome the effects of this harmful influence. The effect of separation from the mother and the consequent disturbances in the formation of friendly emotional relationships were vividly described in cases of children who changed hands repeatedly during their third year of life, or were never looked after by any single person for any length of time. The absence of the father and of the important stimulus his presence gives to social development, was considered to have far-reaching effects upon the child's character and later social behaviour.

Further observations on the influence of the child's separation from his parents and the absence of satisfactory parent-substitutes, were made by Bender (1943). She made a special study of neglected and deserted children raised in institutions without an enduring relationship to any one person during the first three or four years of life. Bender found these neglected children to be characteristically aggressive, psychopathic personalities, totally lacking in anxiety, whose aggression was typically diffuse and destructive and showed little concern for love-objects. This type of institution experience in early years, Bender claims, is not conducive to the development of a strong character or a reliable conscience, but tends to lead toward delinquent or psychopathic development.

Goldfarb (1943, 1944, 1945, 1947, 1949) presented a number of studies on the relation between infant-rearing and problem behaviour, and the effects of institutional care upon personality development. Rorschach study of the personalities of adolescents who had spent a considerable part of their lives in institutions distinguished sharply between children who had experienced deprivation in institutions during infancy and children who had been brought up in families. A basic syndrome of traits was found to permeate the whole personalities of the institution children. Their intellectual achievements were lower, they reasoned less well, were particularly deficient in the ability to perceive relationships, and to act in accordance with the abstract attitude or a conscious intention or goal; they showed reduced drive and application, less emotional maturity and control, less ambition, and tended to be more impoverished, passive and apathetic. The absence of continued individual contact with an adult in the earliest years, and in later years a pattern of life determined purely by group routine, were thought to have an adverse effect on them. Part of the reason for their impoverishment was to be found in the simple absence of normal social stimuli, but more important was the absence of normal identifications in infancy, on which the stimulus for the gradual differentiation of personality depends.

Goldfarb (1945) also studied in detail seventy equated pairs of children from institutions and foster-homes and found that the institution child showed personality traits like lack of initiative, passivity and unwillingness to learn, an unusual curiosity or flightiness of thinking, motility disturbances and extreme social shyness. They were furthermore retarded in learning and showed certain emotional trends such as absence of normal inhibitory pattern, unmitigated affect hunger, emotional imperviousness and superficiality of relationships, absence of normal tension and anxiety reaction, and social regressiveness. Affect hunger in institution children led to demands for excessive displays of affection and sensuality, seeking attention from strangers, wanting to be dressed up and treated like a baby, or 'wanting only to hug and kiss'. Life histories of the institution cases show 'stubbornly maintained patterns of infantilism and passivity', leading to a personality 'congealed on a level of extreme immaturity' with defects in the spheres both of intellect and feeling. The institution child lacks the will to understand or reorganize external experience. He is destructive, disorganized, stubborn, isolated, unable to get along with other children, wanders a great deal, is overtly hyper-active and aggressive in a formless, diffuse, disorganized, and aimless way, and his conduct becomes easily delinquent in unfavourable circumstances. There seems to be no appreciable development of the capacity for identifying with and loving or respecting others, and this results in grave problems in the control of social behaviour. He does not, typically, suffer from neurotic conflicts, but his ego-structure remains primitive, undeveloped, and weak. His need is for the stimulated growth towards a normal character structure rather than the psychotherapeutic amelioration of conflicts and anxiety. For these reasons Goldfarb finds that direct treatment of the institution child is frequently ineffectual, especially when it is offered only belatedly in adolescence.

It is interesting, in the light of this general condemnation of the influence on early psychological development of institutional rearing, to compare a number of opinions about the efficacy of the time-honoured method of institutional treatment of delinquents. Healy and Bronner's 'study in outcomes' of the treatment of delinquents by various methods (1925) showed a 'disconcerting measure of failure' in Chicago, where largely diagnostic and placement work had been done, but greater success was revealed in the Boston follow-ups where considerable use had been made of child placement in carefully chosen and supervised foster-homes which were well followed up after a thorough study of the individual case. Topping (1941, 1943) describes certain types of aggressive pseudo-social boys who are greatly influenced by the gang or social setting, but who are uninfluenced by the life of corrective institutions. Other writers who have been concerned with the long-term treatment of the genuinely neurotic delinquent (Aichhorn, Alexander, Macdonald, Healy, Isaacs, Karpman, Lippman, Friedlander, Powdermacker, Leves and Touraine, *et al.*) are unanimous in recommending that psychiatric treatment for delinquents of this type (and especially for those whose basic mechanism is the guilt-ridden 'need for punishment') can best be carried out under some kind of social and residential supervision or custodial care; for example, in 'hospital schools' or in institutions organized in special and unconventional ways. Healy and Alper (1941), in examining the Borstal system in England, highly praised its use of institutions not as prisons but as training centres. They pronounced that '. . . the Borstal system is truly an attempt at psychological treatment of crime. The approach is highly individual and takes full account of the delinquent's abilities and aptitudes; individual interviews are emphasized; contact with families is maintained. Withal there is insignificant appreciation of psychiatric possibilities both as regards diagnosis and more intimate psychotherapy, and wholly insufficient appreciation of the more basic aetiological factors that can only be obtained through individual psychiatric analysis'. Healy expressed his opinion further (Healy, 1949, p. 317): 'In my opinion the central idea of psychotherapy, treatment of the emotional life, accounts for the unparalleled effectiveness of the celebrated Borstal system for dealing with offenders. . . . Very largely the methods . . . are keyed to mental hygiene principles, although not designated as such. In the usual scheme of highly personalized interview between inmates and selected officials, in the studies of the offender and the subsequent adjustment of him to the different training régimes, the main objective is to deal therapeutically with his inner troubles and offer him deep satisfactions. Although its weakness lies in not having psychiatric advice for special cases, this particular plan for reformation works better than any other that we know about.'

It is interesting to compare with this eulogy of the Borstal system some figures quoted by Mass Observation in a report on

juvenile delinquency (Willock, 1949, p. 129). 'Of 3,367 boys discharged from Borstal during the years 1935-9, 1,389 had been
reconvicted by September 1946—i.e. 41 per cent. Of 2,817 boys
released in 1939 (on the outbreak of war) 1,419 had been reconvicted by September 1946—i.e. 50 per cent. Of the girls, 54 per
cent. of those discharged in 1937-8 were reconvicted by September 1943, 56 per cent. of those discharged in 1939.' Mass Observation also quotes a psychiatrist's opinion that of those sentenced to
Borstal treatment about half would remain unchanged by it and
most of the rest could be treated much more easily and quickly
by other means.

The number of institution children in the present sample is
rather small, but we were interested to note how many of them
had taken the delinquent line of development and how many had
become neurotic. A comparison was made of the number of
children who have lived for any period of time in institutions for
homeless or maladjusted children, in orphanages, residential nurseries, approved schools, or any other kind of children's homes.

HYPOTHESIS: *Periods Spent in Institutions or Children's Homes*
We should expect to find that delinquent children would tend to
have lived part of their lives in institutions, children's homes, etc.,
more frequently than neurotics. (Confirmed.)

Although the number of cases in the present sample is small
the results presented in *Table 22*, Appendix 1, indicate that there
is a significant difference between delinquent and neurotic children
in the numbers who have lived part of their lives in institutions of
various kinds, these children tending to be delinquent more often
than neurotic.

HOME AND FAMILY BACKGROUND CONDITIONS

We examined a number of conditions in the family settings of
delinquent and neurotic children. These included a study of
possible hereditary factors in the child's family history, the structure of the family, the nature of the child's parents, and certain
family relationships.

I. POSSIBLE HEREDITARY FACTORS

Investigations into various types of instability in the immediate relatives and forbears of delinquents have formed an essential part of most of the major investigations into delinquency, although the results of these are by no means conclusive. Healy's account (1949) of the practices prevalent less than forty years ago leaves no doubt that most workers were imbued with the idea that serious antisocial conduct betokened something pathological in the offender. Healy describes his pioneer work as a process of exploring and discarding one after another most of the current theories concerning the essential nature of the individual delinquent. He delved into the theories of the 'born criminal' and the publications upon theories of degeneracy and atavism by Lombroso and the 'positivist school' in Italy; the studies by Talbot in the United States and by Goring in England on reformatory inmates, in search of the 'stigmata of degeneracy' described in current psychiatric textbooks. Healy gives due credit to these 'pioneers in the study of the individual' (Healy, 1949, p. 19) and describes how he examined shapes of head and face, malformed ears, hard palates, enlarged tonsils and adenoids, visual defects, phimosis, cigarette-smoking and coffee-drinking, all of which were claimed to cause refractory behaviour. Healy found no evidence of such influence and early in his pioneer researches discarded these theories, which had, in accordance with the scientific temper of the nineteenth century, continued to grope after some biological explanation of delinquency. He found, too, that no proof was forthcoming for any theory of inheritance of criminalism. Although he had found in his monumental study in 1915 the presence of 'antecedent prior conditions' among which he placed defective heredity, in the history of delinquents, the follow-up studies published in 1925 showed that bad heredity, in general, appeared to contribute little to delinquency.

Burt (1925) gave to inherited and constitutional conditions an important place among various predisposing factors that may bias a child towards delinquency. In assessing causes he found that in approximately 30 per cent of the cases the cause was an hereditary one. Burt found that about 7 per cent of his juvenile delinquents could be classified as 'temperamentally unstable', whilst

'. . . among all the innate psychological characteristics of the delinquent, a marked emotionality is one of the most frequent, as it is one of the most influential'. The importance of hereditary factors has recently been re-emphasized by Mullins (1945).

We examined all cases where morbid or other unfavourable conditions were known to have been present in one or more of the child's parents, grandparents or near relatives. As other authors have done, the writer has had to rely upon reports given by the child's parents or relatives during consultation at the child guidance clinics. Although great pains have been taken to check the accuracy of these reports, there remains the possibility that certain parents may intentionally or unintentionally have given incorrect or unreliable information at certain points. Reference is therefore made to 'known hereditary factors' where the presence of unstable conditions in the family history is known for certain.

Two main groups of conditions were examined:

a. Miscellaneous conditions, e.g. cases of alcoholism, epilepsy, psychosis, temperamental instability,[1] criminality, suicide, or mental defect in the family history.

b. Neurotic conditions.

HYPOTHESES: Unfavourable Conditions in Family History
1. We should expect to find that miscellaneous unfavourable conditions occur more frequently in the family histories of delinquent children than in those of neurotics. (Confirmed.)

2. We should expect to find that neurotic conditions occur more frequently in the family histories of neurotic children than in those of delinquents. (Not confirmed.)

The numbers in each of the sub-sections in *Table 23*, Appendix

[1] Under the heading of 'temperamental instability' (See Burt, 1925, pp. 507 ff.), were included cases which, without being intellectually defective or showing symptoms of neurosis or psychosis, show pronounced emotional instability, frequently allied with a defective moral sense, inability to control impulsive actions, and general lack of emotional control. These include the supposed 'psychopathic personalities' who are typically egotistic, aggressive, recalcitrant and lacking in ordinary guilt and remorse, whose emotional reactions are often grossly and crudely expressed, and who frequently appear to be incorrigible.

1, are too small for conclusions to be drawn about specific conditions, although alcoholism and criminality appear to be more frequent in the family histories of delinquents, and neurotic conditions in the families of neurotics. This table has been regrouped to contrast those families showing neurotic conditions with those showing one or more possibly hereditary factors among the miscellaneous conditions. The results, presented in *Table 24*, Appendix 1, indicate that there is a significantly greater number of delinquent children than neurotic children with histories containing miscellaneous unstable conditions. There is also a positive correlation between delinquency and the existence of such conditions in the child's family history. There was, however, no significant difference between the delinquent and neurotic children whose families showed neurotic conditions.

FAMILY STRUCTURE AND 'BROKEN HOMES'

One of the findings established repeatedly by many kinds of delinquency research is that delinquent children tend to come from broken homes: homes broken by death, separation, divorce, desertion or for other reasons. (Healy, 1915a, 1917; Healy and Bronner, 1936; Burt, 1925; Aichhorn, 1925; Shaw, 1929; Carr-Saunders, Mannheim and Rhodes, 1942; Banister and Ravden, 1945, *et al.*). Aichhorn found that the cases in his institution for delinquents came almost without exception from families where the home was disturbed, broken up or discordant. He writes (Aichhorn, 1936, p. 155): 'It seems as if the shocks the individual received from society are endurable only when he finds a haven, which in our society the family normally offers. Given such a haven, the expression of his instincts is held within bounds acceptable to society. When this is lacking the equilibrium of these unstable individuals is further thrown off balance.' He finds that most of the children were deprived of the affection necessary for normal development, and that the hate which leads to so many antisocial attacks is always a reaction to an unsatisfied need for love. The child's attitude to society gets its imprint from the structure of the family and the emotional relationships set up within the family. The parents, and especially the father, therefore assume overwhelming responsibility for the social orientation of the child.

Healy, in his early studies on the influence of the 'broken home' on young offenders, stressed amongst the sources of mental conflicts which may lead to delinquency certain emotional experience within the family. He describes, for instance (Healy, 1915a, p. 354), '. . . the concealment of family relationships such as the child's actual parentage and the temporary misrepresentative withholding of deep-striking facts from young individuals who eventually learn the truth . . . uncertainty on the part of the child concerning his parentage is a prolific source of deep-seated emotional disturbance.' Being deceived and lied to, and various sexual experiences, Healy found to be the most frequent causes of conflict. In his study of pathological lying, accusation and swindling, Healy (1915b) noted the frequency with which the falsifier had himself—or herself—been misled or been obliged to keep to himself since early years secrets of grave importance, or had been the victim of extensive misrepresentations in the family circle.[1] He stressed the need for confidence between parents and children and deplored lying and misrepresentation to children by older people as harmful and dangerous, even when undertaken for the supposed good of the child. On the troublesome question of adoption, Healy argues (and Anna Freud[2] has expressed similar opinions) that this is frequently badly handled and the child almost invariably learns from others, under traumatic or disastrous circumstances, the supposed secret of his adoption. 'Repression', writes Healy (1917, p. 74) 'in its most vigorous form often takes place with even the slightest suggestion of anomalous parentage. . . . Parental relationship is so vitally connected with the emotional life of childhood that suggestion of irregularity in it comes as a grave psychic shock. . . . The importance of any peculiarity pertaining to parentage is immensely added to in the individual's mind if there is any social derogation on account of it. Innuendos concerning parentage, even of little playmates who

---

[1] Healy (ibid.) cites as 'an extraordinary case' a child brought up to believe that her real mother is not her mother but her sister, and that her grandmother is her mother. In 'Mental Conflicts and Misconduct', he describes a parallel case (Case No. 22) which he also regards as extraordinary. Amongst the cases of our project were two in which the true parentage was concealed in the same way. It seems probable that this subterfuge for young unmarried mothers is by no means as extraordinary as Healy then thought.

[2] Anna Freud, in seminar on 'Adoption', 1950.

hardly know what they are talking about, cut deeper than almost anything else in the world, arouse conflicts and induce definite antisocial attitudes and misconduct. ... To head off in the final place any secret or shock-producing information that almost surely would be imparted, the truth in some form must be declared ... from our experience ... I strongly believe that openness of statement never does as much harm as concealment.'

Silverman (1935) analysed the behaviour of children from broken homes and related this to pathological conditions in their environment, especially the direct effects of abnormal or antisocial behaviour of the parents themselves on the children. He found (Silverman, 1935, p. 11) 'no significant relationship between the broken home which results from delinquency and incompatibility of the parents, and the behaviour of the children from such homes. ... Where problem behaviour occurs it is probably related much more to the subtler emotional relationships within the family group than to the overt delinquency of parents'. Silverman studied the causes of the break-up of the home, e.g. ill-health or death; various mental factors; economic factors; sex delinquency; serious neglect or cruelty or other delinquencies of either parent; cases where the children are aware of the parents' sex delinquency or of extra-marital relationships; where there are illegitimate siblings in the family; where incest has been proven; or where other gross abnormal or antisocial behaviour occurs in the family. Silverman found that only 25 per cent of the children from recognizably noxious homes presented indications of antisocial tendencies, behaviour problems or personality deviation. Study of a control group of normal children showed that the causative factors described above were just as great and in some respects greater in the normal than in the delinquent groups of children. Sex delinquency, theft, serious neglect, desertion and cruelty were found to be just as common in homes of normal as of antisocial children. Silverman compares his own study to one of the findings of Shaw and McKay which also runs counter to the usual claims, in that no significant relation was found between delinquency and broken homes in one area, and that the percentage of broken homes amongst unselected schoolboys was greater than the delinquency in some areas. These results suggest that 'broken home' is probably too loose a concept for any but the most general conclusions to be drawn about its influence in the individual case. Karpman (1948a) maintained that the most important factors leading to delinquency are to be found in the variations of the 'family drama' and the early inter-personal relationships in the formative years. A 'broken home' he regards as important only in terms of the individual's reaction to the situation, or of the conditions—jealousy, sibling rivalry, hostility, rejection or over-protection—involved.

Very few 'objective' studies have been carried out into the specific influences upon character formation of illegitimacy. A study by Kasanin and Handschin (1941) into the psychodynamic aspects of illegitimacy presented rather contradictory evidence about its influence upon the child. Factors found to be important were those affecting the mother's attitude to herself and her child, such as the social stigmata attached to illegitimacy, or its barrier to subsequent marriage. In some cases the influence on the child was thought to be only slight. In others both her attitudes to the father, especially when he is missing, and a history of promiscuity or illegitimacy in the mother's family—however indefinite—play most important parts in the feelings of the unmarried mother, and consequently profoundly influence her child.

Banister and Ravden (1944, 1945) compared the home environment of normal and 'problem' children, and found that the 'nervous' children tended to come from stable 'accord' homes, where parents were frequently fussy and over-protective and gave to the child very little affection. The delinquent children tended to come from homes broken by other factors than the death of a parent or open disharmony such as divorce, desertion, etc., and in which there is open discord, and a similar lack of affection for the child. Unsatisfactory discipline was found in 66 per cent of the problem cases, and was associated with nervousness in the 'accord' homes and with delinquency in the 'discord' homes. Broken homes were found to be associated with other evidences of instability than delinquency, since they occurred very frequently in non-delinquent problem cases also. The well-adjusted children were found to have more strongly developed interests, hobbies and social activities than the problem children.

140

We made a detailed examination of the various ways in which the structure of the normal family circle (i.e. of both parents living together with their own children) was broken. We examined the child's status in the home (i.e. whether foster-, step-, adopted child or the parent's own child); the child's position in the family (to which Adler and others have attached such importance); and the size of the families of delinquent and neurotic children. Under the general heading of 'Family Structure' were included all factual details relating to the child's family situation, as follows:

a. *Stable home.* By this was meant a home in which the parents have lived together with their own children in a relatively settled place over a long period.

b. *Parents separated, divorced, deserted,* e.g. all cases where the marriage has been broken by separation, desertion or divorce, regardless of whether this situation is openly acknowledged or is supposedly hidden from the children.

c. *Irregular unions.* Under this heading were placed all children whose parents are unmarried; whose real father or mother lives with a partner not his or her lawful spouse; or who are children of a bigamous marriage.

d. *Death of mother or father, or child's parentage unknown.* Cases where there is a death of either parent, or children whose parents are unknown, were counted here.

e. *Prolonged absence of mother or father.* Prolonged absences of either parent from the child were included here, as, for instance, cases of absence through desertion or separation, through father's overseas employment or through war service, etc.

f. *True parentage concealed from the child.* In this group were placed all children who had been reared as the child of some person other than their own parents, where there was deliberate secrecy about the child's true parentage, or where the child had been taught to believe that he had no parent, or that someone else was his parent (e.g. a child who is brought up by his grandmother and taught to believe that she is his real mother and that his mother is his sister, Case No. 64, Fred.).

g. *Child of a stable marriage.* This included all children born in wedlock and living with both their own parents, regardless of whether or not the family lived in a settled or a harmonious home.

h. *Step- foster- or adopted child.* This refers to the child's status in the family at the time of referral to the clinic.

i. *Illegitimate child.* All cases where children were born out of wedlock were included here.

j. *The child's position in the family.* We analysed the numbers of children occupying the first-child, the last-child or the only-child position in the family. Certain cases who occupied a quasi 'only-child' position were also included, e.g. a last child born when all other children were already grown up, or a sibling who from birth had been reared away from the family, e.g. with the grandmother, in an only-child position.

k. *Size of family.* An analysis was made of the size of the delinquent and neurotic children's families, including step- and adopted children.

The foregoing material was summarized in order to make a comparison of what could be termed 'stable families' and 'broken families' as well as a comparison of the individual conditions listed. A 'broken family' included cases where the parents were separated, divorced or deserted; where the parents lived in irregular unions; where one partner of the marriage was bigamously married; where there had been prolonged absences of one or both parents from the child; where one or both parents were dead; where the child's true parentage had been concealed from him or where the child was a step-, foster-, adopted, or illegitimate child in the family. A 'stable family' included cases of children born of a stable marriage, and living together with their own parents in a relatively settled home over a long period.

HYPOTHESES: Family Structure

1. We should expect to find that a greater number of delinquent than neurotic children come from 'broken families'. (Confirmed.)

2. We should expect to find that a greater number of neurotic than delinquent children come from 'stable families'. (Confirmed.)

3. We should expect to find that delinquent children have been

deceived as to their true parentage more frequently than have the neurotics. (Confirmed.)

4. We should expect to find that a greater number of neurotic children occupy the first-child, last-child, or only-child position in the family. (Not confirmed.)

5. We should expect to find that the delinquent children come from larger families than do the neurotic children. (Confirmed.)

Table 25, Appendix I, indicates that a significantly greater number of neurotic children come from stable homes and are the children of stable marriages. A significantly greater number of delinquent children come from families where parents are divorced, separated or deserted, where the child's true parentage is concealed from him or where there has been prolonged absence of the father or mother. The numbers are too small to yield any conclusions about irregular unions. The numbers are also rather small for cases where one or both parents are dead or unknown, cases of step-, foster- or adopted children, and cases of illegitimate children, but the tendency seems to be that all of these conditions occur in a small proportion of both delinquent and neurotic children.

The results upon the composite pictures 'broken family' and 'stable family' show a significant difference between the two groups. The delinquent children tend to come from broken families and the neurotic children from stable families. There appears to be evidence that the usual research practice of grouping together homes that are broken for widely divergent reasons tends to obscure the picture with regard to which conditions contribute specifically to delinquency and which might also be found in the histories of other types of maladjusted children. It has been found, for example, that neuroticism occurs in adopted or step-children almost as frequently as does delinquency, and that homes broken by the parents' marital failure appear to be associated with delinquency more frequently than homes broken for other reasons, for instance by the presence of illegitimate children, or by the death of one parent.

The results show no significant difference between delinquent and neurotic children in the numbers occupying first-child, last-child, or only-child positions in the family. Nearly half the children in both groups were first children. There is a significant difference between the two groups in the size of family, the delinquent children tending to come from larger families and neurotics from smaller families. The median number of children in the families from which delinquent children come is four, and the median for neurotic children's families is two. Amongst the delinquent children there are ten families which have from four to ten children, while amongst the neurotic children there is no family larger than five. More than half the neurotic cases belong to families of one or two children.

Examples

The united and unbroken family life of the neurotic children in this study is in strong contrast to the many delinquent cases where the normal home and family ties have been broken repeatedly and in many ways. Amongst the delinquents, examples of broken family life and grossly unstable homes are: Cases No. 17, Monty; No. 13, Paddy; and No. 41, Maureen.

The stable homes (i.e. where the family unit is unbroken) from which some of the delinquents come, are seen on closer examination to abound with social and psychological problems. Even where the family has been free of gross external disturbances, there may be a 'psychologically broken home', which is covered up by the parents' decision to remain together for the sake of the children. This stable but unhappy home which harbours within its walls a multitude of frictions, tensions, quarrelling, and deeper psychological problems, is found very commonly amongst the neurotic children as well. Examples of 'stable' delinquent homes of this type were as follows: Cases No. 39, Rita, and No. 10, Ivor.

Amongst the neurotic children's families there were few cases comparable to the broken families of the delinquent children. There were several where an illegitimate child was subsequently adopted by step-parents, and in the war years there were many prolonged absences of fathers. The three worst examples of broken homes amongst the neurotics, however, each present certain unusual features. These are Cases No. 98, Ruth; No. 53, Colin; and No. 64, Fred.

THE CHILD'S PARENTS

The parents of the children in the neurotic and delinquent groups were studied from three viewpoints: (a) illness or deformity; (b) personality; and (c) parents absent, unknown or dead.

(a) CHRONIC ILLNESS OR DEFORMITY OF PARENTS
Investigations by Burt (1925) upon London children showed that a considerable proportion of delinquents suffered from various unfavourable physical conditions. Mannheim (1948) has emphasized the many practical consequences of this factor in both juvenile delinquents and their parents. Influences upon the family arising from ill-health or deformity of either parent are likely to be both far-reaching and subtle. If, for example, a father's illness or deformity is one that handicaps him as a breadwinner, this is likely to lower the standards of living of the home, to decrease the material and psychological security of the family, or possibly to force the mother into an active position as the breadwinner. This in turn may tend to lessen the mother's close relationship with her children and her control over them, and perhaps at the same time lessen their respect for their father. Such a situation may facilitate delinquent behaviour in the children. Contrariwise if those family ties are already very strong, the sharing of responsibilities under the pressure of adversity may serve to strengthen them. The illness of the mother may lead to a lowering of family standards and general neglect of the children. It is a matter for investigation to determine whether this factor might not tend to produce neurotic conditions associated with the fear of being injured or crippled; a fear of persons who are injured, ill, helpless, or crippled; or conditions related to psychogenic illnesses of the parents themselves. It would be interesting to compare the relative influence of an ill mother or crippled father upon boys and girls respectively[1] and especially upon the neurotic children.

[1] This suggestion was made by Miss Anna Freud. It was unfortunately not possible to include in our project a comparison of the sexes on most of the items, since this would have considerably lengthened the report. Moreover the numbers, which in any case are not very large for such comparisons, would be reduced still further by the need to omit in this particular instance all cases where one or both parents are dead, or the child is reared without one parent.

In the tables showing the results of examining the past and present physical ill-health of both parents and any injury or deformity which either parent had suffered, the data is examined for mothers and fathers (including step-mothers and step-fathers) separately, and for both parents together.

HYPOTHESIS: Illness or Deformity of Parents
We should expect to find that the parents of delinquent children tend to suffer from some form of illness or deformity more frequently than do the parents of neurotic children. (Not confirmed.)

Sex differences with regard to parental illness are shown in *Table 26*, Appendix 1. The results presented in *Table 27*, Appendix 1, show that there is no significant difference between delinquent and neurotic children upon any of the items listed. The composite item 'Chronic Illness or Deformity of Either Parent' is on the borderline for significance and shows a very small positive correlation with delinquency. The results on the whole, however, show that more than one-fifth of the parents of both groups of children suffer from some form of ill-health or deformity, and this appears to be true for both boys and girls.

Examples
The following are some examples of parental illnesses or deformities found in both groups:

Mothers: Pulmonary tuberculosis; rheumatoid arthritis; continued ill-health since rheumatic fever; poor health after a rapid series of pregnancies; goitre; asthma and bronchitis; cerebral malaria (benign tertiary form); blind eye; paralysed arm.
Fathers: Paralysis; rheumatism; diabetes; asthma; duodenal ulcer; migraine; renal colic; kidney trouble; poor health and back injury; chronic arthritis; injured leg; blind eye; crippled foot.

(b) PERSONALITY OF CHILD'S PARENTS
A great deal has been written on the subject of the personalities of the parents of maladjusted children and the role played by the

father or mother in contributing to their children's problems. Aichhorn (1925), Levy (1932b), Banister and Ravden (1944), Bowlby (1944, 1949, 1951), Friedlander (1947, 1949b), and others have investigated various aspects of this problem. The direct effects of abnormal or antisocial behaviour of the parents themselves upon their children was studied by Silverman (1935), who found little evidence that the problem behaviour of the children was related to the overt delinquency of the parents. He thought it was probably related to much subtler emotional relationships within the family, and he found just as much anti-social or delinquent behaviour in the parents of a control group of normal children. Newell (1934, 1936) in a study of the psychodynamics of maternal rejection, related the rejection of the child in most cases to marital maladjustment which usually resulted from unhappiness and psychological instability on the part of both parents. Riemer (1940) also found that mentally ill, mis-mated, unhappy and inadequately adjusted parents were common to a group of 'runaway' children. He found that the basic factor which influenced these children to break with their homes was lack of parental love for the child following upon the parents' own emotional disturbance. Andriola (1946) in attempting to isolate and describe a 'truancy syndrome' found in his cases severe parental rejection, usually by the mother, following serious marital discord and personality maladjustment of the parents, not necessarily apparent to the casual observer. Pictures of disturbed parental emotional life were also presented by Aichhorn (1925) in his studies of the neurotic offender, by Greenacre (1945) in a study of the family life of psychopaths, and by Friedlander (1947) in the case history of a child with 'antisocial character formation' (ibid. pp. 78 ff.).

Preston and Antin (1932) studied the children of committed psychotic patients, and found that such children did not differ materially from other groups of children in the community. They conclude that '. . . the children of psychotic parents contribute only a very small percentage to the future State hospital population . . .'

A comparison of the personalities of the parents of delinquent and neurotic children might lead to significant results, especially

147

if this could include a study of the finer shades of character grading. We could not examine the personalities of the parents as precisely as we wished, but considered only certain limited but important aspects and classified them roughly into four categories: (a) normal; (b) antisocial or morally unstable; (c) neurotic; (d) psychotic.

We made an examination and rating of the personalities of the parents of both groups according to the following scheme. In each case the term 'mother' or 'father' included also the step-mothers or step-fathers, mother substitutes, or persons responsible for the care and rearing of the children, whether these were the real parents or not.

MOTHER'S PERSONALITY

a. *Normal*, i.e. mothers whose personalities are considered to be more or less normal from the social and psychiatric point of view.

b. *Antisocial* or morally unstable, i.e. mothers who are known to steal, shoplift, break the law; to be, or to have been, in gaol; to be promiscuous, alcoholic, or morally unstable; to be of a quarrelsome or dissocial personality, to be 'up against authority', or to protect the child from the legal consequences of his delinquency.

c. *Neurotic*, i.e. mothers who are described by the psychiatrist as having definitely neurotic traits or symptoms, or suffering from a fully developed neurosis.

d. *Psychotic*, i.e. mothers who are diagnosed as suffering from psychotic or near-psychotic disturbances.

FATHER'S PERSONALITY

a. *Normal*, i.e. fathers whose personalities are more or less normal from the social and psychiatric point of view.

b. *Antisocial* or morally unstable, i.e. fathers who are known to steal, to break the law; to be, or to have been, in gaol; to be promiscuous, to be quarrelsome; to be alcoholic or dissocial personalities; to be 'up against authority'; to fail to support or take responsibility for the family; or who protect the child from the legal consequences of his delinquency.

148

c. *Neurotic,* i.e. fathers who are described by the psychiatrist as having definite neurotic traits or symptoms, or a neurosis.

d. *Psychotic,* i.e. fathers who are described by the psychiatrist as suffering from a psychosis or near-psychotic disturbance.

HYPOTHESES: Personality of Parents

1. We should expect to find that the parents of delinquent children will themselves tend to show antisocial or morally unstable tendencies more frequently than the parents of neurotic children. (Confirmed.)

2. We should expect to find that the parents of neurotic children will show neurotic tendencies more frequently than the parents of delinquents. (Confirmed.)

3. We should expect to find that there is no significant difference between the two groups in the numbers whose parents are psychotic. (Insufficient evidence available.)

Table 28, Appendix 1, indicates a highly significant difference between the delinquent and neurotic groups in the number of children whose parents show antisocial or morally unstable tendencies and also in the number whose parents show neurotic tendencies. This held true both for the mothers' and for the fathers' personalities. No significant difference was found between the two groups in the number of children whose parents were found to be normal. The number of cases having psychotic parents was insufficient to draw any conclusions. The results show that about half of the mothers in both groups and more than half of the fathers in both groups have normal personalities. They also indicate that delinquent children tend to have a father or mother, or both parents, whose personality is antisocial or morally unstable more frequently than neurotics, whereas neurotic children tend to have a neurotic mother or father, or both, more frequently than do delinquents. The correlation of delinquency with antisocial tendencies in either the father or the mother is very high. There is also a tendency for a positive correlation between neurotic children and neurotic tendencies in the mother. The numbers were too small to calculate the tetrachoric correlation between neurotic children and neurotic tendencies in the father. There seems to be a definite tendency for many neurotic and delinquent children to show disturbances similar to those shown by one or other of their parents, or by both.

Examples

Examples of children having unstable or antisocial mothers amongst the delinquent children are Cases No. 32, Freda, and No. 35, Maryann. Examples of antisocial or unstable mothers amongst the neurotic children are Cases No. 98, Ruth, and No. 85, Jean. Examples of antisocial or unstable fathers amongst the delinquent children are Cases No. 38, Susan; No. 3, Derek, and No. 32, Freda. Only one case of an unstable or antisocial father has been observed amongst the neurotics, namely Case No. 85, Jean, who has been largely reared away from home.

Examples of neurotic mothers amongst the delinquent children are Cases No. 1, Andrew, and No. 38, Susan. Examples of neurotic mothers amongst the neurotic children are Cases No. 76, Rollo; No. 89, Janice; and No. 57, Bertie. No cases of neurotic fathers were found amongst the delinquents in the present group. Neurotic fathers found amongst the neurotic children were Cases No. 52, Geoffrey, and No. 54, Jackie.

There are only two cases of children with psychotic or near-psychotic parents in the present groups, namely, Cases No. 17, Monty, and No. 5, Thomas. Typical examples of parents who were regarded as normal amongst the present groups were: mothers, Cases No. 52, Geoffrey; No. 82, Laura; and No. 90, Dorothy; and fathers, Cases No. 30, Paul; and No. 70, Ross.

(c) ABSENCE OR DEATH OF PARENTS AND REJECTED CHILDREN

The number of cases where one or both of the child's parents have been absent for long periods, where either parent is dead, or where the child's parents are completely unknown, have been shown in a previous section concerning 'family structure and broken homes'. A further table is appended here, however, to show the number of boys and girls in each group who lacked either mother or father or both, for any of the foregoing or other reasons.

An analysis of *Table* 29, Appendix 1, showed that there was no significant difference between delinquent and neurotic children in the numbers whose parents (one or both) were dead, or whose parents (one or both) were quite unknown. Neither was a significant difference found on the items 'mother absent for prolonged periods', or 'both absent'. There does appear, however, to be a significant difference between the two groups in the numbers of fathers who were absent from their children for long periods, either for legitimate reasons or through rejection of the child. The fathers of delinquent children tend to have been absent for long periods more frequently than have the fathers of the neurotics. This finding is the more significant since the numbers of cases whose fathers were absent were very high in both groups, due to the absence of many fathers on war-service during these children's early years. It is also quite striking that out of twenty delinquent girls studied, fourteen have been reared almost without fathers, or with the father absent during long periods of their lives.

Since neither death nor anonymity of parents accounted for as many cases as parental absence, and particularly absence of the father, we made further study concerning the reasons for these prolonged absences. With the exceptions of absence of either parent on war service, or absence of the father in some profession abroad, the most frequent cause of the absence of one parent was marital incompatibility. As a result of this, without having deserted or divorced their wives, fathers chose to travel, to work in distant places and return home only at rare intervals, to live with a mistress, or to live with relations or friends. A flagrant, quarrel-type of relationship, often reaching violent extremes of sado-masochism and even physical fights, existed between the parents of most of the fourteen delinquent girls whose fathers, while not legally separated from the mother, continued to live apart from her for long periods. In some of these cases there was a continuous and monotonous history of quarrels, estrangements, reconciliations, followed by more quarrels and fighting (and occasional drinking bouts) at the end of which the father would again leave home for an indefinite period (e.g. Cases No. 47, Sarah, and No. 38, Susan). Almost inevitably there was an involved history in which the respective parts played by disturbed sex relations, infidelity, and alcoholism were very difficult to assess. It seems clear, however, that sado-masochistic relationships between the parents, in which a regression to the anal-sadistic stage has taken place, with exaggerated hatred, hostility, pleasure in fighting, cruelty and spiteful interchanges, are almost invariably associated with sado-masochistic or perverse relationships between parents and children also.

In several of the neurotic cases where the father was absent for long periods, he either complained that the mother 'drove him away' with her complaints, nagging, dissatisfaction and hostility, or confessed in psychiatric interviews that the reason for his desertion and neglect of his family duties was lack of a satisfactory sexual relation with his wife, the reasons for which were as varied as the personalities of the parents themselves. In several of the neurotic cases this appeared to be a result of the wife's hysterical or frigid, male-rejecting attitude (e.g. Case No. 87, Penelope), or related to the father's abnormal sexual life (Case No. 85, Jean).

In many of the cases of disturbed marital relationships the parents live under a constant strain of estrangement, retaliation, mutual blame and dissatisfaction, much open quarrelling and frequent prolonged absences from each other. In such cases one parent's relation to the child often appears to become over-intense, jealous, rejecting, fault-finding, and loveless ('She's growing more like her father every day', 'She'll be an absolute rotter like her Dad', are typical of the bitter complaints of such frustrated and disappointed mothers). It is interesting to compare observations upon cases of this type with several studies of rejected children where the authors have reached similar conclusions. Newell (1934, 1936) studied the psychodynamics of maternal rejection and the influence of this upon a group of child guidance clinic cases compared with a control group of non-clinic cases. He found that the rejection of the child was, in most cases, primarily due to marital maladjustment which usually resulted from emotional instability on the part of father or mother. Unhappiness amongst the mothers was especially marked, and their handling of the child was frequently inconsistent, wavering between over-protection and overtly hostile behaviour. The children in turn showed a mixture of aggression and antisocial behaviour, as well as submissive or neurotic symptoms. Aggressive behaviour was found to occur more frequently when the parental handling was consistently hostile, whereas submissive behaviour occurred when the parental handling was consistently protective. The normal group showed a striking correlation between constructive parental handling and stable behaviour on the part of the child.

Levy (1937) took up the work of Ferenczi (1929) on the unwelcome child and his death instinct and of Newell (1934) on rejection. Levy found a high percentage of instability among rejected children and developed the concept of 'primary affect hunger' which he found to be typical of rejected children. He described the rejected, unloved child's difficulty in establishing social relationships as 'a personality deficiency comparable to a vitamin deficiency at the organic level'. Rosenheim (1942) described the character structure of the rejected child and stressed the relation of the fantasy content of the early rejection experiences to later behaviour and development. The rejected child he found to be unloved and to maintain an attitude of complete justification for antisocial behaviour at all times. He never confesses his thefts, indignantly complains of the injustice of the accusations of stealing; feels persecuted by all and hated by everyone; in some phases he even appears to simulate hostility in order to keep people at a distance; and by deliberately unfriendly means provokes punishment.

Lippman (1943), also following Ferenczi's paper upon the fate of the death instinct in unwelcome children (1929), finds that in rejected children the absence of love in early life is responsible for the emergence of aggressive hostility and hate. An excess of early acceptance and warmth is then required to neutralize these destructive forces, and this, Lippman suggests, is the reason why problems of the treatment of rejection occupy much of the work of children's social services. Glover (1933) stated this position more strongly when he said that not only is hate an indication of aggressive tendencies but it can be used as a protection against inner anxiety. The inception of destructive aggression expressed in war and delinquency can be traced, he thinks, to the relationship between the young child and his neurotic parents and their actual behaviour towards him. 'The truth is', he states (Glover, 1933, p. 96), 'that the human environment of the child is charged with feelings of anxiety and hate, with envy and jealousy, with tyrannical impatience and with aggressive and sadistic impulses which seldom stop short of psychic cruelty and sometimes . . . physical cruelty.' At times these are mixed with or disguised by parental love, solicitude or over-protection which cover concealed attitudes of hate, anxiety and guilt towards children.

Parental rejection played an important part among the psychiatric factors causing stealing in child cases examined in detail by Tiebout and Kirkpatrick (1932). Goodman and Michaels (1934) in a study of the incidence and interrelation of enuresis and other neuropathic traits in children found that the highest percentage of enuresis was in the rejected or neglected children, and the lowest in over-protected children. Bender and Paster (1941), in a study of the factors determining homosexuality in boys, found that in certain cases of rejected children living in foster-homes, the unfavourable results of neglected early infantile emotional needs and the later fixation upon homosexual and perverse goals, favoured the development of the psychopath. A number of writers, including Levy (1934, 1943), Bender (1943), Lowrey (1940b), Goldfarb (1943, 1944, 1945), Greenacre (1945), and Burlingham and Freud (1942, 1943), as well as earlier investigators like Aichhorn, Healy and Bronner, and the Gluecks, have agreed unanimously, but with varying degrees of emphasis, upon finding experiences of rejection, deprivation, misery, neglect and early emotional disturbance in delinquents and psychopaths. Benedict (1939) also maintains that delinquency is a way of life which is offered to the delinquent 'faute de mieux' and which is, at base, 'rooted in deprivations'.

Examples

Two examples of the fate of such rejected children are the following:

Case No. 49. Daisy, was an illegitimate, unwanted baby, deserted by her mother, and little is known of her early history, except that it was spent in several institutions. She was adopted at the age of two years by an elderly, eccentric couple, and spent a very troubled childhood, which led to several court convictions and a sentence of three years in an approved school from the age of eleven to fourteen years. This was followed by two domestic jobs in country schools from each of which she absconded and returned to her steadily deteriorating home. Both adoptive parents are in a senile condition, the home is overcrowded and dirty, the child frequently runs away and has once more been placed on probation for continued offences.

Case No. 14. Keith, is a docile, apathetic, and miserable-looking little boy of nine and a half who looks more like a boy of five. He is an orphan whose parents are unknown, and his history is one of general neglect and haphazard upbringing. He has lived in a succession of public assistance committee 'homes' since early babyhood.

All traces of his earlier foster-homes appear to have been lost, but it is known that changes were frequent, and that his stay in each of his many homes was very short until the age of five and a half, when he settled down in his present foster-home. He had previously been evacuated and billeted in several different places. After four years in this home his ignorant, easy-going, middle-aged foster-parents appeared to know little about him, and he had not established a close relationship with either of them. He appears unhappy, does not play like a normal child, is passive and shy with outbursts of boisterousness with other children; he frequently runs away from home and tells lies about where he has been; and his lack of interests and lack of effort and wish to learn at school had so puzzled his teachers that they had thought him to be defective.

FAMILY RELATIONSHIPS

The recognition of defective family relationships as one of the most important causes of delinquency has steadily increased throughout the past forty years. This was repeatedly stressed by Healy who concluded an early study (1917, p. 313) with the penetrating observation '. . . there is one common feature that belongs to what may be termed the psychical environment. The misdoers with mental conflicts never had anyone *near* to them, particularly in family life, who supplied opportunities for sympathetic confidences. Repression . . . (of mental conflicts) . . . has gone on largely as a result of this need'. Healy and Bronner (1936) later compared the families from which delinquents come with a control group of families that were free of delinquency. This was a research of considerable significance as regards the nature and paramount importance of good family relationships, especially between the child and the mother or person caring for him. The authors were able to group the families according to the degree of liability to delinquency, and to make fairly reliable prognoses of the probable outcome. Their results emphasized the importance of emotional factors such as frustration, insecurity, feelings of inferiority and rejection, denial, jealousy, guilt and manifold reactions to family disharmony. A significant finding was that of two siblings who grew up in the same environment, the one who did not become delinquent had been able to form a good relationship with the mother or with another person in the family, whereas the delinquent child frequently had either a severely disturbed relationship or none at all. Healy and Bronner described the problem as one of lack of emotional satisfaction in the home and inability to find gratification elsewhere, as a result of which the delinquent approaches the world with an attitude of having been socially maltreated and feels that only by violence can he obtain justice.

Aichhorn (1925) stressed the danger of unhealthy family relationships which fail to permit a normal adjustment to social life; e.g. emotional influences in the home, such as insufficient love from one or other parent, parental quarrels, and unequal relationships where the father or mother is weakly, inconsistent in discipline, and unstable. Family patterns which he found frequently amongst delinquents were those where the mother is dominant; where the father is brutal, tyrannical and a drunkard; where there are open conflicts or divorce, or where the mother is a nagging, quarrelsome, abusive woman of an aggressive, masculine type, given to continual fighting.

Levy (1937, 1943) worked out in considerable detail the influence of maternal over-protection upon the child. He held that maternal over-protection allows a freer unbridled expression of instincts, whilst rejection may heighten the individual aggressiveness and hostility which are so frequently behind delinquent acts.

Lowrey (1936) studied the influence on the child of various inter-family relationships, and maintained that parent-parent relationships in particular are reflected in parent-child relationships. Certain types of relations between parents he thought to be harmful to the child, such as being over-engrossed in each other to the exclusion of their children; or unequal relationships where the child is pulled between the parents, or is permitted over-indulgence, which makes adaptation to reality difficult and fosters extremes of rebellion. Certain emotional factors in the parent-child relationship such as parent fixation upon the child, rejection, and identification of him with others in extreme forms have most pernicious effects upon the child's personality. Over-protection or over-valuation of the child may also lead to an infantilizing of the personality with an inability to meet the practical problems of life and very commonly to difficulties in all forms of group relationships.

Greenacre found, as Aichhorn had done, that certain configurations of parent-child relationships among problem cases occurred with considerable frequency. She described (Greenacre, 1945, p. 499 ff.) as a typical 'family constellation' one with 'a stern, respected and often obsessional father who is remote, preoccupied and fear-inspiring in relation to his children; and an indulgent, pleasure-loving, frequently pretty but frivolous mother who is often tacitly contemptuous of her husband's importance . . . and a marked discrepancy or definite conflict between parental ideas and attitudes towards the child's immediate experiences, with a conspicuous conflict between a brave family façade and the conflict and misery behind it'. There is a basically poor relationship between the parents and the infant from earliest days, and 'pride and shame are frequent substitutes for a counterfeit love'. These children were not greatly loved, and what might

157

appear as an excess of love was generally an excess of indulgence or solicitude and thinly disguised narcissism. 'Both the inner and outer psychic situations of the parents with their over-valuation of external appearances, tend to promote a kind of shop-window display role for the child, with a premium on formally good behaviour for the sake of reflecting favourably on the parents . . . This family situation . . . tends to increase very much the exhibitionistic component of the child's narcissism'. He becomes emotionally impoverished, with poor sense of reality, fantastic ideas of omnipotence and magic, and an attitude of intense ambivalence towards the father and all authority. Behind a façade of emotional attachment to both parents, and protected from frustrations by the mother, the child receives a mockery of education, is defrauded of the sense of reality, and acquires a charming, opportunistic versatility of the psychopathic type which, nevertheless, may have been 'the best possible adjustment to a world consisting only of the rigid, exacting parents'.

Karpman (1948a) found that the delinquents he studied tended to seek only personal and egocentric pleasures and to lack consideration for others; to have no genuine sense of guilt and moral or ethical values; to blame others for their own difficulties; and to have a carping, critical attitude towards others. He considered that important factors leading to delinquency were hostility, egocentricity, and lack of consideration for others. These may depend primarily upon abnormalities of constitution, or upon the effects of early thwarted or disturbed relationships in the family or its substitutes.

Bowlby (1940, 1944) linked together several chains of research into the early development and early experiences of delinquents. The Freudian theory of character formation had led many psychoanalytic investigators to examine closely the nature of the child's first relationships with its parents, and to expect disturbances in the child's personality according to the nature of the parents' (especially the mother's) personality and methods of handling the child in his early years. The continuity of the mother–child relationship is an essential ingredient in Freud's theory of the interweaving of object cathexes and identifications in normal super-ego development and character formation. Some of the effects of separation from one or other parent have been summed up by Flugel (1921), Fenichel (1934, 1945) and Burlingham and Freud (1942, 1943). Bowlby (1944) has performed the service of putting to simple statistical test the frequency of certain early experiences in the lives of delinquents. He compared a group of juvenile thieves with a control group of other (non-stealing) maladjusted children from a child guidance clinic, and claims that prolonged separation of the child from its mother during the first five years of life bears a specific aetiological relationship to later delinquency and particularly to a certain form of persistent stealing. He found that fourteen of his group of forty-four juvenile thieves, and none of his control group, could be described as 'affectionless characters'. This, he argues, constitutes a true psychiatric syndrome hitherto only partially recognized, but which it is often possible to diagnose as early as the fourth year. The affectionless thieves were significantly more delinquent than the other thieves, and together constituted more than half of the more serious and chronic offenders. A high percentage of the thieves (1) had suffered complete and prolonged separation from their mothers or mother-substitutes in the early years; (2) had ambivalent, unconsciously hostile mothers; (3) were openly hated by their fathers; and (4) had experienced recent traumatic events. He concluded that prolonged separations from the mother in the early years of life are a specific and frequent cause of chronic delinquency. Bowlby (1949) stresses the complexity of the conscious and unconscious factors determining the mother's attitude to her child and suggests that two factors are frequently present in the history of delinquents and persons 'susceptible' to antisocial conduct. These are (1) a prolonged separation from or frequent changes in the relation with the mother in the first five years, and (2) being a more or less unwanted child of parents who are themselves unstable and unhappy people with ambivalent, hostile, criticizing and punishing attitudes towards the child. Bowlby states that these two factors will be found in most but not all cases and will together account for a majority of the more intractable cases, amongst whom he includes the 'constitutional psychopaths' and 'moral defectives'.

The main emphasis in studies of the influence of defective

family relationships on character development has fallen upon two aspects of these early object-relationships, namely, (a) upon *interruptions* in the child's emotional or psychological relationship with its parents, often in consequence of separation at an early age (Burlingham and Freud, 1942, 1943; Bowlby, 1944; Friedlander 1947); and (b) upon *disturbances* in the emotional relationship between parent and child (Burt, 1925; Aichhorn, 1925; Healy & Bronner, 1929; Alexander & Staub, 1931; Levy, 1943; Friedlander, 1947; Bowlby, 1949, 1951, *et al.*). We examined both these aspects in our project. Interruptions in the psychological bond or emotional tie between mother and child were specially studied by Friedlander in her work with delinquent children and our work was based largely on her previous formulations. The *age* at which the interruptions in the relationship with either parent occurred was also carefully investigated. Disturbances in parent-parent relationships, as well as in parent-child relationships, and disturbances in sibling relationships were also examined.

INTERRUPTED MOTHER-CHILD RELATIONSHIP

Following current psychological and psychiatric practice, the term 'mother-child relationship' is used to emphasize *one* of the various meanings of the word 'relation', namely, 'that which one person or thing has to do with another person or thing',[1] or the 'kind of connection or feeling that prevails between persons or things'. The relationship between mother and child is truly a psychological entity involving the child's inner situation as well as that of his environment. Strictly speaking, it includes more than an emotional relationship, since parental attitudes towards care, responsibility, physical and material solicitude, etc., are also involved. The interruption in this inner psychic bond between parent and child is also clearly distinguished in this investigation from the physical separation or absence of the child from its mother or father (as studied by Bowlby, 1944). A physical separation and a break in the psychological bond between parent and child do not necessarily coincide, as Burlingham and Freud have shown (1942, 1943) in their war-time studies of children separated from their parents. In most families there are occasions such

[1] *The Concise Oxford Dictionary.*

as the birth of a new baby, or the child's illness in hospital, when the mother has to be separated from her child for a long or short time. Separation in such cases may be inevitable; it may be managed in more or less benign ways, and it does not, apparently, *always* have profoundly adverse effects upon the child. In most cases the psychological bond between the mother and child has been preserved (albeit under strain) and a contact between them has been maintained by various means. In the sense in which the term is used here this would not be termed a broken or 'interrupted' mother-child relationship. Physical separation does not necessarily mean an interrupted emotional relationship, but neither does staying together necessarily ensure an uninterrupted psychical relationship.

An example in point is Case No. 20, Ian, whose behaviour is perhaps the most violent of all the delinquents in this study. Ian is believed to be a (secret) illegitimate child of the husband, a middle-aged Air Force officer. Ian had suffered in infancy a long period of gross mishandling and neglect, and had been reared to the age of five years by a young stepmother who was ignorant of his paternity and who had believed (after five years of childless marriage) that she could not have children of her own. After the births in rapid succession of three babies, including twins, and her great preoccupation with them, Ian's behaviour deteriorated in alarming fashion as a reaction to jealousy, neglect and rejection, and this deterioration led to further rejection. In this case there can be no doubt that the relationship of mother and child had been broken irreparably; the step-mother had rejected her role as mother and the boy had accepted the role of outsider in the family, with great consequent damage to his personality. In this case, admittedly rare, there is ample evidence that the child had experienced an interruption in his emotional relationship with his mother without there being any physical separation. It appeared that this break coincided with the young mother's discovery that Ian was her husband's child and her withdrawal and turning away from him to her own children.

In most of the other cases the interruption was one of two

kinds. Sometimes the relationship was broken off and the child lost his true mother, or first mother-substitute; for example, when he was reared in an institution or with foster-parents who did not take the role of parent substitutes. In this case the child may form no genuine relationship with any substitute mother at all. In other cases the child was passed from one relative to another and from one home to another with frequent changes of persons handling and caring for him, so that whatever relationships he formed were repeatedly broken off. A very close and detailed knowledge of each case is necessary before the history of the child's mother-relationship can be traced, and very often this can only be studied in the transference during therapy. The designation given in the present research, however, is in all cases the result of very careful inquiry by the child guidance clinic staff, who were concerned with special research in this subject, and who were dealing with children who were mostly in long-term psychotherapeutic treatment, or under prolonged periods of observation. In each case the child's history was examined for the age levels at which interruptions in the mother-child relationship occurred. Particular care was paid to the period up to the age of seven years, since this was held to be of primary importance. The child's reaction after the separation, or other cause of the interruption in the relationship, was also carefully studied. Children of one to three years in the war-time nurseries who cried and screamed on the return or reappearance of the mother, were thought to be probably less disturbed than the infants and toddlers who did not know or refused to recognize their mothers again and reacted to them with indifference and apathy. It is possible that the expression of grief and anger in the former case is more normal and indicates that the relationship, though severely strained, has not been interrupted, and the more disturbed reactions are those of the many children who no longer knew their mothers, or were indifferent to them on their return. Only a scrutiny of the inner world and experiences of each case can determine whether such an interruption has occurred.

HYPOTHESIS: Interrupted Mother-Child Relationship
We should expect to find that interruptions in the mother-child

relationship have occurred more frequently in delinquent children than in neurotic children. (Confirmed.)

The results presented in *Table* 30, Appendix 1, indicate that there is a highly significant difference between delinquent and neurotic children in (a) the total number of cases showing an interrupted mother-child relationship, and (b) the number of cases showing an interruption in the mother-child relationship at each age level up to the seventh year. Delinquent children tend to have experienced a greater number of interruptions in the mother-child relationship before the age of seven and throughout the whole of their childhood than have neurotic children. This result is most marked during the period of the second year, when there is a very high correlation between delinquency and an interrupted relationship with the mother or mother-substitute.

INTERRUPTED FATHER-CHILD RELATIONSHIP
In similar fashion we examined the interruptions in the father-child relationship for each child. This also proved to be a task requiring the most careful inquiry, particularly for the children whose fathers had been absent over a long period during the war. In some cases of older children it was clear that in spite of fairly long absence as, for example, absence overseas, the father still played the role of the rightful, effective and permanent head of the family. Memories were kept alive by photographs, by letters and in family consultations and decisions, and there had been no question of a break in the dependent emotional or psychological relationship with the father. Such cases were not included under this heading but were classified under 'prolonged absence of the father from home'. The remarks on the psychological bond between the mother and child apply also to the father-child relationship.

The importance of the father-relationship, especially in the re-education of delinquent children, has been demonstrated in the therapeutic work of Makarenko (1935), Aichhorn (1925), and Slavson (1943c), all of whom worked on the basis of establishing a relationship of tolerant, infallible paternal friendship with delinquent boys and girls; using this relationship both as a model for
163

identification and for the focusing of filial attitudes; and exerting a parental-educational influence over the child on the basis of this emotional tie. Burlingham and Freud (1942, 1943) have also demonstrated the importance of the father-relationship in evacuated children and the role of its absence in fatherless children. They have shown that children who had no fathers tended to invent fantasy father-figures whose primitive and diabolic aspects on the one hand and all-loving, forgiving tender care on the other, unchecked against the educational influence of a real father, were exaggerated to a remarkable extent.[1] The articles of Macdonald (1938) and of Menaker (1939) have thrown considerable light on the role of the absent father in the case of criminally aggressive boys with a passive-effeminate type of character structure.

HYPOTHESIS: Interrupted Father-Child Relationship
We should expect to find that interruptions in the father-child relationship have occurred more frequently in delinquent than in neurotic children. (Confirmed.)

The results presented in *Table* 31, Appendix 1, show that there is a highly significant difference between delinquent and neurotic children at all age levels in the number of cases who experience interrupted father-child relationships. The delinquent children have experienced a greater number of interruptions in their relationship with their fathers than have neurotic children. The correlation between delinquency and broken relationships with the father is high and positive throughout childhood and especially marked at ages seven to eleven years and in the second and third years.

It is interesting to note that a greater number of interruptions occur in the father-child relationship than in the mother-child relationship. The psychological interpretation of these statistical results is not straightforward. Probably the interruption of the relationship with the father operates powerfully but indirectly on the child at the early ages, since a normal father-relationship usually provides the guarantee of security in the mother-relationship and in the home. The relationship with the mother probably has more direct influence, since she assumes the intimate physical

[1] See also a case described by Bennett and Hellman (1951).

care and psychological contact with the child and undertakes his first social and emotional education. It is also possible that factors which cause a break or interruption in the father-relationship (e.g. desertion) also tend to cause indirectly the interruption in the mother-child relationship (for instance, the mother may be obliged to put her child in an institution or foster-home while she goes out to work).

It has been pointed out earlier that an absence of the father from the home does not necessarily involve an interruption in the father-child relationship, although this sometimes does occur, particularly in the case of younger children who cannot be expected to remember their fathers or to have the father-relationship kept alive by letters, photographs and other psychological links. Such a case is Case No. 52, Geoffrey, where the relationship has been broken through war-time absence of the father. It might be expected, since the subjects of this study were all fairly young children during the war years, that the incidence of interrupted father-child relationship would be very high in both groups. It is interesting to note, however, that a clear distinction exists between the fathers of the delinquent children and the fathers of the neurotic children. Many neurotic children's fathers were also in the Services or overseas, but the complete interruption in the relationship with the child is by no means as common as it is in the delinquent cases. It seems that the good father from a stable home was able to find ways of maintaining the relationship in spite of separation.

The results in both these sections throw overwhelming emphasis upon the association between delinquency and interruptions in the parent-child relationship. They point in one direction to the problem of the *causes* of broken homes (of which the child's broken family life is very often only the consequence), and on the other hand to the original *dislocations* in the child's early social and emotional education which lie behind the faulty character development of the delinquent.

Examples
Relationship with mother. There are many examples of children who have had frequent changes of mother-substitute, so that each

time the new relationship has been attempted it is broken again within a very short time by the next change of maternal care. (Cases No. 1, Andrew, No. 20, Ian, No. 21, Bobby). In other cases, under similar or less favourable circumstances, the child does not appear to have made a relationship at all to the persons who care for him, or the original satisfactory mother-relationship has been broken and no substitute ever provided. (Cases No. 14, Keith; No. 35, Maryann; No. 13, Paddy; No. 41, Maureen; and No. 39, Rita.)

Relationship with father. In the majority of cases, an interruption of the mother-child relationship implied that the father-child relationship had already been interrupted by the same circumstances, e.g. evacuation, placement in foster-home or institution, adoption, illegitimacy, and so on. Because of this each of the foregoing cases can also be regarded as an example of an interrupted father-child relationship. In addition to these, however, there are a number of cases where the child has been reared without a father or father-substitute, or where the father has been totally absent, or has died very early in the child's life. Examples of this are Cases No. 6, Ernest; No. 17, Monty; and No. 87, Penelope.

DISTURBED EMOTIONAL RELATIONSHIPS
WITHIN THE FAMILY

We next examined four types of disturbed family relationships: i.e. emotional disturbances between:

(a) mother and child;
(b) father and child;
(c) mother and father;
(d) and between siblings.

(a) DISTURBED MOTHER-CHILD RELATIONSHIP

This section refers to the child's psychological relationship with his mother, his stepmother, or the person who has served as his permanent mother-substitute. Included here were all cases of relationships between the mother and child which were emotionally disturbed to the extent that they did not allow the child's emotional development to proceed normally. Examples included mothers who had extremely rejecting, over-protecting, over-gratifying, ambivalent, sado-masochistic, irresponsible, indifferent or grossly inconsistent attitudes towards the child, or any other type of abnormal emotional attitude between mother and child (cf. Aichhorn, 1925, Friedlander, 1947).

(b) DISTURBED FATHER-CHILD RELATIONSHIP

We examined the child's relationship with his father, his step-father or his father-substitute, and all cases were counted as disturbed where the father did not support the family and was disinterested in the child, where the father-child relationship was completely lacking, or where the emotional relationship itself was disturbed, or of such a type that it did not allow the child's emotional development to proceed normally. Examples included fathers who had extremely rejecting, over-protective, over-gratifying, ambivalent, sado-masochistic, irresponsible, grossly inconsistent, or any other abnormal attitudes towards the child (Cf. Aichhorn, 1925; Friedlander, 1947).

(c) DISTURBED MOTHER-FATHER RELATIONSHIP

Under this heading we included all cases where there was an unsatisfactory or unhappy marriage, where there was discord rather than harmony, open hostility or evidence of hidden hostility, where one parent was unfriendly, belittling, disapproving, or critical towards the other or failed to support the other in matters important to the child. Also included here were all parents who had open or hidden quarrel relationships with each other, or where there was a disturbed sexual relationship, or any abnormal emotional relationship.

(d) DISTURBED SIBLING RELATIONSHIPS

In this group were included all cases of disturbed emotional relationships between the child examined and his siblings. Examples were cases of extreme rivalry, jealousy, or competitiveness between the children, or quarrel relationships of a sado-masochistic type, or sexual relationships of various types between siblings.

HYPOTHESES: Disturbed Emotional Relationships within the Family

1. We should expect to find that disturbed emotional relationships between mother and child occur more frequently in delinquent than in neurotic children. (Confirmed.)

2. We should expect to find that disturbed emotional relationships between father and child occur more frequently in delinquent than in neurotic children. (Confirmed.)

3. We should expect to find that disturbed emotional relationships occur more frequently between the parents of delinquent children than between the parents of neurotic children. (Confirmed).

4. We should not expect to find any significant difference in the frequency with which disturbed sibling relationships occur among delinquent and neurotic children. (Confirmed).

The results presented in *Table* 32, Appendix 1, show that there is a significant difference between delinquent and neurotic children in the number of cases showing disturbances in the (a) mother-child relationship (b), the father-child relationship, and (c) mother-father relationship. There is no significant difference between delinquent and neurotic children in the numbers showing disturbed sibling relationships. Correlation between delinquency and disturbed family relationships is moderately high and positive in all cases (except in sibling relationships). From these results one may conclude that delinquent children tend to show disturbed emotional relationships within the family more frequently than do neurotic children. It is worthy of note, however, that the frequency of disturbed emotional relationships is also fairly high in both groups, and disturbed sibling relationships occur in both. Both delinquent and neurotic children tend to quarrel, to make disturbed relationships, and to have difficulty in getting on with their siblings. It is interesting to note the high proportion of delinquents as compared with neurotics who have disturbed relationships with their fathers.

Examples

Examples of disturbed family relationships occur in the following cases:

Disturbed Mother-Child Relationship: Cases No. 6, Ernest; No. 38, Susan; No. 39, Rita; No. 2, Peter; No. 87, Penelope; No. 76, Rollo.

Disturbed Father-Child Relationship: Cases No. 32, Freda; No. 38, Susan; No. 5, Thomas; No. 3, Derek; No. 4, Reginald; No. 54, Jackie; No. 52, Geoffrey.

Disturbed Mother-Father Relationship: Cases No. 5, Thomas; No. 3, Derek; No. 38, Susan; No. 27, Jeremy; No. 47, Sarah; No. 88, Daphne; No. 85, Jean; No. 54, Jackie.

Disturbed Sibling Relationship: Cases No. 34, Ellen; No. 20, Ian No. 90, Dorothy ; No. 80, James; No. 40, Minnie.

CHAPTER V

The child himself:
his development and personal history

This chapter describes how we examined the groups of delinquent and neurotic children on a selected set of conditions concerning their development and their educational and personal experiences. These included the child's health and physical conditions, a number of items from his early history, evidences of earlier difficult behaviour, the type of discipline he had received, traumatic experiences he had undergone, and a survey of his present interests and achievements.

HEALTH AND PHYSICAL CONDITIONS

We examined the health and physical conditions of the children under the following headings, past as well as present physical conditions having been as far as possible taken into account.[1]

Undergrown, including all children who were underweight or undersized for their age on referral to the clinic.

Overgrown, including all children who were over-sized, over-tall, or grossly fat for their age on referral.

Chronic illnesses in the past. Under this heading were placed all children who had suffered during their development from a number of chronic or acute physical illnesses, or who had suffered

[1] This section has been adapted from Burt (1925) who found a considerable proportion of the London delinquents in his survey to be suffering from ill-health and various other unfavourable physical conditions. The numbers of puberty cases were too small for comparison with those in Burt's groups, and were the same for both groups, since age formed one of the bases of their selection.

from the usual childish illnesses more frequently or in a more severe form than usual.

Chronic illnesses at present. All children who were suffering at the time of examination from poor health or from any chronic or acute illness were included here.

Special defects. In this section were included all children suffering from any of the following physical defects:

   i. Defective hearing.
   ii. Defective vision.
   iii. Speech defects.
   iv. Any other physical disability or disfigurement (e.g. flat feet, facial paralysis, disfiguring scars, deformed limb, etc.).

Accidents and injuries. Included here were the numbers of children who had incurred during their lifetime some form of grave accident or injury (e.g. broken leg, street accident, assault, injuries in air raids, etc.)

Many operations. Under this heading were included all children who had, during the past, had to undergo several major or minor operations.

HYPOTHESIS: Physical Conditions
We should expect to find that delinquent children suffer, or have suffered from a greater number of unfavourable physical conditions than have the neurotics. (Not confirmed.)

The results presented in *Table* 33, Appendix 1, showed no significant differences between the delinquent and neurotic children upon any of the foregoing items. There was a small negative correlation between delinquency and chronic past illness on the one hand, and being undergrown on the other, but this tendency was not large enough to be significant on the chi-square test. A high proportion of the children in *both* groups tended to have suffered from chronic illnesses in the past, and about one-quarter of the children in each group suffer from some special physical defect at present.

Examples
No unusual conditions were found amongst the cases of children
171

who were undergrown or overgrown, or who suffered from defects of vision, hearing, etc. The considerable number of children who had suffered from severe illnesses in the past had undergone such illnesses as pyloric stenosis, dysentery, whooping cough, mumps, tonsillitis, eczema, bronchitis, chicken-pox, German measles, scarlet fever, a long series of severe chest colds, bad reaction to diphtheria immunization needles, rheumatic fever, measles, pneumonia, chorea, influenza, and bronchial catarrh. Three neurotic children were found to be suffering from chronic illnesses at present. These were cases of prolonged poor health, with heavy colds; infected tonsils; and a case of asthma, headaches, pains, and abdominal symptoms.

Accidents and injuries were found to have consisted mostly of broken limbs, cuts or falls, and in several cases severe burns. One child drank inhalation fluid; another was attacked by a dog which savaged him. Among the cases of physical disability or disfigurement were found the scar of an infantile facial burn (which occurred in three out of the twenty delinquent girls); disabilities such as flat feet; and disabilities left by illness, such as a leg paralysed by poliomyelitis, or a paralysed half of the face and weak left leg which were the outcome of encephalomyelitis. Operations including the removal of tonsils, or tonsils and adenoids, mastoid operations, removal of a birth mark, appendicectomies and two cases of operations following unsatisfactory circumcision.

These results are in consonance with those of Healy and Bronner (1925) who found little evidence to show that malnutrition, physical stigmata, developmental deviations or physical defects contributed specifically to delinquency rather than to other forms of childhood maladjustment. In view of Burt's (1925) findings it would be interesting to compare the general health of the children in a London area with that of children in this and other rural areas, and with that of children in other countries.

THE CHILD'S EARLY HISTORY

Under this general heading were included a group of conditions concerning the child's earliest years which, according to almost all dynamic psychological theory, exert a most important influence upon later development. These included breast-feeding; early habit-training with regard to sleeping, feeding, and bowel and bladder control; and the changes in home and maternal care experienced by those children who were separated from their mothers or mother-substitutes and frequently changed from one person's hands to another's during their formative years.

Period of Breast-feeding
The subject of breast-feeding has been given considerable prominence in psycho-analytic theory, especially by Abraham (1927) and Glover (1925). More recently the subject has again been examined empirically by Childers and Hamil (1932), by Goldman (1948a and 1948b) and by various anthropological writers who claim that the nature and duration of breast-feeding has a deep and permanent effect upon character formation.

Childers and Hamil (1932) studied the relation of emotional problems in children to the duration of breast-feeding in infancy. Their results showed that the percentage of disturbed behaviour was highest among those children weaned between the first and fifth months of infancy; next highest among those not breast-fed at all; considerably lower than both these groups in those breast-fed for the 'normal' time (sixth to tenth month); and lowest in the groups breast-fed beyond the eleventh month, although the difference between this and the 'normal' group is not marked. The explanation offered for the highest percentage of abnormal behaviour manifestations in the children weaned between the first and fifth months was that this group were called upon to make emotional adjustments in the changed feeding situation to which the other groups were not subjected in the same degree. The emotional traumata might not necessarily be based entirely on physical difficulties but on the conditions in the family necessitating the changed type of feeding.

Goldman (1948a and 1948b) studied the influence of breast-feeding on character formation in normal adult subjects, and her results were found (1) to support Glover's theory that the shortening of the period of breast-feeding must be regarded as a traumatic factor; and (2) to coincide with anthropological observations that a long period of breast-feeding tends to be associated with such characteristics as imperturbable optimism, generosity, bright social conduct, sanguinity, etc. Goldman, following Ribble, took as the critical period for weaning the fourth month, and the end of the fourth month was chosen as the dividing line between 'early' and 'late' weaning. Early weaning was defined for the major part of the investigation as weaning at ages up to the fourth month and late weaning as weaning at five months of age or more. Since the average breast-feeding time for the group was approximately five and a half months, it is difficult to see how this can be taken to mean 'late' weaning. This interesting study would have been more valuable if Goldman had set the problem of breast-feeding in its cultural context. To speak of weaning at five months plus as 'late breast-feeding' is to concentrate upon local breast-feeding customs which are probably very different from those Central European cases upon which Freud's original observations and Abraham's first concept of 'oral character' were formulated. Comparison with Childers and Hamil's figures (1932) suggest that even for a pathological group the breast-feeding time is longer in some parts of the United States than in Goldman's English cases.[1] This is probably also true for some Australian conditions[2] where four to five months would be regarded as 'early average' weaning time, with 'average' falling about six to eight months, and 'late' weaning somewhere between nine to fourteen months. There seems to be no doubt that breast-feeding periods differ considerably in different cultures. They are influenced by many social and economic factors, by local tradition and custom, by the role played by women in the community, and the mother's own attitude towards breast-feeding. The wording of Goldman's English study (1948b, p. 7) that a rejecting mother would have 'thrown off the burden of breast-feeding' by the third or fourth month 'rather than drag on further' suggests the hidden bias of a culture pattern where breast-feeding is regarded as a burden, mothers are not expected to enjoy it and are

[1] The writer is grateful to Dr. Goldman for permission to use her table of weaning periods (Goldman 1948b, p. 7) which are compared with the findings upon breast-feeding in delinquent and neurotic children in *Table 35*.

[2] Data supplied by Dr. Irene Sebire, Director, Child Guidance Clinic, School Medical Service, New South Wales (private communication, 1950).

very rarely seen feeding the child in public. More important probably than any of these considerations for such an investigation would be the mother's attitude to the baby while she is feeding it.

Levy (1934) presented an interesting series of experiments on the sucking reflex and social behaviour of dogs. He has shown that animals whose movements are restricted develop tics, and that excessive sucking activities in puppies result from inadequate sucking activity at the appropriate time. A similar finding resulted from individual case studies of children who were pronounced thumb-suckers. In the experimental situation he observed the dogs' social activities, and drew certain inferences which are of interest for the possible effects on the human infant of separation from the mother for short periods (Levy, 1934, p. 223)' . . . from the human point of view both the mother-dog and returned pups were strange to each other. The powerful conditioning of continued lactation, care and general contact, physical and social, has been broken. The natural relationship . . . was never restored. The same biological considerations would apply to humans . . . a break in early mother-child relationship would disturb profoundly the natural impulses of one or the other for some time, i.e. a special problem in mutual re-adaptation would arise.' Levy also observed that the difficulty produced by the sucking deficiency enhanced certain personality responses in puppies, such as aggressive behaviour in one case, and estrangement, isolation and submission in another.

A group of character traits, later referred to in psycho-analytic literature as 'oral characteristics' were first described (in various writings) by Abraham and Freud, and later by Glover, as characterizing persons fixated, under the influence of early traumata and feeding frustrations, to the 'oral' stage of libidinal development. Reich (1925) traced the significance of these character traits and of certain parallel anomalies of the super-ego, e.g. of their relation to the super-ego in the 'instinct-ridden characters'. Alexander (1930), in his study of the group of 'neurotic characters', also described orally-fixated patients who tend to 'act out' their neurotic conflicts in impulsive ways, and Fenichel (1945, Ch. XVI) has brought together a great deal of psycho-analytic literature on the 'impulse neurotic', who, being fixated to the oral phase, tends to react to frustrations with violence. The case histories of juvenile delinquents (e.g. those of Healy, 1915a, and of Aichhorn, 1925) give abundant illustration of such 'oral' character structure and distorted super-ego development. Goldman (1948a, b) attempted to construct tests for the measurement of such 'oral' traits' in normal adult subjects, and correlated their occurrence with the period of breast-feeding these subjects had experienced.

In the present study a number of 'oral' traits are examined, such as wilfulness, impulsiveness, demandingness, inability to tolerate frustrations, 'redress-demanding' attitudes, lack of concern for consequences of actions, etc., and found to be characteristic of the behavioural picture presented by delinquents (See Chap. III); while others such as selfishness, greedy, insatiable behaviour, and inability to wait for satisfactions have been found to characterize both neurotic and delinquent children. In view of these findings it was interesting to compare the duration or total absence of breast-feeding with delinquency and neuroticism respectively. The lack of breast-feeding is, in itself, no indication of the occurrence, or the extent, of feeding frustrations, nor does it tell us anything about a predisposition towards subsequent oral fixations. It is, however, probably an indirect indication of the lack of maternal care and general neglect typical of the early histories of many delinquents. The case histories were examined in order to determine (a) whether the child had been breast-fed at all, and (b) the duration of breast-feeding in those children who had experienced it. The period of breast-feeding in the latter case was counted to the nearest month at the *end* of weaning (i.e. regardless of the child's diet being supplemented with other foods before and during weaning).

HYPOTHESES: *Breast-feeding*

1. We should expect to find that a greater number of delinquent children have been bottle-fed (i.e. have not been breast-fed at all) than neurotics. (Confirmed.)

2. We should expect to find that neurotic children tend to have been breast-fed for longer periods than delinquent children. (Confirmed.)

The results presented in *Table* 34, Appendix 1, indicate a highly significant difference between delinquent and neurotic children in the periods for which they have been breast-fed, the delinquent children tending to have been breast-fed for shorter and neurotic children for longer periods. There is a similarly significant difference between the two groups in the number of children who have not been breast-fed at all. A greater number of delinquents tended to have been entirely bottle-fed than had the neurotics. The Null hypothesis that there is no necessary relation between breast-feeding for less than four months and delinquency, and between breast-feeding for more than four months and neuroticism, is confidently rejected. A tetrachoric correlation between delinquency and breast-feeding for a period of three months or less on the one hand, and breast-feeding for four months or more on the other, showed that there is a positive correlation between short-term breast-feeding and delinquency, and a substantial negative correlation between delinquency and average and longer breast-feeding. These results indicate that there is also an association between average and longer breast-feeding and neurotic conditions. (We might also expect to find an association between average and longer breast-feeding and normal conditions.)

NEW SOUTH WALES CHILD GUIDANCE CLINIC CASES

For the purposes of cross-cultural comparison, data were obtained concerning the duration of breast-feeding for ninety-nine cases selected at random (but excluding mental defectives and certain organic cases, e.g. epilepsy, etc.) from the files of the child guidance clinic of the Department of Public Health, Sydney, N.S.W[1]. Strictly speaking, these cases were not readily comparable with our selected English cases, since their classification rested on different theoretical grounds, but it was possible to group them, largely on the basis of their histories and symptom-pictures, into roughly comparable groups of: (a) delinquent children (forty-one cases); (b) neurotic children (thirty cases); and (c) children with various behaviour difficulties and certain types with mixed delinquent and neurotic tendencies (twenty-eight cases.) The difference

[1] This information has been kindly supplied by Dr. Irene Sebire (private communication, 1950).

between the delinquent and neurotic children in the length of time for which they had been breast-fed, was then tested by chi-square and found to be significant. These results are presented in *Table* 35, Appendix 1, and indicate that the New South Wales delinquent children also tend to have been breast-fed for shorter and the neurotic children for longer periods.

COMPARISON WITH OTHER INVESTIGATIONS

It was interesting to compare the results on this problem from our English rural subjects (a) with those obtained by Childers and Hamil (1932) upon a sample of United States children referred for various types of maladjustment to a neuro-psychiatric clinic; (b) with those obtained by Goldman (1948b) upon a group of English normal adults (university students); and (c) with the aforementioned group of Australian child guidance clinic cases. Direct comparisons were not possible, since the populations from which the samples were drawn, and the methods of tabulating and presenting the data differed in each case. If, however, the tables are regrouped according to the arrangement adopted by Childers and Hamil, and if the frequencies throughout are expressed as percentages of the respective totals, a table may be drawn up which throws these four groups into contrast (see *Table* 36, Appendix 1). The variation in the numbers of cases in these investigations makes it difficult for any precise conclusions to be drawn, but it seems clear that the tendency shown by the three English groups is for the delinquent child to be bottle-fed, or breast-fed for short periods, more often than the neurotic or the normal cases. The neurotic children tend to lie very much closer to the normal children than to the delinquents. The normal children are breast-fed for the longest period of all, and this group contains the smallest number of bottle-fed babies. In contrast with the other three groups, relatively few delinquent children are breast-fed for more than five months. The trend of the American figures (1932) does not appear to follow closely that of any of the English groups, since the cases are very evenly spread over the four periods of breast-feeding. The distributions most resembling those of Childers and Hamil, although the comparison is relatively poor, are those of the combined totals of the Australian maladjusted

178

group and those of the English normal students. There appears to be a general tendency for the Australian delinquent children to be breast-fed on a pattern similar to that of the English neurotics, and the Australian neurotic children appear to be breast-fed for longer periods than the English normal children. The fact that there appears to be some kind of sliding relationship between the Australian and English groups under discussion suggests that factors other than breast-feeding are also involved, and these might be expected to lie somewhere in the different cultural fabric in which the respective groups of children have been reared. It might be found, for example, that breast-feeding customs are related to social class differences, although a comparison of class differences in the English, American, and Australian groups would be by no means easy in view of the different social and cultural significance of class divisions in these societies. In our rural clinic cases the fact that the groups were found to be fairly evenly matched for social class points to the validity of the conclusion that breast-feeding was in fact one of the important aetiological factors operating in the early lives of delinquents.[1]

It was interesting to note, among Sebire's figures, that out of the six Australian children who had been breast-fed longest (eleven to eighteen months) five were delinquents. This finding is consistent with Glover's (1925, 1926) contention that over-indulgent breast-feeding might also lead to oral fixation, in view of the subsequent frustration of weaning (and possibly of sudden or traumatic weaning, as at the arrival of another child) being more unbearable because of the heightened oral gratification resulting from over-satisfaction of oral drives.

A number of further studies might usefully be made on this important and complicated question, one of which might be a detailed study of both the social and psychological reasons *why*

---

[1] It is possible that the results of the present investigation have been thrown out of line with those of previous sociological investigations of the class level of delinquents because the majority of such studies have been concerned with the legal rather than the psychological meaning of delinquency, i.e. with cases convicted before a juvenile court, whereas in the present definition of delinquency the presence or absence of a court charge was irrelevant. The finding that many delinquents come from the middle as well as from the working classes is, however, in line with the findings of some psycho-analysts, e.g. Aichhorn, Karpman, and Greenacre.

the delinquent children, in general, tend not to have been breast-fed.

DIFFICULTIES IN EARLY HABIT-TRAINING

Considerable importance is attached in psycho-analytic theory to the methods of handling the child and the attitudes shown towards the child's instinctual manifestations while training him to acquire normal, civilized habits with regard to sleeping, feeding, bowel control, and bladder control. The methods of achieving the child's habit-training are thought to have considerable direct influence upon his later social behaviour and character development. During the preparation of the case histories special attention was paid by the psychiatric social workers to the child's behaviour associated with each of these bodily functions and the regulation of habits related to them. We examined all children in both groups who had experienced difficulties beyond those normally encountered in the establishment of such habits. This included all cases where, for constitutional or other reasons, the child had been particularly 'difficult' or resistant to training; cases where there had been frequent or severe breakdowns in control during the child's training; where the mother was known to have been overstrict in her methods of training; where normal habits had been established only after a prolonged series of 'battles' or a 'clash of wills' between mother and child; or when the child showed marked defiance and rebellion over these matters.

Breakdowns in the child's bodily habits may result from any number of influences, especially in periods of strain or after traumatic events. Typical examples among young children are the cases of regression on the birth of a sibling, or after learning in traumatic circumstances the fact of adoption. No attempt was made to assess the actual numbers of difficulties under each of these various headings, since this would have required the study of numerous special conditions peculiar to each case. A record was made simply of those cases where the habit-training had only been accomplished with great difficulty owing to the child's obstinacy, to the mother's mishandling, or to any other cause whatever.

Disturbances in sleep habits. These included all cases of night terror, sleep-walking, sleep-talking, insomnia, pronounced difficulty in going to sleep or in waking up, bad dreams, nightmares, pavor nocturnis, etc.

Disturbances in feeding habits. These included anorexia nervosa, gluttony, food fads, refusal to eat, having to be coaxed to eat, abnormal feeding habits, or any abnormal attitude towards food.

Disturbances of habits of bowel control included cases where there were breakdowns in habit-training, episodes of smearing or eating faeces, encopresis, severe constipation, and so on.

Disturbances of habits of bladder control included all cases of diurnal and nocturnal enuresis and frequency of micturition.

These difficulties referred throughout to the past, and particularly to the very early, development of the child, rather than to his present symptoms, which were included in Chapter III. This section was meant to refer to difficulties encountered during the process of early socialization, i.e. the development towards normal adaptation to social standards.

According to psycho-analytic theory, difficulties in early habit-training may be expected in both delinquent and neurotic children. Both types of children are likely to express early difficulties in the form of sleep disturbances, feeding disturbances, or disturbances in bladder or bowel control. However, a symptom even at a very early age may have very different meanings for different children. If the same children were examined at a later stage of development, it might perhaps be shown that the delinquent's rebellion against habit-training, or simply his failure to acquire socially desirable habits, was a forerunner of other types of aggressive reaction against the environment, such as stealing or running away from home.

On the other hand, the neurotic child, at a later stage of development, will probably have suppressed or repressed his early tendencies and developed a neurotic symptom that causes the child himself much internal suffering but does not necessarily trouble those about him. Other children with similar early difficulties may have resolved them by more normal mechanisms. For these reasons, early difficulties might be expected to occur in both our groups, but the fate or outcome of the early tendencies will probably be seen in different sequelae in each group.

HYPOTHESES: Early Habit-training
1. We should expect to find no significant difference between delinquent and neurotic children in the frequency with which difficulties occur in early habit-training. (Confirmed.)
2. We should expect to find that the numbers of children showing difficulties in early habit-training would be fairly high in both groups. (Confirmed.)

The results in *Table* 37, Appendix 1, show no significant differences between delinquent and neurotic children on any of the foregoing items. There is a slight tendency for neuroticism to be associated with early feeding difficulties, but in all other respects there is no difference between the two groups with regard to difficulties experienced in habit-training. Such difficulties occurred very frequently in both groups, and the totals for sleep disturbances, feeding disturbances, and difficulties in bowel and bladder control are in each group very high. We should have to compare our results with those from a normal group before we could conclude that these difficulties in early development might be indicators or forerunners of later disturbances in both delinquent and neurotic children. However, in almost all cases where these difficulties caused concern in later years, they had already made a pronounced appearance much earlier in the child's life.

'INFANTILE WANDERINGS'
Fenichel (1945) has described a situation in the early life of 'instinct-ridden' characters where lack of lasting object-relationships in early childhood, allied with other unfavourable conditions such as traumatic experiences, make the complete establishment of an effective super-ego impossible. He cites, for example, (ibid., p. 373) cases where 'the parent figures may have changed in such rapid succession that there was objectively no time or opportunity to develop lasting relationships and identifications.

However, persons of this kind also experience frustrations and develop reactions to them. Their super-ego is not lacking but incomplete or pathological, and the reactions of the ego to the pathological super-ego reflect the ambivalences and contradictions which these persons felt towards their first objects.' A paper by Anna Freud (1951) suggested the possibility of measuring yet a further aspect of the general neglect and the lack of opportunity for establishing emotional roots within the security of a normal family unit which appears to be the destiny of so many delinquent children. Miss Freud in her lectures and teaching has stressed that the emotional attachments of the child who repeatedly loses or is disappointed in his infantile love-objects tend to become increasingly superficial and shallow, the child withdrawing after each new rejection experience, into more and more embittered narcissistic isolation. As I have described in earlier chapters, a child's character normally develops through a series of identifications with his early love-objects in which he gradually assimilates of their approved standards of behaviour, at the same time becoming more independent. This process depends on a constantly repeated series of interactions between the child and his love-object rather than on isolated occurrences of the identification mechanism. It follows that the child who suffers from repeated changes of mother-substitute, or from 'infantile wanderings'[1] from one temporary home or family to another, so that he never establishes an unbroken and enduring emotional tie with one person, lacks the very fabric of psychological experiences out of which growth and adaptation to normal social life are made.

We compared the numbers of delinquent and neurotic children who, in their first five years, had 'changed hands' or 'changed homes' a number of times, or who completely lacked emotional roots in any home. This section refers to children who suffered several changes of maternal care and handling in infancy or in the earliest childhood years. Cases where a child is handed over temporarily to the care of a grandmother or aunt during the mother's illness or when a new baby is born, were excluded; so too were those cases where the upbringing of the child is given entirely into the hands of the grandmother when the child is still very

---

[1] This expression was coined by Miss Freud in a seminar discussion.

young, so that after the one interruption in the child's mother-relation, the grandmother becomes, as far as our purpose is concerned, the child's enduring mother-substitute and accepts the responsibilities attached to this role. Also excluded were cases where, through hospitalization or evacuation, the child is temporarily cared for by persons other than his mother, but loses neither his contact with her nor his rightful place in the home. Our cases are, rather, that fateful band of infantile wanderers, neglected, unwanted, or bereft, who pass continually from one person's hands to another's in a long-drawn-out search for an ordinary, normal home.

HYPOTHESIS: 'Infantile Wanderings'
1. We should expect to find that delinquent children tend to have undergone a series of changes of home and maternal care more frequently than have neurotics. (Confirmed.)

The results presented in *Table* 38, Appendix 1, indicate that there is a significant difference between delinquent and neurotic children at each of the age levels examined, the delinquent children tending to have experienced frequent changes of home and maternal care very much more than the neurotics. Forty per cent of the cases had already changed hands a number of times before the age of two years, and almost half the cases had experienced repeated changes before the age of five years. Many of the children had changed hands five or six times, and in a few instances twelve or fifteen times, within a few years.

Examples of 'Infantile Wanderings'
A number of examples occur in the early histories of adopted children prior to the finding of their adoptive home, e.g. Case No. 20, Ian, an illegitimate baby who had already passed through the hands of *nine* foster-parents before he found an adoptive mother at the age of eleven months. Other cases frequently occurring are those of illegitimate children who spend the first five or ten years of life supported, with tremendous hardship to herself in many cases, by a mother who has to work to maintain herself and the child and to look after him at the same time. Very

often the mother seizes on the nearest solution and places the child in an unsuitable home. Often the child lives in a series of foster-homes or residential nurseries, more or less out of touch with the mother, until the passing years bring a change in her fortunes, a subsequent marriage, perhaps, and the child's belated adoption into the mother's and step-father's home. Such a child's early life is spent 'muddling along' through a series of unplanned, make-shift arrangements, often never meant by any of the parties concerned to be anything but temporary expedients. In other cases the unmarried mother, or the unhappy mother, whose marriage has foundered, is forced to leave her child with some person who assumes physical care of him without accepting the responsibilities of parenthood, and when the child shows difficult behaviour, he is passed on once more. Then there are institutions that offer the mother or child a home for a limited space of time. Some mothers' and children's homes, in many respects very good, insist that the mother should find herself and the baby a home within a stated period after its birth, and some nurseries refuse to keep children, whom they have cared for from birth, after the age of two, when the child's wanderings must begin again. In some of the saddest cases (e.g. No. 41, Maureen, and No. 35, Maryann) the child has had so many changes of milieu, such a completely loveless environment, and such grossly inconsistent educational influences, that he has never learned to develop object-relations—friendly or otherwise—at all.

TYPE OF DISCIPLINE IN THE HOME

Healy (1915a) has pointed out the variation in standards of conduct required in the homes of delinquents and normal children, and Burt (1925) presented figures showing conclusively that delinquency is frequently associated with defective discipline in the home. More recently, similar findings have been obtained by Banister and Ravden (1944, 1945). Aichhorn (1925) and Fried-lander (1947, 1949b) have put forward the view that delinquency is specifically related to a certain type of discipline which makes normal character development extremely difficult for the child.

This has been described as 'inconsistent discipline', and includes inconsistency shown towards the child in a number of ways; e.g. in the parents' own behaviour, in the standards of behaviour demanded of the child, in the giving of rewards and punishment, in the sharing of discipline between various members of the family who are in disagreement about it, or in constantly making threats or promises that are never fulfilled, or following impulsive and unpredictable whims in handling the child. Greenacre (1945) found a similar type of capricious discipline in the early lives of psychopaths whom she treated psycho-analytically.

From the earlier literature, containing only an armchair, speculative type of approach to problems of misconduct, one would expect to find that it is the child who is over-leniently treated and for whom discipline is lax or non-existent, who is likely to become a law-breaker or a rebel. According to the observations and theory behind the present investigation, however, this is not the result which would be expected if this method were applied over a long period of the child's development. A lack of disciplinary standards may give rise to many personality problems but these are likely to be of a type other than those shown by the typical delinquent. According to psycho-analytic theory also, laxity of discipline is not, by itself, likely to produce delinquency (Aichhorn, 1925, Friedlander, 1947), and over-indulged children are frequently those whose parents are typically selfish, capricious and inconsistent as well as indulgent. The delinquent is thought to be typically the child who has been submitted to grossly inconsistent discipline, in which periods of over-gratification of early instinctive drives alternated with severe frustration of these drives. In such cases educational pressure on the child to acquire desirable social habits and to develop a strong character has not pursued a consistent line, and its influence has therefore been steadily undermined.

One might expect to find a different picture if the child has been over-strictly disciplined. From the earliest days of psycho-analytic study of the repressive forces involved in neurotic fears, phobias, and obsessions, psycho-analysts and others have been aware that, of all the important environmental influences, the one most frequently and constantly present is over-strict or rigid handling of the earliest manifestations of the child's instinctual impulses. The educational demands made during the early years of the life of a neurotic person are frequently found to have been not merely strict but harsh and implacably opposed to the primitive nature of the child's instinctual life. Under the influence of one aspect only of these early and often misconstrued findings, many educators (e.g. A. S. Neill and Homer Lane) went to extremes in allowing free expression of impulses in young children. Their 'gospel of freedom', applied to the education of young children, chiefly involved allowing free play to the child's aggressive instincts and a policy of *laissez-aller* in sexual matters. This policy would be regarded by most present-day educationists as mistaken. A more reasonable statement of psycho-analytic educational policy gained from insight into neurotic and other conditions is to be found in the teachings and writings of Anna Freud, Susan Isaacs, Aichhorn, and others. The first aim of early education should be to achieve modification of instinctual drives by working with a minimum of fear or threats and keeping to a middle way between too much frustration and too much gratification. This would allow, on the one hand, sufficient time and scope for the sublimation of antisocial instinctive drives and, on the other hand, for the gradual development of a strong and healthy character. This does not mean, of course, that over-strict discipline alone necessarily causes neurosis, since multiple psychological factors may combine to produce neurotic behaviour in even the most progressive and lenient homes.

We examined all cases from the point of view of the discipline the child had received at home and classified them according to the following scheme.

Normal discipline. Here we included all cases where the parents used ordinary restrictive and educational measures applied within normal limits. The methods, moreover, were consistently followed by both parents, who were in agreement about the main lines of education for the child. In such homes the standards of discipline were more or less fixed and consistent in themselves, good behaviour usually being followed by reward and bad behaviour by censure, punishment, or threatened loss of the parents' love. To be termed normal, disciplinary measures should have some reasonable relationship to the nature and degree of the offence and be applied in such a way that the child understands the justice of his punishment. For example, a child who is beaten for a small offence like breaking a plate, or for unknown offences, or for speaking out of place before a drunken father, receives punishment disproportionate to the offence.

Over-lenient discipline. Here we included all cases where the parents were lax in discipline, or where the child had been allowed to 'run wild' without adequate supervision, or had been consistently indulged.

Over-strict discipline. This included all cases where the parents were harsh, rigid, or repressive, enforcing a very high standard of conduct upon the child with consistent severity. This applied in particular to restriction of the child's instinctual manifestations and his normal pleasures and enjoyments.

Inconsistent discipline. This included all cases where either parent or both were inconsistent, e.g. gratifying or restricting the child according to temper or whim instead of making a consistent demand according to the child's capacities. Examples would be a child who is gratified one moment and frustrated the next for the same behaviour; or a child whose parents disagree with each other's methods, and do not support each other's decisions; or cases where one parent undermines the authority of the other. There may be inconsistency in the justice of the punishment for the offence (e.g. cases where breaking a plate will bring severe censure whereas encouragement and sweets are given to the child who keeps his mother's secrets or tells a 'white lie' for her). In many cases there may be dual control of the child, for example by mother and grandmother, with consequent changing and unequal standards for the child to follow. Inconsistency in the parents' own behaviour and conduct has, of course, the greatest influence upon the discipline of the child.

HYPOTHESES: Discipline in the Home
1. We should expect to find that a greater number of neurotic

than delinquent children have experienced normal discipline. (Confirmed.)

2. We should expect to find no significant difference between the numbers of delinquent and neurotic children who have received over-lax or over-lenient discipline in the home. (Confirmed.)

3. We should expect to find that a greater number of neurotic than delinquent children have received over-strict discipline. (Confirmed.)

4. We should expect to find that a greater number of delinquent than neurotic children have experienced inconsistent discipline in the home. (Confirmed.)

The results presented in *Table* 39, Appendix 1, indicate that the difference between the two groups was significant in the case of normal discipline, over-strict discipline and inconsistent discipline, but was not significant in the case of over-lenient discipline, where the number of cases is very small. The results show that neurotic children have experienced normal or over-strict discipline in a significantly greater number of cases than have delinquent children, whereas inconsistent discipline has been applied to a significantly greater number of delinquent than neurotic children. There is a positive correlation between delinquency and inconsistent discipline, and a negative correlation between delinquency and normal or over-strict discipline. It is interesting to note that Comfort (1950) in his analysis of authority and delinquency in the modern State, and Adorno, Frenkel-Brunswik, Levinson, and Sanford (1950) in their study of the authoritarian personality, found a similarly defined inconsistency or 'capriciousness' of discipline to be characteristically present in the early lives of the authoritarian type of personality (with whom the delinquent is considered to have much in common).

EARLIER 'DIFFICULT' BEHAVIOUR

Writers upon the treatment of delinquency have stressed the fact that the chances of therapeutic success are greatly increased if the child can be brought for treatment as far 'upstream' (Healy and Bronner, 1936) in his delinquent career as possible. They are agreed that we should detect as early as possible the first symptoms of abnormal development and attempt to remedy them before undesirable habits have become deeply embedded in the child's character. I feel this to be as true for the neurotic child as for the delinquent. How far back these symptoms originated and how much greater would have been the chances of curing them at their onset is not perhaps always realized.

In this section an examination is made of children who had shown a history of difficult behaviour—whether of a neurotic, delinquent, or merely a generally 'difficult' nature—some considerable time before their present referral. Children were included who had shown difficulties in the early years of childhood, or during a period of not less than two years before the onset of the present trouble.

HYPOTHESES: Earlier Difficult Behaviour

1. We should expect to find that in both neurotic and delinquent children the numbers of cases that show earlier difficulties is very high. (Confirmed.)

2. We should expect to find that there is no significant difference between the two groups in the numbers showing earlier difficulties. (Confirmed, except for the first two years.)

The results presented in *Table 40*, Appendix 1, show a significant difference between delinquent and neurotic children upon one item only, i.e. difficulties experienced before the age of two years. Delinquent children are shown to have experienced fewer difficulties before the age of two than neurotic children,[1] though more than half the children in both groups experienced difficulties during this period. The total number of cases showing difficult behaviour in their earlier development is very high in both groups, i.e. 96 per cent of the total number of cases in this investigation, and the numbers are very high in both groups at each age level.

[1] It is possible that the mothers of neurotic children may have been more anxiously observant in their general care and concern for the babies.

Examples of Difficulties Earlier in Development
We found a history of difficult behaviour in almost every child
we examined and in most cases this had appeared much more
than two years before the present problems. Difficulties before
the age of two years usually took the form of feeding or sleeping
disturbances, refusal of the breast or of the bottle, difficulties in
finding a correct diet for the children, difficult weaning, or pronounced difficulties in habit-training. In some cases there were
problems over crying, temper tantrums or night terrors, and in
several cases specific difficulties associated with pyloric stenosis,
'acidosis' and failures to gain weight. Convulsions occurred in
only one (neurotic) child (Case No. 94, Juliet) during the first
three days, and these were not subsequently repeated. Other
difficulties concerned screaming attacks and inability to get the
baby to sleep, and a number of infantile illnesses. Difficulties in
later years covered the whole range of symptoms, in both delinquents and neurotics, for which the children were later referred
to the clinic.

TRAUMATIC EXPERIENCES
After Freud's early papers on hysteria and on the traumatic neuroses (1893a–1905b), psychological theory placed increasing emphasis on the part played by traumatic events experienced during
childhood and early youth in adult psychological disturbances.
The influence of traumata on the neurotic has been more widely
recognized than their influence on the delinquent child. Certain
neurotic conditions are ascribed to traumata alone, whereas close
examination often shows that it is the attitude with which a person faces and deals with the experience (i.e. its inner psychic
meaning) rather than the severity of the traumatic event itself,
which determines whether his reaction will be of a neurotic or
another type. More recently Fenichel (1945) has emphasized that
the delinquent child no less than the neurotic has frequently
suffered from traumatic events during his formative years.

Aichhorn (1925) stressed the significance of traumatic experiences allied to a state of 'latent delinquency' where the child's
delinquency is basically due to faulty character development and
the emotional trauma is merely the precipitating factor which

results in the delinquent act. Powdermacker, Leves, and Touraine (1937) describe a form of delinquency, thought by them to be rare, where the child fails to meet social demands because of his preoccupation with the memory of painful events. Friedlander (1947) also describes a type of character structure constituting a predisposition to delinquency, which may or may not become manifest depending on a number of constitutional and environmental variables which may be traumatic, accidental, or merely circumstantial. Mowrer and Mowrer (1938) have described the occurrence of enuresis in delinquents as a regression in response to traumatic experiences, and Levy (1932a, 1943) has found certain traumatic responses intensified by sibling rivalry. Lander (1941) presented a valuable study of traumatic factors in the background of 116 delinquent boys. He holds the view that delinquency results from no single causal factor, but from the sum total of many predisposing, aggravating and precipitating causes. Among the 'predisposing causes' one most frequently found is the presence of a 'traumatic environment' in the child's early years. Emotional traumata very early in life frequently lay the foundation for subsequent emotional and social maladjustment, but whether in a specific case certain early experiences will have a harmful effect upon the child is determined by later incidental factors. Of the delinquent boys studied, 84 per cent were found to have suffered grave traumatic experiences. Many subtle traumata other than those originally studied were also revealed. Removal from home, for example, even from the most deficient and diseased home, was often found to be one more intolerable blow for the child.

We studied our two groups for the incidence of such obvious traumatic experiences as accidents, frights, death in the child's family, experience of assault or of attack by animals, the witnessing of births, air-raid experiences, evacuation or hospital experience. We also noted more subtle factors where only a close examination of the individual case can determine whether or not any particular event was traumatic. A visit to a dentist, for example, for a child who is prepared for it by a matter-of-fact parent, who is not himself unduly concerned or fearful, may not be traumatic at all. In the case of a more timid and sensitive child who is threatened, or forced to go to the dentist as a punishment, the experience itself may be so exaggerated as to be highly traumatic. Similarly, the birth of a sibling in certain circumstances may be traumatic to the child (e.g. when associated with the mother's illness or other factors), and in others it may be taken very naturally. For theoretical reasons we thought it of interest to study the age at which traumatic events occurred in the lives of these children.

HYPOTHESES: Traumatic Experiences
1. We should expect to find no significant difference between the numbers of delinquent and neurotic children who have suffered traumatic experiences. (Confirmed.)
2. We should expect to find that the numbers of children having had traumatic experiences will be very high in both groups. (Confirmed.)

The results presented in *Table* 41, Appendix 1, indicate that there is no significant difference between the delinquent and the neurotic children in the number of cases who have experienced traumatic events at any of the respective age levels. The numbers of children who have suffered traumatic experiences are very high in both groups, and comprise a little more than three-quarters of all the children in our project (delinquents 74 per cent and neurotics 82 per cent).

An interesting result was obtained from the comparison of the numbers of boys and girls who had suffered traumatic experiences. *Table* 42, Appendix 1, shows that the delinquent girls had suffered a significantly greater number of traumata than delinquent boys, but there is no significant difference between neurotic boys and girls on this point.[1]

Examples of Traumatic Experiences
0–2 *years.* The traumatic experiences suffered by children in these groups are surprisingly varied, and some of them very severe.

[1] The explanation for this difference is a matter for speculation. The observation that three out of twenty cases of delinquent girls have suffered from a severe facial burn in infancy points once more to general neglect of the delinquent child in infancy, and perhaps indirectly to parental ambivalence towards the girl.

193

Several cases were grossly ill-treated in babyhood by the father (Cases No. 38, Susan, No. 3, Derek, and No. 20, Ian). In other cases, sudden weaning produced a traumatic reaction before the age of two years (Cases No. 60, Irving, and No. 65, Julian). The sudden loss of the mother, whether owing to her rejection (No. 60, Irving), or desertion (Case No. 49, Daisy), or to mother's treatment in hospital (Case No. 71, Gregory) in many cases produced a traumatic and frequently depressed condition.

2–5 years. Examples include 'blitz' experiences; an attack by a dog; the mother's illness and sudden separation from her; the death of a parent; the witnessing of violent scenes between parents; witnessing of sexual scenes; abrupt transfer to a new foster-mother; death of a beloved grandmother or other member of the family; accident to the head; the dismissal of a beloved nannie in a sudden and spiteful way; frequent evacuation changes; quarrels between the parents; a practical joke at the hands of other children which had serious consequences; car accident; broken leg; drinking of inhalation or noxious substances; the loss of beloved animals; birth of siblings under traumatic circumstances; facial burns; hospitalization; unfortunate evacuation experiences; and severe beating and rejection by a new step-father.

5–7 years. Examples include air-raid and evacuation experiences; accidents; hospitalization; death in the family; sudden changes of foster-mother; parental rejection; death of a school friend; operation; witnessing suicidal attempt of mother; learning of adoption from strangers; reaction to appearance after many years of injured and ill father; the advent of a new stepmother; accident with a car; cruelty of the father; being sent away from home; and the occurrence of a birth in the home in unusual circumstances.

7–11 years. Examples include air-raid experience; death of siblings or of parents or other members of the family; experiences in riots in India; intensely unhappy evacuation; learning of adoption; sex episode with an elderly man; being suddenly sent away from home; confinement to bed with paralysis; hospitalization; internment camp experiences; the birth of parents' own children for a rejected, adopted child; father's disgrace and imprisonment;

a new and unsympathetic stepmother; separation from parents; witnessing the death in the 'blitz' of an only brother; hospital operation; and the tragic death of a brother, allied with the mother's prolonged depressive mourning for this.

11 *years plus.* Traumatic experiences include air-raid experiences; periods in hospital; witnessing a woman's death; accidents; witnessing a case of assault and interference by a man; evacuation experiences; being sent away from home; death of father; desertion by father; learning of adoption and being sent into a children's home; being sent to a mental hospital.

INTERESTS AND ACHIEVEMENTS

We found this field a particularly difficult one in which to obtain systematic information or to establish any form of reliable measurement. We wanted to find out whether or not there are significant differences between delinquent and neurotic children in their achievements, fields of interest, or the development of skills and attainments in various directions. These might indicate differences in strength and integration of the ego, personality differences in ego-skills, in the capacity for sublimation, and in the readiness to find satisfactory fields of expression for impulses. It is well known that the character structure of the delinquent tends to be weak, that he is likely to be dominated by pleasure-seeking impulses and that he lacks the persistence necessary for outstanding achievement. It is also well known that the delinquent tends to be backward; or, perhaps more accurately stated, that backwardness makes for delinquency by limiting the resources of the ego and lessening the degree of mastery over environment. The delinquent may find it difficult to gain his desired ends by socially accepted ways since he lacks skill and persistence and the ability to defer satisfactions. On the other hand, the neurotic child, although frequently highly intelligent, imaginative and sensitive, is sometimes too withdrawn and reserved to have achieved a great deal of external mastery. Limits are placed on the choice of the neurotic child's activities by his fears and inhibitions, rather than by any genuine incapacity for external mastery. Banister and Ravden (1944, 1945) have shown the problem child to be inferior in interests and attainments to the normal child. Both Burt (1925) and Rose (1949) found the delinquent child to have poor school achievements and a poor employment record, and Yarnell (1940) found educational backwardness and learning disabilities to be characteristic of his group of juvenile fire-setters. The present comparison of the achievement level of delinquents and neurotics is of especial interest because the intelligence of the children in the two groups has been equated, thus ruling out the factor of the duller intelligence of many delinquents.

In order to compare the interests and achievements of children of different age groups, it was necessary to find some guide, however rough, to the relative success of delinquents and neurotics in various fields. A crude index was found by making an examination of three areas of the child's achievements:

    (a) School attainments;
    (b) Reading interests;
    (c) Interests and activities.

In each of these groups a rating was made into three categories: below average, average, and above average. In the case of *school attainments*, it was possible to do this from school reports or by an assessment made by the educational psychologist at the clinic.

As regards *reading interests* it was found possible to ascertain in most cases:

(1) The teacher's opinion of the child's reading level and the amount of his general reading;

(2) A child's membership of a club or library;

(3) The child's own preferences and the approximate number of books which he had read, or types of books which he specially liked. Certain children, for example, had followed a special line of reading such as scientific subjects, or preferred to read an encyclopaedia;

(4) Whether the child reads with only average interest—i.e. does not ask for books, or seek out books on special subjects;

(5) Whether the child dislikes books or reads only what is required of him in school, or only children's books and comics;

(6) The children who are virtually non-readers.

From this survey it was possible to grade the children into the following rough divisions:

Above average. Children were placed in this group who showed a membership of and attendance at a library; an excellent or very good grade in reading at school; who showed marked or sustained pleasure and interest in books, seeking out and asking for them; who followed a special line of interest in reading; who in general read voraciously; children who owned many books; who chose reading as a hobby; asked for books as presents, or saved money to buy books.

Average. i.e. the average reader on his school records, or a child who has read only the usual school books and children's journals, or books and comics; who reads moderately but not excessively at home; who owns a few books but does not ask for or save money for books.

Below Average. A child who is backward or below average in reading at school; who reads only comics; who has no interest in or possession of books; who never finishes a book or who has read very few books.

In allotting our cases to each of these groups, account had to be taken of the children's age level. For example, Case No. 52, Geoffrey, aged six and a half, who had read encyclopaedias about the life history of newts in order to give a 'lecture' on the subject at school, was certainly above average, whereas a boy of fourteen, who has done so in accordance with class-room requirements, is not necessarily above average. Special interest in reading women's magazines or detailed interest in film-star annuals was unusual in girls of seven, but in a girl of fourteen this was judged as average. An attempt was made to work out criteria systematically but the grading on this item was necessarily subjective.

In the case of 'interests and achievements' grading was even more difficult. Under this general heading we included all club memberships, group activities, skills, hobbies, and sports, and any other interests spontaneously developed or pursued by the child. We considered activities in which the child had taken a lively degree of interest over some time, and in which he had established some degree of skill (e.g. playing the piano, making model aeroplanes). Also included as an 'interest' was a child's planning and being consistently interested in whatever he wanted to do when he was grown up. The distribution and range of the children's interests were then listed and a rating-scale was worked out setting limits for the grading 'above average', 'average', and 'below average' according to the number of interests and activities steadily pursued.

HYPOTHESES: Interests and Achievements
1. It was expected to find that delinquent children will tend to be inferior in their interests and achievements in comparison with neurotics. (Not confirmed.)

2. It was expected to find that the interests and achievements of both neurotic and delinquent children will tend to be below average. (Confirmed.)

The results presented in *Table* 43, Appendix 1, indicate that there is no significant difference between the delinquent and neurotic children in the level of their school attainments, reading interests, or leisure interests and activities. The tetrachoric correlations showed a slight tendency for delinquents to be associated with sub-average interests and attainments and for neurotic conditions to be associated with better than average reading interests, but these tendencies are very slight and inconclusive. It is interesting that in both groups the number of cases falling below average is very much higher than that falling above average. The general conclusion seems to be that both groups of children tend to rank low in interests and achievements of the type examined here.

Examples of Children's Interests and Activities
We found the interests and activities of the children extremely varied. Fields of expression included music and singing, scientific
198

interests, 'a practical bent for making things', or for painting, or story-telling, drawing, making things out of wood, and carving, writing stories, modelling, art-work, dancing, elocutionary and histrionic activities, dramatic art, dressing up, writing, miming and play-acting. We found their sports and pastimes included football, swimming, cycling, boxing, fishing, cowboys and Indians, gymnastics, riding, playing on the beach and fishing, cross-country running, tree-climbing, jiu-jitsu, hockey, tennis, jumping. Clubs which children attended included the Young Farmers' Club, a dress-designing club, girls' club and school dramatic society, boys' club, church choir, ambulance classes, Salvation Army Junior Brigade, boy scouts, first-aid classes and Christian Science clubs.[1] Future occupations which children had elected included 'joining the Navy like father', being an artist like father, being an engineer, joining the Air Force as an engineer, painting, 'going to Oxford or on the stage', being a 'bus-driver, taking matriculation examinations, working on a railway, being a carpenter, learning about radio, being a waitress, a nurse, a domestic science teacher, a children's maid, doing domestic work, being a dressmaker, being a nursemaid, teaching in nursery school, doing kennel work, 'looking after babies', working in an office. Others wanted to be a plumber, a veterinary surgeon, a sailor, 'an office boy or engineer', a music or dancing teacher, a missionary, a physical training instructor, a tractor-driver, a civil engineer, a gardener, 'a pirate' (girl), to undergo university training, to be a teacher, to be a cinema usherette, an air hostess, or 'to do one of six things—to be a film-star, a mannequin, do domestic work, nursing, teaching, or hairdressing'.

Other activities and interests described as favourites were: going to church and choir, playing games, selling primroses, driving a car or a motor-bike, caring for animals, having a paper-round, collecting stamps, doing homework, having one's own garden, helping father to mend a lorry, talking with a girl-friend, making gadgets, 'playing weird animal games', 'pretending to be tough', earning money, sewing, designing dolls' clothes, games with dolls, all kinds of domestic work, cooking, sketching, having

[1] One child (Case No. 20, Ian) organized a gang with himself as leader for the purpose of whipping other boys.

boy friends, playing with the dog or the kitten, having elocution lessons, making aeroplanes and soldiers, 'collecting fish and bulbs for nature study', being a form captain, learning ballet, learning handicrafts, keeping chickens, pressing flowers, 'having mother read to me', making a kite, 'just talking', and 'just doing nothing'.

CHAPTER VI

Discussion and summary of results

My chief reason for undertaking this project was that I wished to test certain aspects of psycho-analytic theory about the development of neurotic and delinquent children by using some of the systematic methods and tests of general psychology. I hoped that such a verificatory study might contribute in some measure to bridging the gap between academic psychology and psychoanalysis and facilitate communication between the social sciences generally. The combination of methods used in the investigation has, without doubt, proved extremely valuable. The strict procedures of general psychology used in the planning and organization of the research have yielded very interesting results when applied to hypotheses derived from earlier investigations, and in particular from psycho-analytic studies of children's emotional development. My fellow-workers in the Child Guidance Service and I feel confident that we have effectively demonstrated the need for combining the outlook of dynamic psychology with the technical methods of modern research work. I do not wish to under-estimate the many difficulties which lie in the way of such team collaboration; but rather to claim that the combination of methods used to obtain and to analyse our data has provided special and important information about a wide variety of influences affecting neurotic and delinquent behaviour which are often ignored in social planning and administration.

Our findings support the general psycho-analytic dictum that the major influences determining a child's development and behaviour are to be sought in his very early years and that the main lines of his character development are laid down in this period. The child's reactions to influences from his inner and outer environment inevitably have a more far-reaching and permanent effect at this period than at any other. The importance of determining those factors in his environment which are essential for normal emotional growth and which may lead to various disturbances in development cannot be over-emphasized.

In the following pages I shall attempt to assess the extent to which our results offer support for various tenets of psycho-analytic theory, and to consider the implication of these findings for the personality development and emotional education of the child.

We have been able to demonstrate that certain types of beha-viour, not always recognized as indicating abnormal develop-ment, in fact do. The commonly used definitions of neurotic behaviour, for example, might well be extended to include some of these items: excessively good, quiet, and easily controlled behaviour; pronounced envy or jealousy of other children; diffi-culties in special subjects at school; exaggerated fantasy and imagination, especially where there is failure to distinguish be-tween fantasy and reality; unemotional, apathetic and lethargic behaviour; marked tendencies to imitate the behaviour of the opposite sex.

Our analysis of the miscellaneous group of behaviour items yielded some 'unexpected' results in that certain items commonly regarded as being typical of either neurotic or delinquent beha-viour were found equally in both groups of children. The exami-nation of the social relations of *both* groups showed, for example, that the delinquent as well as the neurotic group contained a considerable number of children who were unsociable and lacked relationship with others. We also found that the delinquent child tends to get bullied, teased, or victimized in more cases than he bullies or intimidates other children, and in this he is comparable to, rather than the opposite of, the neurotic child. There are relatively few cases in either group of children who are easily led or choose bad companions. We found that both neurotics and delinquents are retarded in school, and have many difficulties in adjusting to school life. It is also interesting to note that the num-bers in the two groups are comparable in the sections dealing with persistent nervous habits, such as thumb-sucking and other bodily habits, and also in the sections dealing with queer habits and odd behaviour and with children who are unchildlike and humourless. Many neurotic children were shown to be as dirty and untidy in habits as were delinquents, and with regard to disorders of organ function, delinquent children showed as many feeding disturbances, sleep or speech disturbances, or disturbances of bladder or bowel control as did the neurotic children. Enuresis and encopresis, which are likely to prove grave symptoms in the case of older children, constituted an obstinate problem in about 30 per cent of the total group of delinquent and neurotic children.

Certain other character traits commonly associated with delinquent behaviour, such as unreliability and irresponsibility at school or at work, inability to keep jobs, selfishness, lack of persistence, and laziness, were also found very frequently in the neurotic child. The same is true of greedy, demanding behaviour, of frequent feelings of unhappiness and dejection, and of feeling unwanted, rejected, and disliked. Both delinquent and neurotic children tend to have temper outbursts and 'nasty' or irritable tempers. Both also are frequently stubborn, obstinate and negative in behaviour. It is interesting to note that 16 per cent of the total group of delinquent and neurotic cases show tendencies towards self-punishment, either hurting themselves or getting hurt or provoking punishment. In Case No. 20, Ian, the child's delinquency arises largely from a sense of guilt which leads him to behave in a manner that will lead to punishment. (In few other cases is this mechanism so unmistakably clear.)

We found that precocious sex games and offences, which are commonly regarded as delinquent characteristics, occurred also in neurotic children, especially at certain stages in the child's early development. It is possible that under certain traumatic or repressive conditions these may lead to neurotic disturbances. It was also found, as Bender and Blau (1937) have indicated, that the child who is usually supposed to be the 'innocent partner' in the sex games is sometimes more disturbed than his or her seducer and is not always as passive as might at first appear. In our view indications of future neuroticism lie less in the actual practice of sex games or offences than in the incipient inversion; that is, attempting to take over the role of the opposite sex, or masochistically submitting rather than fighting or running away.

If the common definition of delinquency were extended to

cover a wider understanding of some of the emotional characteristics referred to in our investigation, this might influence educational policy and help to determine what types of treatment are
likely to suit individual cases. We found the delinquent lacks a
sense of guilt or shame, or any impulse to make good his misdeeds; he is wilful and has poor control over his impulses, being
unable to wait for satisfactions. His emotional characteristics
present a picture that is consonant with the psycho-analytic explanation of the delinquent's arrested or distorted conscience formation; i.e. he is unable to tolerate frustration or to defer his
immediate satisfaction in favour of more distant goals because his
conscience development remains at a level similar to that of the
small child. Even where his conscience has developed, it fails to
control his behaviour in the face of temptation and moral choice.
The conscience development is faulty because it fails to arouse
guilt or shame, and does not lead the child to adapt his behaviour
to the demands of reality. This condition may be expected to
develop where the child's education has been carried out with
great inconsistency and where he has been alternately over-
stimulated and harshly rejected. Such treatment leads to confusion
in his values and standards of behaviour so that he cannot judge
what is the right thing to do. Didactic moral training has no
meaning for him, since it is not rooted in imitation and emotional
identification with a person to whom he is attached by recipro-
cally deep and loving emotions. Such a child has no incentive for
giving up his egocentric aims and selfish pleasures, and his emotional development becomes arrested at a 'narcissistic' stage. His
emotional attachments tend to be shallow because they have been
frequently interrupted and mishandled, each new relationship
becoming more superficial and impoverished than the previous
one. For this reason he genuinely does not care, or even resents,
what others think or say, and it is often impossible to influence
him by ordinary methods. Often he presents an impenetrable
armour towards those who seek to change him by appeals to his
feelings or moral sense. He seeks chiefly for direct gratification of
his wishes without thought of the consequences and without the
mature person's capacity to consider other people's feelings. We
found that the delinquent child's distrust of adults and fear of

authority goes with a compensatory attitude of bravado and un-concern and acting the part of a 'tough guy'. In certain cases this characteristic approaches the hard emotional core of some 'affec-tionless characters',[1] or so-called psychopathic personalities; in other cases it amounts only to uncommunicativeness, evasiveness, and an obstinate denial of all difficulties.

According to psycho-analytic theory, such attitudes result from a failure in normal, friendly social and emotional relationships, the basis for which is laid down early in the child's relationship to his mother. This first human relationship is so important and satisfying for the child's security and self-esteem that he is pre-pared to give up his uncivilized ways in order to maintain his mother's approval and his security. In cases such as we have des-cribed the child seems callous, affectionless and emotionally hardened to the point of refusing to admit to normal friendly feeling or concern for others at all. Such children have frequently suffered severe emotional traumata, or had parents who from very early years have deceived or rejected them. In other cases early emotional relationships have repeatedly failed or been in-terrupted, so that the child now appears to have a vested interest in being 'tough' and hard and denying all emotional ties or feel-ings for others so as to pursue his aggressive, vengeful, or selfish goals. These children are severely disturbed, with 'warped' characters, and a long-standing history of antisocial disorder. Because of the child's lack of any enduring friendly relationship in the past, this type of case is particularly resistant to re-education or treatment, as many probation officers have been forced to ad-mit after their painstaking efforts have been constantly rebuffed. Such character traits, when they occur in association with a his-tory of delinquent behaviour, are so unmistakable that they should certainly be borne in mind as a supplementary diagnostic criterion and be given a particular weight when the type of treatment required for an individual case is under consideration.

Delinquent children were found to be unable to bear frustra-tion; to be greedy, demanding and extravagant with money; to resent strongly criticism and correction from others; and to be 'up against authority'. The fact that on these items they differed

[1] As described by Bowlby (1944) and Bender (1943).

greatly from the neurotic children supports the psycho-analyst's theory of the delinquent's defective super-ego formation. Further traits shown by delinquents were revengeful, spiteful, tell-tale behaviour, and a mischievous incitement of other children to join them in misconduct; they were both the ringleaders in making trouble and the scapegoats for group misdeeds. These characteristics indicate failure to make satisfactory social and emotional relationships and inability to take a normal model as a standard for group behaviour. Just as the child's failure in early emotional relationships with the parents leads to a failure in conscience formation, so his lack of identification with the standards of his social group makes it impossible for him to adapt his behaviour to suit theirs; he becomes an 'outsider' and avenges himself on the group by immature, teasing, quarrelsome behaviour, which sometimes gives him perverse pleasure.

What we found out about the children's home and family background supports the psycho-analytic theory that certain conditions in the environment of the young child are essential for normal growth. We found substantial evidence that the child needs a stable and united home for his adaptation to the social group to be accomplished slowly and gradually. Psycho-analysts have always held that within this stable framework of the home the child must have a satisfactory and uninterrupted relationship with the mother or substitute mother during the child's early life, and especially during the first six or seven years. This relationship must be mutually loving, steady and secure, neither interrupted by external disturbances nor distorted by an emotional attitude on the part of the mother that prevents the child's emotional and social development from proceeding normally. The most favourable attitude in both parents is one that allows for the maturation of instinctual urges without an arrest of development at any point or tendencies towards immaturity or regression. Friedlander (1946b) has stressed the need for the child's earliest training in control of his bodily habits to be carried out with an understanding of the child's needs at the time. She stresses the need for timing early educational demands according to his stage of development, so that he can adapt his behaviour to them without undue difficulties or battles of will. Such conflicts will lead to an arrest of development at a certain stage and to disturbed relationships with whoever cares for the child. Parents should steer a course between too much frustration and too much gratification, and treat their children consistently both as regards their demands and their own behaviour and example. All exponents of psychoanalytic theory are agreed that the normality of the parents' own emotional life and the warmth of their response to the child are of fundamental importance to him. These are reflected in the way in which each parent is able to make a genuine relationship with each successive child in the family, and sincerely to enjoy the children without making the sort of exclusive and intense emotional demand that often results in a disturbed relationship, and a dwarfing of the child's personality. They should allow sufficient time and scope for the sublimation of antisocial instinctual drives which will further the gradual development of a strong and healthy character, and the growth, without undue difficulties, of an independent conscience that will provide an *inner* guide and control for the child's behaviour.

We found that the delinquent children lacked those conditions essential for normal emotional development at points in their lives, where the neurotic children did not. Lack of stable home life may be due to gross environmental disturbances or to immaturity, instability or incompatibility in the parents, or to other factors responsible for breaking up the family unit. The child who is thus deprived of the primary requirements for his normal social and emotional development also has to face additional problems that are extremely difficult for him to overcome.

We found manifold evidence that delinquent children suffered from the absence of, or interruptions in, a secure emotional relationship with their mother during their crucial formative years. Where an enduring relationship with the mother existed, it was frequently found to be emotionally disturbed, or rejecting, or in some way not conducive to healthy emotional growth. The neurotic children, in contrast, had not suffered from interrupted or broken relationships with their mother to any comparable extent; but we often found in their histories exclusive and intense emotional relationships between mother and child that were harmful to normal development. The frequency with which interruptions in the psychological relationship with the father occur in delinquent children's lives points to the same lack of a stable background. The extent to which the broken relationship with the father in the delinquent's life precedes and sometimes causes the breaking up of home life and an interruption in the child's relationship with his mother has not been determined. It happens with monotonous regularity that external gross environmental disturbances are mirrored in psychological frustrations for the child.

We have also been able to show that the methods of handling or disciplining the delinquent throughout his development have not been such as to modify his instinctual drives without arrest of development at certain stages, or establishing tendencies to regression; nor have they been applied with a minimum of fear and a maximum of consistency. The delinquent's emotional education, in contrast with the neurotic's, has typically been carried out with the greatest inconsistency, extremes of impatience and harsh frustration alternating with indulgence and spoiling. The parents' own emotional life frequently sets the child a bad example and this, allied to the insecurity and interruptions in his relationship with his parents, leads to faulty and incomplete identification with them, or to an arrest at infantile, narcissistic levels of emotional development. Thus he has not been able to develop a strong character, an independent and reliable conscience, or the capacity for making friends.

We found that the delinquent child's relationship with his parents was usually resentful and of a sado-masochistic type, i.e. one involving an arrest of libidinal development and a regression to the anal-sadistic stage of emotional life. This produces either fixation or regression (often remarkable in extent, intensity and obstinacy) to hostile attitudes, hatred and cruelty to others, and extremes of provocation and sado-masochistic interchanges with the parental partner (e.g. Cases Nos. 20, 21, and 55). This type of relationship is later transferred from the parents on to the child's elders and to society in general, and may be so skilfully and subtly provocative that he invariably arouses similar responses from teachers, foster-parents, probation officers, other children, the police, or wardens of hostels and remand homes. There are many varieties of this type of relationship and we found substantial evidence that inconsistent handling of the child's early emotional and instinctual manifestations is aetiologically linked with the delinquent's repetition-compulsion to form, with striking regularity throughout his later life, a type of intense, quarrelsome and tormenting relationship from which he derives power and perverse satisfaction.

The infantile origin of tendencies towards antisocial behaviour, and the consequent need for recognizing them early, have been emphatically stressed by all writers on delinquency, from both the psychodynamic and the sociological schools. If we had been able to get help for our delinquents at least two years, and in some cases as much as five or ten years, before they actually came to the clinic, we could have recognized and possibly corrected the incipient or pronounced difficulties in their behaviour.

With similar finality we have been able to show that both delinquent and neurotic children tend to have suffered from numerous traumatic experiences in their early years, and thus to confirm one of the earliest psycho-analytic theories, namely that severe traumatic experiences, especially in very early childhood, are unfavourable to a child's psychological development and may form the kernel of much future psychopathology.

The psychological value of breast-feeding is also a point on which psycho-analytic opinion has been unanimous since the first systematic observations on libidinal and character development were made. The theory that the deepest roots of the child's emotional relationship with his mother lie in the feeding situation has been championed by many other writers. This, however, is not the place to assess the influence of breast-feeding on character formation. In my opinion what we found from our comparison of the duration of breast-feeding in our two groups should be interpreted with due caution and in relation to many other factors, such as the personality of the delinquent child's mother; disturbances in the external environment; certain special conditions that have brought about an interruption in the mother-child relationship; or in the general conditions of neglect and haphazard circumstances in which many delinquent children are shown to have passed their early years. Quite apart from breast-feeding being a vital, warm and secure life-experience that the delinquent child tends to lack in his earliest babyhood, it is probably the general attitude of the mother while she feeds her child, either by breast or by bottle, that is of importance in character development. Lack of breast-feeding is probably crucial only when it coincides with a lack of warmth and security in this mutual relationship. It is also possible that in many cases constitutional factors in the child may be partly responsible for early feeding difficulties, at the breast or in general.

It has been of great interest to see from the results of our project which conditions held by psycho-analytic theory to be essential for normal social and emotional development were absent in the lives of delinquents, and which were missing in delinquents but were present in neurotics. Of the latter, the most important appear to be: first, the rich complex of psychological conditions, reliable and enduring, which are present in a stable home; and second, a consistent attitude, patient, kindly, and firm, in handling the child's instinctual manifestations, as opposed to an inconsistent discipline. Though we found that the neurotic child had a stable home, he had to contend with many degrees of disturbance in his parents' personalities, as well as many subtle types of disturbed or immature relationships that have not yet been analysed in detail.

SUMMARY OF RESULTS

The conditions that we found to be associated with delinquency or neuroticism cannot be said to *cause* these disorders in the sense that a certain result may be predicted from the fact that one or another of them is present or absent; all we have been able to demonstrate is that certain factors tend to occur together with certain types of behaviour. The question must inevitably arise whether there is not a more fundamental cause for delinquency or neuroticism. For example, the well-proven finding that delinquent children come from broken homes does not prove that the broken home has 'caused' the delinquency. Our method of comparison cannot give any indication of whether some other factor, such as instability in the parents or some unknown demoralizing influence in the family, has not 'caused' both the broken home and the associated delinquency as well. We cannot answer such questions and the conclusions are for this reason stated in cautious terms. All that we can claim is that in the small samples of English clinic cases actually compared, the original division into delinquent and non-delinquent, i.e. neurotic, is not fortuitous but is in some way related to the corresponding divisions that we found in the various conditions we examined. Where the actual observations were found to differ significantly from those expected on the basis of a given hypothesis, then they may perhaps agree with the findings expected on the basis of some other hypothesis. Where the actual observations agree with the expected findings, then it may be claimed that the results favour the given proposition, but do not 'prove' it. What has been shown in each case is that the differences are too great to be accounted for by chance.

Bearing in mind these reservations, the significant findings of the present investigation may briefly be summarized as follows:

1. *Broken home life.* The findings of almost all previous investigators[1] that delinquents tend to come from broken homes, or from unstable homes broken by gross environmental disturbances has, in general, been confirmed. Our results suggest, however, that the term 'broken home' is very obscure and indefinite, and that the psychological reasons for the home being broken should be investigated as well as the sociological facts. Although the number of present cases is small, it has been shown, for example, that in homes that are 'broken' owing to the child's being step-, foster-, adopted or illegitimate, the children tend to be neurotic as frequently as they are delinquent. Delinquency occurs much more commonly in homes that are broken for other reasons, e.g. by parental absence, or by broken marriages.

2. *Neuroticism and stable homes.* We have shown that neurotic children (in common probably with normal children) tend to come from 'stable' homes in contrast to the 'unstable' homes of delinquent children. This finding is in accord with a statement by Friedlander (1949b) that the homes from which neurotic children

[1] With the noteworthy exception of Shaw; see Shaw (1929) and Shaw and McKay (1942).

come are often apparently 'good' (i.e. stable, unbroken) but that certain so-called 'stable' homes in fact contain psychological disturbances that tend to make a child neurotic. Banister and Ravden (1945) also agree that 'nervous' children tend to come from 'accord' homes and delinquent and aggressive children come from 'broken' homes. The implication that 'stable homes' (i.e. homes with an unbroken family circle) are not synonymous with psychologically healthy or normal homes, merits further research into the problem.

3. *Social level of the home.* Among our present cases we found no difference in the social level from which delinquent and neurotic children come; and delinquents come as often from middle-class as from working-class families. The reason for this is possibly that the county has few industrialized, crowded factory areas, or slums. The interesting thing about this finding is that it is at variance with most previous studies on the home background of the delinquent. It is consonant, however, with Aichhorn's division (1925) of delinquents into three main types which include the narcissistic, 'spoilt' or over-indulged and mis-educated child from the middle-class home.

4. *Possible hereditary factors.* We found little conclusive evidence about the influence of hereditary conditions in the causation of delinquency or neurosis, although there is some evidence of the presence of various unfavourable conditions in the family histories of delinquents. This finding is in line with earlier statements by Freud (1905b), Healy (1915a, 1917, 1925), Burt (1925, 1935), and Mannheim (1940, 1942) that neither hereditary nor environmental conditions can be regarded as decisive, but that a combination of both factors is always present.

5. *Physical illness of parents.* We showed that chronic physical illness is common in the parents of both delinquent and neurotic children.

6. *Physical illness of child.* We found that chronic physical illnesses appeared very frequently in the past histories of neurotic and delinquent children. Similar results were also found by Healy (1915a) and by Burt (1925 and 1925a).

7. *Personality of the parents.* We found that delinquents very often had parents who showed antisocial tendencies, while neurotics tended to have neurotic parents. Our investigation of the parents' personalities supports the early postulates of Freud, Aichhorn and others that normality of the parents' own emotional life is essential for healthy emotional development in the child, both from the viewpoint of providing a suitable 'model' for the child to imitate and for the satisfactory handling of the child's own instinctive and emotional drives.

8. *Early ascertainment.* Our material offers abundant evidence in support of the necessity for early ascertainment of delinquency. That earlier ascertainment is possible is demonstrated by the fact that almost all the cases examined showed difficult behaviour at least two years, and very often up to five or ten years, before the present offence. This finding was also true for the neurotic children, whose difficulties had usually been evident for very considerable periods.

9. *Heterogeneity.* Our findings fully support what Levy and Karpmann have stressed: that the time is overdue for a recognition of the fact that 'delinquency' is not a clinical entity and should not be used as a diagnostic term; that so-called delinquents belong to a varied group of recognizable personality types. We propose to use criteria for separating 'neurotic delinquents' from children who become delinquent through lack of adequate social training, or from institutional, deprived children who become delinquent. We also established criteria for distinguishing the sporadic aggressive behaviour of the passive-effeminate type of boy from the habitual aggression of the so-called 'psychopathic delinquent', and from that of the unstable, dull, or borderline defective, as well as other types. The methods of treatment suitable for the different types vary considerably.

10. *Inconsistent discipline.* Our figures support Aichhorn and Friedlander who both found that inconsistency in the handling and discipline of the child's instinctual and emotional needs (over-frustration alternating with over-gratification) is one of the specific features in the aetiology of the delinquent character. We

H   213 found very few cases of over-lenient discipline in either group, and found that over-strict or normal discipline was characteristic of the histories of neurotic children. This finding is partly in agreement and partly at variance with Burt's results (1925a).

11. *Parent-child relationship.* The importance and the nature of a satisfactory parent-child relationship, described by Freud and also by Healy, White, Burt, Aichhorn, Friedlander, Levy, Greenacre, and many others, has been emphasized by our results. A very high proportion of delinquent children tend to have an emotionally disturbed relationship with one or both parents. This relationship is often of a quarrelsome, aggressive, sado-masochistic type. There is evidence that this same kind of perverse, immature relationship is formed in association with inconsistent discipline during the early years of the child's life.

12. *Intra-family relationships.* The parents of delinquents tend frequently, through immaturity, instability, or mutual incompatibility, to have a severely disturbed emotional relationship with each other, often of an outspoken, quarrelsome, and sado-masochistic type . Overtly disturbed relationships between the parents of neurotic children occur less frequently and follow a variety of other subtle patterns. Both delinquent and neurotic children tend to have disturbed relationships with their siblings. Disturbed relationships with grandparents, aunts, lodgers, etc. also tend to occur frequently in delinquents.

13. *Interruptions in the emotional relationship between parent and child.* Careful and prolonged inquiries into the nature and history of the emotional relationship between mother and child, and between father and child, have shown a striking difference between delinquent and neurotic children in the frequency with which a break or interruption occurred in this relationship. Delinquent children tend to have experienced frequent interruptions in the mother-child relationship before the age of seven years, and interruptions in the father-child relationship at all age levels, much more frequently than neurotic children. The most significant age for a break in the mother-child relationship appears to be in the second year. This finding agrees with statements of Burlingham and Freud (1942, 1943, and in their seminars and teaching) that

214

interruptions in the mother-child relationship between six and eighteen months have the most serious adverse effects upon socialization and emotional development.

14. *Parent-child separations.* Separations of the child from its home and parents, or absences of the parents, occurred more frequently in delinquents than in neurotics, especially in the early years. This finding supports Bowlby's observations (1944, 1951). The delinquent children appear to have suffered from repeated separations rather than from one single, traumatic separation.

15. *Breast-feeding.* We found that delinquent children had been breast-fed less often than the neurotics, and when breast-feeding did occur, they were weaned much earlier than the neurotics. This is supported by similar findings on Australian cases.

16. *Specific experiences in early childhood.* Our research under this heading offers factual evidence in support of Healy's contention (1915a) that children who have been deceived during their early childhood, especially those who have been deceived about their true parentage, are likely to become delinquent. The evidence also supports Freud (1893a, 1905a), Friedlander (1947a), Lindner (1944), Lander (1941), and others, on the frequency with which delinquent and neurotic children have undergone various traumatic experiences in their early years. And it confirms the observations of Lowrey (1940b), Burlingham and Freud (1942, 1943), and Goldfarb (1943, 1944, 1945) on the influence of a lack of satisfactory mother-child relationship in the earliest years, the lack of an enduring friendly relationship with one adult throughout childhood and of various deprivations and isolation experiences in infancy. The results also support the psycho-analytic theory of the importance of handling the early drives and habit-training of the young child in a way that will avoid the kind of upheavals and abnormal difficulties that tend to have occurred in the early years of both delinquents and neurotics. There is also abundant evidence that the quality and the vicissitudes of the child's psychological relationships with various members of his family in his earliest years have a very great influence on his later social and emotional development.

17. *Infantile irritability.* No evidence has been found in support of Karpman's theory of the exaggerated infantile irritability of certain delinquents. Over-aggressiveness, irritability, and similar difficulties before the age of two years were found more frequently among neurotic children than among delinquents.

18. *Social relations and achievement level.* We found a marked failure in the sphere of social relationships amongst both neurotic and delinquent children. Allied with this, both types of maladjusted children were markedly retarded in school and below average in general interests and attainments. Neurotic children also tended to show learning inhibitions with regard to specific subjects.

19. *Conscience development.* We found failures in conscience development in almost all the delinquents, more rarely in the neurotics. These were frequently associated with lack of a satisfactory parent-model, lack of an enduring relationship with a loved adult, and lack of consistency in discipline. The lack of an independently functioning conscience has been variously described by Freud, Aichhorn, Friedlander, Greenacre, Levy, Karpman, and others. We suggest that this may be one of the paramount factors, as yet little understood, which is inherent in what Mannheim has called 'susceptibility to delinquency', Aichhorn 'latent delinquency', and Friedlander 'the antisocial character'.

20. *'Over-good', well-behaved children.* We found that neurotic children were often 'over-good', obedient, and well behaved, whereas delinquents tend to be disobedient and aggressively defiant. This finding offers indirect support for the theories of Freud, Friedlander, Glover, Gordon, and others, with regard to neuroticism being a 'moral' conflict psychologically internalized within the individual, whereas delinquency represents an open conflict between the unsocialized individual and the environment. It also suggests that teachers should be aware that 'over-good', tractable children, who never present problems in school, may nevertheless be suffering from a serious psychological disturbance.

21. *Imitation of the opposite sex.* We found in many of the neurotic children trends in their behaviour, interests and activities contrary to their biological role and sexual disposition, and indicative of

confused identification patterns within their characters. This finding offers indirect support for Freud's theory of the sexual aetiology of the neuroses and of the tendency towards inversion that lies behind many adult neuroses.

22. *Emotional characteristics of the delinquent.* At a certain stage in the normal child's early development, he will tend to be wilful, impulsive, unable to bear frustration, shameless, greedy, and over-demanding; this cluster of immature conditions is found in delinquents, though not in neurotics. Our figures in this section support the findings of such writers as Freud, Aichhorn, Reich, and Friedlander, and demonstrate that these characteristics may persist unmodified throughout the child's later years. Our results also suggest that much delinquent behaviour should be regarded less as something bizarre or abnormal in the personality, than as an immaturity in emotional and social development leading to a distorted, 'crippled' character, calling less for intensive psychotherapy than for long-term re-education of the character and the emotions.

23. *Size of family.* We found that delinquent children in our survey tended to come from larger families than did the neurotics. There was no difference in first-child, last-child, and only-child position. We have no evidence for comparison with the size of families from which normal children came.

FURTHER OBSERVATIONS CONCERNING PATTERNS OF FACTORS IN HOME AND FAMILY BACKGROUND

As Healy (1915a) and Burt (1925, 1925a) pointed out, delinquency is caused by a plurality of factors, and the balance between various conditions is more important than any special circumstances or individual 'cause'. The complexity of this interweaving and interplay of forces is abundantly illustrated in our cases and it may seem from many points of view a hopeless matter to attempt to disentangle the relations and combinations of these factors. However, a beginning may be made in this direction by examining which factors or sets of environmental influences tend to be combined together with any degree of frequency. I was repeatedly struck, during the statistical analysis of the results and the writing of the case histories, with the frequency with which certain 'patterns' or clusters of factors tended to recur. Although I realized that many special problems would arise in such an undertaking and that this kind of further analysis of the results would be rather unwieldy and time-consuming, I decided to go part of the way in analysing some of the most striking of these patterns and will now give a brief account of this attempt.

Table 44 CONDITIONS AFFECTING DELINQUENT BEHAVIOUR

	Delinquent	Neurotic	χ^2
1. General morbid conditions in family history	20	8	9.51**
2. Unsettled home, frequent moves	31	13	11.70**
3. Interrupted mother-child relationship	36	11	23.12**
4. Interrupted father-child relationship	40	11	31.37**
5. Disturbed mother-father relationship	26	15	5.22*
6. Antisocial or morally unstable personality of father or mother	30	7	16.80**
7. Disturbed mother-child relationship	42	31	5.07*
8. Inconsistent discipline	36	14	17.60**
9. Breast-fed three months or less	31	17	12.39**
10. Broken family, i.e. one or more of the following conditions: Parents separated, divorced, deserted, irregular unions Child step-, foster- or illegitimate, Mother or father or both dead Prolonged absence of mother or father Child reared in ignorance of his true parentage	22	11	4.52*
11. Period spent in institution or foster-home	12	2	6.72**

* P = ·05; χ^2 > 3·841   ** P = ·01; χ^2 > 6·635 (see p. 487)

Table 45 CONDITIONS AFFECTING NEUROTIC BEHAVIOUR

	Delinquent	Neurotic	χ^2
12. Neurotic conditions in family history	10	21	9.51**
13. Stable family	28	39	4.52*
14. Neurotic personality of mother or father	10	24	5.72*
15. Over-strict discipline	7	19	6.29*
16. Chronic past illnesses	23	33	3.29
17. Normal discipline	4	14	5.49*
18. Feeding disturbances	21	34	2.85
19. Difficult behaviour before the age of two years	21	34	5.82*
20. Breast-fed four months or more	7	25	12.39**

I examined the factual conditions in the second section of this study, namely in Chapter IV, 'The Child at Home: His Family Background and Social Setting'. I selected the conditions which showed a significant difference between delinquent and neurotic groups. Certain items of borderline significance, but of special theoretical interest, were also included. I arranged these items in two groups (*Tables* 44 and 45), representing the items by numbers.

Tables were then drawn up for the incidence throughout the 100 cases of each of the foregoing conditions, and then searched for the number of times in each group that certain 'patterns' or 'clusterings' occurred in the children's histories. Patterns of three factors were counted at first, and then the patterns systematically enlarged to a group of nine conditions in the case of delinquents and a group of six conditions in the neurotics. A chi-square test was then made of the significance of the difference between the two groups upon the incidence of each of these 'patterns' or clusters of conditions. Our results are represented in a very condensed form in the relevant tables and a tentative discussion follows.

For example, the data in *Table 46* (Appendix 1) should be read thus: 'Three factors, viz. items number 3, 4, and 10 from *Table* 44 occurred together in the family history of thirty-four delinquent cases and of only seven neurotics', and so on. By treating each pattern as a unit, a 2 × 2 table was constructed (i.e. the group of children have or have not experienced the given pattern of influences or experiences) and the significance of the difference between the groups upon this pattern was tested by chi-square technique.

In these tables it is clear that the various conditions overlap to some extent, rather than occurring as separate experiences. 'Broken family', for example, frequently 'causes' interruptions in the mother-child relationship; interruptions in the father-child relationship often tend to accompany a breaking up of the family, or vice versa; or the break in the mother-relationship may follow as a consequence of the desertion of the father, and so on. However, such patterning tends to show up more clearly by keeping the items separate rather than by regrouping them under some more general heading.

An examination of the results in these tables shows that certain patterns of conditions accounted for a great number of the cases in the respective groups, i.e. that certain conditions tended to appear regularly with certain others, particularly in the delinquent group. The chi-square test shows all of these differences to be significant, and in most cases highly so. The inclusion of further conditions, i.e. enlarging the size of the patterns, however, has not increased but consistently decreased the size of the chi-square, especially in groupings of more than five conditions in the case of delinquents, and three conditions in the case of neurotics.

There is a consistent tendency in the delinquent group for disturbance in the child's relationship with either parent, or inconsistent discipline, to be bound up with a broken family and an interruption in the child's parent-relationships. These conditions in turn are frequently associated with unsettled homes, frequent moves, or over-crowding.

Among the neurotics, there is a tendency for neurotic conditions in family history to be combined with the following factors: a neurotic personality either in the mother or the father; a stable family circle; breast-feeding for a period of four months or more; problems arising before the age of two years; feeding difficulties and a tendency towards chronic ill-health.

Within the framework of the stable neurotic family there are many subtle and dynamic factors which are hinted at but are outside the scope of our present research. To understand the causes of neurotic development, a further study is needed parallel to the present one but involving a rather different and more psychiatrically specialized approach.

It is very interesting to bear these constellations of factors in mind when considering the detailed life stories of our one hundred socially maladjusted children.

OUTCOME OF TREATMENTS: A COMPARISON

A final project was the comparison of the relative success of child guidance treatment methods (a) in the two groups and (b) in our total sample of maladjusted children as a whole. Such results are always extremely difficult to assess; the three categories used, which describe the outcome of treatments as 'satisfactory', 'inconclusive', or 'unsatisfactory', were arrived at only after careful deliberation by the clinic staffs and are based on follow-up reports from the child's home and school as well as continued observation of his behaviour in the clinic.

In general, mere disappearance of symptoms was not, in itself, considered sufficient evidence to describe a case as satisfactorily treated. Nor does one think any longer in terms of 'cure' in relation to neurotic disturbances or behaviour disorders. In the psycho-analytic treatment of adult patients it has long been customary to think of a successful therapeutic outcome in terms of the restoration of normal functioning, particularly as regards the basic adult capacities for work and for love. In child analysis one must seek elsewhere for an indication of when the treatment should come to an end. Even in those cases where the response has been maximally favourable the child analyst takes into consideration a network of internal and external indices of psychological well-being. In most cases one speaks not of 'cure' of isolated conditions but of degrees of improvement in the child's functioning in relation to his whole personality and emotional life. Anna Freud has repeatedly stated in her lectures that the success or failure of a child's response to psycho-analytical treatment can only be judged in relation to the processes of his *inner development*; i.e. the crucial question to be decided is whether or not as a result of our therapeutic intervention the child is now freed to

221

move forward undisturbed into the next phase in the normal sequence of his psychic development. Treatment is not normally terminated until the child has been accompanied safely into this new phase of his development.

In the following condensed summary of the results of treatment of our 100 cases, it should be borne in mind that while the three terminal gradings can offer only approximate accuracy they have been applied stringently and with very detailed knowledge of the cases under consideration.

Satisfactory cases. These included those cases where, in the opinion of the clinic staff, the outcome of the clinic's intervention in the case (whether this involved individual psychological treatment, change of environment, supervision of probation work, remedial teaching or a variety of other measures) had resulted in a satisfactory response in terms of the child's personality and development. The term 'satisfactory response' implied a radically improved adjustment within his home life and steady evidence of normal progress in his emotional development plus the capacity to maintain these gains without support when followed up for some considerable time.

Outcome inconclusive. This grouping included those cases where the recommended treatment had been offered or applied but where the results were incomplete or inconclusive for reasons not always within the control of the clinic staff. There were cases, for instance, where treatment was satisfactorily begun but was broken off because of the family going away; or because of a juvenile court ruling for a child to be sent elsewhere; or where a long-term programme of emotional re-education had been begun (e.g. in a hostel for maladjusted children or an approved school) but insufficient time had elapsed for a reliable assessment of the child's full response to be made; or when treatment was broken off because the parents were satisfied by purely superficial improvements; or when treatment was interrupted because of the parents' resistances or lack of sincere cooperation; or where the outcome of treatment still in progress remained doubtful.

Unsatisfactory cases. These include a mixed group where the outcome was unsatisfactory for a variety of reasons: where the response to psychological treatment was negligible; where treatment was offered but was refused or discontinued by an uncooperative parent or foster-parent (or sometimes by a probation officer); where practical difficulties such as distance or lack of special school vacancies made it impossible for the child to be treated.

It is obvious that this third group of 'unsatisfactory cases' contains a wealth of problems for research work. There is much that we should learn from their detailed examination concerning the failure of effort or organization, the wastage or uneconomical use of community services, and a host of inadequacies in our professional understanding and techniques.

It is stressed that this assessment is fraught with ambiguities and uncontrollable variables. Not the least daunting of these is the knowledge that the statistical assessment of 'failures' in psychological treatment very often measures only the size, number and persistency of the obstacles in the way of establishing the conditions under which our therapeutic operations may be safely carried out, rather than measuring success or failure in the serious application of the techniques themselves. The same problem arises in assessing the long- and short-term results of endeavour in many of the fields of preventive medicine.

A summary of the findings from this examination of the outcome of our treatment procedures is presented in the following table:

Table 48   OUTCOME OF TREATMENT PROCEDURES

Treatment Outcome	Delinquent			Neurotic			Combined Totals
	Boys	Girls	Total	Boys	Girls	Total	
Satisfactory	15	6	21	21	13	34	55
Inconclusive	7	9	16	6	4	10	26
Unsatisfactory	8	5	13	3	3	6	19
Totals			50			50	100

It will not be surprising to psycho-analytic readers to find that the proportion of successfully treated neurotic cases is higher than the proportion of delinquent cases. The psycho-analytic method was evolved by Freud for the treatment of neurotic disorders and it remains true that this class of case still responds better than any other to orthodox psycho-analytic techniques.

Modifications of psycho-analytic technique have led to considerable success in the treatment of certain classes of disorder, as Aichhorn and others have demonstrated with delinquents. Psycho-analytic understanding and insight have shown themselves to be powerful tools when applied to the educational and emotional problems of many disturbed cases who cannot strictly be classified as neurotic at all and they are being increasingly applied to the baffling and difficult 'borderline' cases. These applications and extensions of technique, however, will not work so easily or directly as with the 'purely neurotic' child who already has a reasonable and cooperative ego-structure ready to ally itself with the analyst against the unconscious conflicts which overburden and restrict its functions. The conflict in which the child's psychic life is enmeshed is an internalized, intrapsychic one, and its roots are unconscious. In the delinquent child, the conflict tends to be still externalized, goes on between a primitive and defective ego (and super-ego) structure and a constantly provoked and punishing environment. There is often a difficult preparatory phase in the psychotherapeutic treatment of delinquents which involves arousing in the child a sense of concern about and recognition of his problem; if this is not carefully handled the delinquent child is very likely to give up attendance. This preliminary phase in the treatment of delinquents will take all the analyst's skill and resource as well as a great deal of time, and it is interesting that many of the 'unsatisfactory' and 'inconclusive' cases were those which really broke away—or were taken away from the surveillance of the clinic—before reasonable conditions for treatment could be established. In a number of the latter cases there was hope that patient work over a longer time might have brought about or might yet bring about a more hopeful outcome. It is significant that the most frequent reason for a case to be rated 'unsatisfactory' was the failure of the parents to concern themselves fully in the child's treatment, or even to let the child attend the clinic regularly.

One further consideration helps us to understand the lesser demonstrable success in treatment of the delinquents. For fairly obvious reasons, many chronic delinquent children do not fall into the class of case suitable for child guidance treatment or even for individual psychotherapy. In the great majority of cases a distortion in character development has taken place very early in the child's life and a long-term programme of psychiatrically supervised emotional re-education (rather than intensive psychotherapy) is indicated. This tends both to be more difficult to put into practice and to take *very much longer* periods of time to carry out adequately than the so-called 'lengthy' transference analysis of the neurotic. We know from our attempt to analyse those forces and conditions which go into the making of a delinquent child that it has taken a very long time for his emotional development to get set into its characteristic twisted and embittered course and we must expect that it will also take us a long time to undo this faulty pattern and to transform the child into a happy and socially healthy being again. When normal home-life has for one reason or another failed to achieve its socializing functions, the substitutes we offer in the way of foster-homes, special hostels or institutions, etc., can only operate under a treble handicap; namely, that their socializing and corrective influence, even when most wisely and kindly administered, comes *after* there has been a deeply inscarred original failure, often publicly recognized; that these 'secondary homes' to which the child is transplanted operate at best within a second-hand authority system which has weakened human attachments and diluted emotional meaning and is therefore a shallower soil for the child's roots than his 'own' home; and thirdly that very often this 'second chance' in social adaptation is offered *so many years too late*.

INDICATIONS FOR FURTHER RESEARCH

The value of this research would have been immensely increased had we been able to include comparable material from a group of normal children. Practical difficulties made this impossible; besides which a similar amount of research upon a normal group would have taken a great deal of time and money. It is hoped to investigate such a third group at some time in the future. It may not always be as difficult to obtain psychiatric observations upon normal children as we found in our project. One child guidance clinic[1] has already begun, and will continue, to make detailed psychiatric observations on a group of normal children over a period of years. Such research programmes should in time make it possible to compare the histories of normal children with those of delinquent and neurotic or other groups.

We took great care to exclude as far as was possible the 'mixed' cases of delinquent children who are mildly neurotic, or neurotic children who are also delinquent. This distinction, however, was by no means easy to make. Inevitably certain delinquents were included who showed mild neurotic trends which are not regarded as the basis of the delinquent conduct, nor sufficiently pronounced to account for the long-standing history of delinquency. These trends often became evident only after intensive and continued observation of the child's character structure, or during a period of psychological treatment. The exclusion of delinquent neurotic children was on the whole an easier matter.

For many reasons, I have reached the conclusion that a fruitful method of research in this field (under ideal conditions and with suitable time and staff available for the routine labour involved in such large-scale psychological case-indexing) would be to investigate five groups of children, selected in the manner similar to that described in Chapter II and divided into the following groups:

(a) Delinquent children.
(b) Delinquent children with neurotic tendencies.
(c) Normal children.
(d) Neurotic children with delinquent tendencies.
(e) Neurotic children.

Before her untimely death, Dr. Friedlander had begun to plan a large-scale research of this type on a group of selected child guidance clinic cases. This might have uncovered a host of new problems (and new complexities in social patterning) in the areas concerning the less well understood 'borderline cases' which bulk so large on our clinic waiting-lists.

One of the 'side-effects' of our investigation has been to open up new avenues of research. For example, the finding that neurotic behaviour tends to be associated with stable homes, is ambiguous and by no means indicates that stable homes 'cause' neurotic behaviour. All that the results suggest is that the neurotic, and probably also the normal, child tends to come from a stable and unbroken home, in contrast to delinquents who tend to come from broken homes. Why some children become neurotic in apparently stable homes is a question that cannot be satisfactorily answered by external observational means, or by these alone. An understanding of the way neurosis-producing forces operate in the child's psychological life and early environment would involve the addition of very different methods. The dynamic causation of neurosis in particular cases can probably only be found out by undertaking the gigantic labour of sifting the complete records of a long-term psycho-analysis. Although it is not impossible to find both the material and the methods for such investigation, Burt (1935, Part V) has shown that in order to unravel the genesis of the neurotic disturbance, a new research project is necessary for almost every case. It is clear that comparable 'objective' research into the home conditions that foster neurotic development would be concerned with many complex and subtle psychological factors, many of them unconscious, such as those which give rise to intrapsychic conflicts; to abnormal emotional relationships; to interplay with neuroses in the parents; to special attitudes toward the handling of the child's emotional and instinctual behaviour, and many historical factors.

A further subject for research would be to find out more about the tendency for neurotic—and some delinquent—children to imitate and take over the behaviour of the opposite sex. An important beginning would be to investigate the roles of the parents towards each other. We found that in many cases the mother's role in the family may be dominant, quarrelsome, and aggressive, showing little femininity or tenderness for the child. Such mothers are sometimes the breadwinners for the family, or they may compete with their husbands in professional fields or in the earning of money. Others openly despise and reject, or criticize and patronize, their husbands, and are nagging and bullying towards them. In many such 'family constellations' the fathers appear to take the opposite role and to be submissive and passive personalities who are loving and gentle towards the children and non-aggressive towards their wives. They appear content to be henpecked or regarded as a failure and they sometimes undertake to do the housework and shopping, or to handle the babies, or they expect a great deal of 'mothering' themselves. It would be of great interest to discover to what extent this reversal of parental roles is associated with a child's tendency to imitate and identify with the parent of the opposite sex, and to what extent it is associated with subsequent neuroticism. Aichhorn (1925) and Greenacre (1945) have suggested that other family constellations tend to occur with special frequency in delinquents, such as, for example, the presence of a vain, self-indulgent, frivolous mother and a remote and feared, but bigoted, righteous and stern father in the case of the 'spoiled' delinquent child or the plausible psychopath.

The results on breast-feeding are, for many reasons, difficult to interpret. It would be interesting to undertake a retrospective investigation into the total feeding situation as it was experienced in large groups of delinquent, neurotic, and normal children, respectively. A parallel inquiry into the psychological aspects of this situation might focus attention upon conditions as they currently occur in the feeding of both breast- and bottle-fed babies, with regard to the mother's emotional attitude while she is feeding the child, her handling of the feeding situation in general; and in relation to special difficulties as they occur. Psycho-analytic studies of many types are being made on normal babies, with observations which accompany their feeding situations throughout at least the first year. The results of such studies might very well be coordinated with results of further investigations into the incidence of 'oral character traits' (as assessed by psycho-analytically trained observers). This might involve an examination of both oral character traits which have positive emphasis (self-assurance, optimism, generosity, confidence, security, 'bright sociability', etc.) and those which have negative emphasis (greed, dependence, 'demandingness', vengefulness, depressive pessimism, a tendency to take things by force, inability to wait for satisfactions and a sadistic 'redress-demanding' attitude) as they occur in delinquent, normal, and neurotic children respectively.

I should also like to see further investigations made into the general behaviour of the neurotic child at school. It would be important to determine the degree to which backwardness and inability to develop normal interests *result from* rather than *contribute to* faulty social adaptation and personality disorder. This was undoubtedly the case in both groups of children studied here. Although not lacking in native capacity, many of them gave the impression of being as effectively separated from the world of the normal by their restricted energies and generally impoverished psychological functioning, as they would in fact have been by deafness or ignorance.

In collecting the histories of these 100 'problem' children and getting to know their circumstances and their life stories intimately, it was a saddening experience to realize again and again how many of them tended to be gravely inferior in attainments and limited in their 'mental furniture' compared with the average child. Moreover, when recognition and real help became available for them (i.e. psychological understanding coordinated with the services of both school and community), this usually reached them so many years too late that many had missed the main stream of their educational opportunities. Although not differing from the normal in their primal instincts, their modes of instinctual expression had become so channelled into negative habit patterns that many of these 100 children could not respond to or make use of their native abilities, even when surrounded by opportunities to develop them. Lacking the vital securities of childhood or crippled by neurotic inhibitions, the minds of these children remained rooted in doubt and narrow suspicion, resentful, unenterprising, discontented both with themselves and with others and unable to trust in other human beings. The abundance of rich and carefree experiences of a happy childhood was not for them.

PART THREE

CASE HISTORY SUMMARIES

CHAPTER VII

Collecting the case history material

Sources of Referral

The 100 children in this study were referred to the child guidance clinics from the sources indicated in *Table 1*.

Table 1   SOURCES OF REFERRAL

	No. of cases referred
School Medical Officers	27
Friends and relations	21
Courts and Probation Officers	17
School teachers	15
Private doctors	5
Maternity, Child Welfare, and Health Clinic	4
Speech therapists	3
Hospitals	3
Social agencies	3
Police	1
Child himself	1
	Total 100

The information available about the children in compiling the case summaries included the following:

1. A social and family history, usually obtained by the psychiatric social worker in the clinic at the time of referral, from the mother or father of the child.

2. Reports on home visits and on subsequent guidance or treatment interviews carried on by the psychiatric social worker with one or both parents.

3. The results of psychometric examinations carried out by the educational psychologist, usually at the time of referral. In some cases of very disturbed children, the intelligence tests were postponed, or repeated, or supplementary tests were given when sufficient progress had been made in psychological treatment for the child to cooperate fully.

4. The results of scholastic and educational achievement tests given, where necessary, by the educational psychologist.

5. A report on school behaviour and progress that was usually made by the educational psychologist in consultation with the child's teacher.

6. A report from the school medical officer about each child's health and physical development. In relevant cases specialist medical reports were also available.

7. In juvenile court cases reports from the probation officer on the child's family conditions, his past and present offences or other matters; and proposals for dealing with the child in the future after discussion of his case with the clinic staff.

8. Reports on a few children who had been referred to a mental hospital or who had spent some time in a mental hospital were available from the medical officer responsible for treating the child, together with the hospital social worker's report.

9. Reports from the warden of a hostel for maladjusted children on cases sent to him for observation or for residential treatment.

10. Detailed case notes of diagnostic observational interviews carried out by the psychiatrist in charge of each clinic.

11. In cases taken on for psychological treatment, detailed notes of each interview with the child by the psychiatrist or child psychotherapist undertaking the treatment; quarterly progress reports by them; and closure reports summarizing the views of the therapist and of the staff conference held at the termination of the treatment.

12. Reports and discussions on individual cases at the local clinic conferences and at combined inter-clinic conferences. These were attended regularly by the writer throughout the period when the majority of the children in this study were current cases.

13. Regular follow-up reports on the child's adjustment at home, at school, at work, or in hostel or foster-home, and on his progress on probation, his present interests, activities and friends. The follow-ups are normally carried on for many years. In most of the cases in the present study there has been time only for one to three years' follow-up.

14. For research purposes a statement was drafted by the psychiatrist and therapist on the outcome of treatment in each case. A comparison was then made between the outcome and the treatment goal formulated at the time of diagnostic examination.

15. In addition, the writer was able to make use of private discussions about the aetiology and treatment of more difficult cases with the psychiatrist and other staff members, and to consult the psychiatric social workers as frequently as necessary on points which were not obvious from the history records.

From this mass of information 100 case histories were compiled and all the important factual information for each case was summarized and carded. A systematic method of social history taking[1] was followed. This was intended to serve as a general guide that could, however, be elaborated or considerably altered in individual cases where this seemed necessary. A skeleton of the record form used for the collection of data about each case is given below:

RECORD FOR SOCIAL HISTORY TAKING

NAME   I.Q.   Sex

Birth date   Age (at diagnostic interview)

                                                 Religion

PROBLEM

Referred by   Reason for referral

Statement of problem

Problem as diagnosed

---

[1] This scheme was adapted from that followed by Burt (1925) and from a series of recording systems developed by Dr. Friedlander and the author.

INTELLIGENCE and SCHOOL PROGRESS

Results of intelligence tests

Results of special tests

School history (including age of commencing and changes of school)

School progress

Educational attainments

Results of attainment tests

Special problems or special abilities

Social adjustment at school, (a) in the class
                                  (b) in the playground

FAMILY BACKGROUND

Father's occupation (including war record, period spent in Services, whether abroad, etc.)

Mother's occupation: (a) before marriage
                             (b) state periods she has worked outside the home since marriage

Family structure

    Parents married, unmarried, second marriage, adoptive, foster- or step-parents, etc.

      Mother dead

      Father dead

    Parents separated, divorced, or deserted

    Illicit sex relationships of parents (whether known to child)

    Child step-, foster-, or adopted

    Illegitimate child

    Father's absences

    Mother's absences

    Child reared in ignorance of his true parentage

Siblings and sibling position

    Sibling relationships

    Special problems, special friendships, etc.

    Marked physical differences in health, size, looks, etc.

    Marked differences in I.Q. or in special abilities

    Jealousy problems

    Parental preferences

Hereditary conditions
   Cases of instability or 'neuropathic diathesis' in family history
      (a) general
      (b) neurotic conditions
Presence of other adults in the home (Grannies, nannies, lodgers, ayahs, uncles, aunts, etc.)
   Their relationship and influence upon the child
Parents
   Mother's age   Father's age
   Mother's personality (social and psychiatric description)
   Mother-child relationship (social and psychiatric description)
   Interruptions in mother-child relationship
   Father's personality (social and psychiatric description)
   Father-child relationship (social and psychiatric description)
   Interruptions in father-child relationship
   Marital relationship

HOME CIRCUMSTANCES
   Social status
   Economic and material circumstances
   Poverty, over-crowding, frequent changes, etc.
   Psychological factors (attitude in the home to matters of religion, sex, family standards, etc.)
   Discipline (over-strict, over-lenient, inconsistent, normal)
   Recreation (facilities for leisure, etc.)
   Other (alcoholism, companions, etc.)

CHILD'S HISTORY
   Pregnancy and birth
   Wanted or unwanted child
   Habit-training
   Feeding habits (including breast- or bottle-feeding, weaning, early feeding difficulties, etc.)
   Toilet-training (bowel, bladder control)
   Sleeping habits

Physical and psychological development
    Infancy (teething, sitting up, crawling, walking, talking)
    Two to five years
    Five to ten years
    Puberty
    Adolescence
    Child's physical appearance and bearing
Health history
    Past illnesses, operations, accidents, etc.
    Periods spent in hospital
    Present physical condition
    Special defects or disabilities
Social development
    Any earlier delinquent or neurotic behaviour
    Onset of present problem and method of handling it
    Separations from mother (state duration, child's age, and his
                             reactions)
    Separations from father („   „   „   „)
    Periods at boarding school(„   „   „   „)
    Periods with friends and („   „   „   „)
      relatives
    Periods spent in institu-
      tions, foster-homes, etc.(„   „   „   „)
    Evacuation   („   „   „   „)
    Air-raid experience.
    Traumatic events (e.g. accidents, deaths, air-raids, frights,
      assault, traumatic family experiences, etc.)
    Sexual behaviour and sexual knowledge
Data not available about child's history (state reason)

CHILD'S PERSONALITY

    Emotional characteristics
    General temperamental stability
    Moods and affections
    Habits
    Attitudes (to parents, to discipline, obstinacy, humour, rebel-
      lion, etc.)
    Friendships, sociability, etc.

INTERESTS AND ACTIVITIES

Hobbies, club membership, sports, dancing, etc.
Games preferences
Reading interests
Constructive achievements or field of expression
Attendance at cinema
Ambitions for future

CHILD GUIDANCE CLINIC TREATMENT

Summary of psychological treatment
Recommendations and disposal
Vocational guidance

CAUSATIVE FACTORS (psychiatric assessment)
PROGNOSIS
OUTCOME OF CASE
FOLLOW-UP REPORTS

SUMMARIES OF CASE HISTORIES

Summaries of our 100 case histories are presented in the two
following chapters. These have been very highly condensed in
order to allow examples of as wide a variety of cases of delinquent
and neurotic children as possible to be included. The amount
of data presented was necessarily restricted on account of considerations of space in this section. The unabridged account of the
detailed stories of these 100 children would have filled a large
volume on their own. What is included here is meant to be, in
each case, a digest of the essential facts taken from the dossiers
containing all the information which is available upon each child.
These thumbnail sketches of individual children are included as
an essential supplement and qualitative background to the factual
results presented in Part Two.

A brief and inevitably limited statement is made of the causative
factors that were thought to contribute to each child's disorder.
These are stated rather bluntly, without adequate qualifying
remarks, and with chief reference to psychological facts. It is

239

always assumed, however, that the predominant causes in any psychological disturbance may depend upon actual experiences, or may be constitutional, and that in any case these causes will produce their greatest effect when constitution and experience work together in the same direction. Freud (1905) has stressed this fundamental concept when he stated his view of the relative

Table 49 NAMES AND DETAILS OF PAIRED CASES: BOYS

	DELINQUENTS				NEUROTICS		
Case No.	Name	Age in years and months	I.Q.	Case No.	Name	Age in years and months	I.Q.
1	Andrew	5.10	103	51	Maurice	4.11	110
2	Peter	6. 2	139	52	Geoffrey	5.10	143
3	Derek	7. 1	96	53	Colin	6. 2	100
4	Reginald	7. 2	103	54	Jackie	6. 7	108
5	Thomas	7. 8	115	55	Billie	6.11	123
6	Ernest	7.10	105	56	Roger	7. 6	105
7	Felix	7. 7	83	57	Bertie	7.11	89
8	Frankie	8. 6	88	58	Anthony	8. 1	89
9	Philip	8.10	79	59	Clifford	7. 1	85
10	Ivor	8. 9	99	60	Irving	8. 9	105
11	Patrick	9. 1	116	61	Richard	8. 1	110
12	Carl	9. 1	101	62	Phineas	8. 3	105
13	Paddy	9. 3	137	63	Charles	8. 5	130
14	Keith	9. 6	88	64	Fred	8. 9	89
15	Donald	9. 7	111	65	Julian	8. 4	109
16	Jonathan	9. 8	98	66	Mark	9. 2	96
17	Monty	9. 4	100	67	Portland	10. 1	110
18	Percy	10. 0	92	68	Roy	9. 7	99
19	Leonard	10.10	125	69	Matthew	9. 9	122
20	Ian	10. 6	90	70	Ross	11. 3	93
21	Bobbie	11. 8	100	71	Gregory	10. 8	98
22	Clive	11. 3	111	72	Alexander	13. 2	108
23	Martin	12. 0	134	73	Malcolm	13. 4	137
24	David	12. 3	97	74	Denny	12.11	100
25	John	12.10	132	75	Angus	14. 7	138
26	Christopher	13. 2	111	76	Rollo	13. 4	118
27	Jeremy	13. 7	87	77	Rupert	11. 9	96
28	Steven	13. 7	106	78	Preston	14. 3	115
29	Alfred	16. 3	114	79	Pierre	16. 2	109
30	Paul	16. 9	131	80	James	15. 7	129

Table 50 NAMES AND DETAILS OF PAIRED CASES: GIRLS

| DELINQUENTS | | | NEUROTICS | | |
Case No. Name	Age in years and months	I.Q.	Case No. Name	Age in years and months	I.Q.
31 Alice	6. 5	101	81 Joanna	4. 5	102
32 Freda	6. 8	93	82 Laura	5. 6	100
33 Petula	7. 0	93	83 Gertrude	8. 2	86
34 Ellen	8. 9	86	84 Ruby	7. 1	89
35 Maryann	8. 7	101	85 Jean	9. 9	103
36 Florence	9.10	122	86 Elspeth	9. 4	133
37 Caroline	10. 4	90	87 Penelope	10. 8	100
38 Susan	11. 7	81	88 Daphne	12.11	88
39 Rita	11. 9	132	89 Janice	12. 3	138
40 Minnie	11.10	84	90 Dorothy	11.11	94
41 Maureen	12. 2	120	91 Patricia	13. 5	124
42 Meg	13. 3	109	92 Pamela	12. 5	99
43 Peggy	13. 6	124	93 Eva	12.10	133
44 Doreen	13.11	94	94 Juliet	12.10	98
45 Bertha	13.11	110	95 Edith	13.10	108
46 Joyce	14. 6	104	96 Juanita	13. 2	107
47 Sarah	14. 6	81	97 Theresa	14. 5	85
48 Monica	14.11	97	98 Ruth	13. 0	100
49 Daisy	15. 4	103	99 Jane	15. 7	105
50 Joan	16. 4	104	100 Frances	15.11	103

aetiological importance of what is innate and what is accidentally experienced. He states (ibid. p. 116 ff.) that the relation between these two is a cooperative and not a mutually exclusive one. 'The constitutional factor must await experiences before it can make itself felt; the accidental factor must have a constitutional basis in order to come into operation. To cover the majority of cases, we can picture what has been described as a "complemental series", in which the diminishing intensity of one factor is balanced by the increasing intensity of the other; there is, however, no reason to deny the existence of extreme cases at the two ends of the series.'

Tables 49 and 50 present the names and the details of ages and Binet I.Q.s of the 50 delinquent and 50 neurotic children in this study. The equated pairs of delinquents and neurotics are arranged parallel to each other, and the pairs, as also the case history summaries following, are presented in approximate order of age, from the youngest upwards.

Pseudonyms are used throughout and the identities of these children have been very carefully veiled by the use of a variety of minor subterfuges which effectively screen them without destroying the value of our scientific records.

CHAPTER VIII

Fifty delinquent children

Case No. 1: Andrew. *Age:* 5 years, 10 months. I.Q. 103.

Andrew is a good-looking boy, active, cheerful, and responsive.

Referral: by mother, on account of restlessness and uncontrolled behaviour, truanting, romancing, lying, disobedience, petty pilfering, and staying out late at nights.

Family background: illegitimate; adopted at 3 years after his mother's marriage; lives with mother, adoptive father, adoptive paternal grandmother. Household crowded when other relatives have lived there for certain periods.

Mother: attractive, unstable, and insecure; hysterical symptoms of long standing; parents separated, brought up strictly by grandmother. Nervous breakdown in puberty caused her to develop acute fears and temporarily to lose speech. At 14 years, left school, looked after mother, who was then separated from her husband and pregnant by another man. After trouble between her and her mother, she left and took various jobs. Became pregnant with Andrew by a naval man who left her before the baby was born in a Home. When he was 3, she married. Relationship with child is inconsistent; she has high and restrictive standards, is unable to tolerate aggression from him. When told she herself was in need of help, she was willing to have treatment.

Adoptive father: clerical worker. Mother describes him as unsympathetic and moody; not very strong. Gives more attention to his mother than to his wife. Sees little of Andrew, as he leaves for work early and returns late. Discipline is divided between him, the mother, and the grandmother. Many family quarrels; wife has threatened to leave him.

Adoptive paternal grandmother: hypochondriacal, nagging; antagon-

243

istic and rejecting towards Andrew, restrictive and abusive towards the mother. During the boy's treatment, attempted suicide and was admitted to a mental hospital where she died.

Material conditions in the home are fairly good, though probably mother is not a good manager.

History: an unwanted child. Pregnancy and birth normal. Mother remained in the Home with child for 9 months. Good-tempered baby; breast-fed for 3 months during which time mother was unhappy in the Home. No weaning difficulties. From 9 months until 3 years, mother kept him in small private Home where, as far as she knows, treatment was satisfactory; mother saw him every fortnight, and he always recognized her. At 3 years, left the Home, as mother had married. He was then timid, anxious to please. Not told of true paternity. Between 2 and 5, severe temper tantrums and temporary breakdown in habit-training; sleep restless. Temper tantrums continue; he is nervous, afraid of dogs, pilfers, and has run away from home and school. In early years had bronchial trouble, acidosis, pneumonia, and measles. A year ago had diarrhoea, and had tonsils and adenoids removed. Now quite healthy.

School record and intelligence: Nursery school until 4½, which he liked; made no special friends. At 5, went to big school, where he was always in trouble; bullied by other children. Head teacher says it is invariably Andrew who starts the trouble by threatening the children. Work in all subjects below average. Because he cannot be controlled by ordinary methods of discipline, mother asked to remove him. Boisterous and unmanageable.

His I.Q. was assessed as 103. Comprehension and reasoning good, memory poor. Responsive and self-assertive.

Personality and behaviour: According to mother, an affectionate, sensitive child, imaginative but tense and cringing, always expecting reproof. Makes personal contacts easily, acts impulsively, is popular and likes adventurous, highly imaginative exploits; easily led. Good at drawing and plasticine modelling. Produces fantasies easily, and during treatment developed imaginary companion. High-spirited and untruthful.

Clinical summary: diagnosed as a case of primary antisocial conduct disorder. He and his mother taken on for treatment. At first, Andrew was provocative, aggressive, and destructive. After defensive motive of aggression was analysed, he made efforts to cooperate with the therapist. Underlying passive-effeminate tendencies then emerged and were satisfactorily dealt with as far as possible within limits of short-term treatment. He was helped towards understanding difficulties in his relationship with other boys, and arrangements were made for transferring him to a more suitable school. Mother's hysterical symptoms decreased. Grandmother's death and Andrew's response to mother's altered methods led to improvement in the home situation, while her confidence in handling the boy increased. Prognosis thought to be good if present improvements in home situation can be maintained.

Causative factors: mother's neurotic personality; interrupted mother-child relationship; lack of settled home in infancy; inconsistent handling; marital discord; crowded family life. The follow-up shows that the improvement in Andrew's behaviour has been maintained.

Case No. 2: Peter. *Age:* 6 years, 2 months. I.Q. 139.

Peter is a fair, healthy boy of sturdy appearance.

Referral: by mother, on account of backwardness at school, where he is difficult and destructive. At home, he lies and is disobedient.

Family background: the elder of two boys from a stable, middle-class home.

Mother: pretty and intelligent, emotional, talkative, over-anxious about children. Intensely loving with disturbed relationship with Peter. Jealous of his attachment to her. Punishes him harshly for destructiveness; confides in him, likes him to share her hobby, which is painting. The nature of her rather childish personality made it doubtful whether or not she would cooperate in treatment.

Father: a professional man. Over-anxious; fails to take much responsibility for the children and prefers Peter's brother, who resembles him. Relationship with wife is disturbed and sado-masochistic; frequent quarrels between them followed by fervent reconciliations. Peter is interested in father's work, but father expects too much of the boy; talks to him about doing well at school, going to the university, and puts much pressure on him to learn. Opposed to Peter being brought to the clinic.

History: a longed-for child. Pregnancy and birth normal; breast-fed for one month. Habit-training strict, clean early on a conditioned response basis. Punished harshly by mother for destructiveness, and even more harshly when, at 18 months, habit-training broke down and he began soiling and smearing furniture with faeces. Walked and talked early. At $4\frac{1}{2}$, mother became pregnant, which displeased both parents, who were ambitious for Peter to have university education. Peter led to believe he would have a sister; when boy was born, mother shared disappointment with Peter, made him believe he would now be deprived of a university education. Peter ignored the baby, resented the attention given to it by the mother, who insisted he must love it and was intolerant of any hostility he showed.

School record and intelligence: sent to a strict, old-fashioned school following brother's birth. After first term, teacher informed mother that Peter was dreamy and lazy; no wish to learn to read; prevented other children from learning and ignored the teacher. Mother taught him to read and says she was successful within one week, though he still refused to learn at school. Hates sums; bored, except in drawing lessons; good at acting and telling stories; appears to be absorbed in religion. Since going to school, seems to be constantly worried; sleep restless. Day-dreams a lot.

His I.Q. was assessed as 139. Good knowledge of words, excellent memory. Seems not to listen unless particularly interested. Friendly and unreserved about likes and dislikes; casual and uncritical about his performance. Admitted hatred of school, said it was because there was too much religion.

Personality and behaviour: described as being extremely sensible and able to be talked to as a grown-up. Loves painting, and goes off on expeditions with mother when they are 'feeling fed up'.

FIFTY DELINQUENT CHILDREN

Told the psychiatrist that he did not want to go to college, wanted to be an engine-driver. Play activities restricted, full of fantasies and day-dreams about killing; liked to stage a quarrel so as to convince himself that he was the stronger. Enjoys horror stories on radio. Aggressiveness and antisocial behaviour in the playground make him unpopular with other children.

Clinical summary: diagnosed as a case of primary antisocial conduct disorder. First interviews gave clear indication of Peter's dissocial character. Only in single instances did he establish a relationship, usually at the end of an interview, when he would suddenly be destructive or quarrelsome. For most part, he tried to remain polite and friendly but suspicious and aloof. Talked a little about fantasies and preoccupation with religion, but discontinued this after the psychiatrist showed readiness to enter into the fantasy. Interpretation of polite, friendly behaviour as a defence resulted in an admission of suspiciousness, feeling of helplessness, and wish to be helped. After 12 interviews, an awkward but more positive relationship was established, and he then expressed fear that his jealous mother would forbid his coming, asked to be helped in this. Began to discuss sado-masochistic relationship with parents, admitted his previously denied jealousy of brother. At this point, mother ceased attending, left letters unanswered. After two further interviews, boy ceased to come. The prognosis is therefore considered to be poor. Follow-up shows that behaviour at school remains difficult and he has stolen money.

Causative factors: primarily, personality of mother, her ambivallence, strict methods of toilet-training, inconsistency of handling, and her pronounced sado-masochistic relationship with both husband and boy. Secondary factors exaggerating this disturbed relationship were birth of brother, father's dissatisfaction with Peter and his openly expressed preference for younger boy.

Case No. 3: Derek. *Age:* 7 years, 1 month. I.Q. 96.

Derek is an anxious, insecure boy who lives in a world of fantasy. He has one of the worst records of delinquent conduct in this study.

Referral: by Ministry of Health on account of uncontrollable and aggressive behaviour, enuresis, encopresis, speech and sleep disturbance, sexual offences, jealousy, truanting, stealing, lying, wandering at night, exaggerated masturbation, destructiveness, and retardation at school.

Family background: elder of two children from unstable, broken home.

Mother: aged 30. Pathetic, tearful woman of average intelligence; is small and thin, has suffered from gastric upsets since she was 19. At 21, married; husband deserted when Derek was 6. Two years before this had obtained legal separation, but poverty had forced her to return to him with her two children. Admits she is unable to manage Derek, and adopts a fatalistic attitude. Her attempted control is feeble and ineffective. Derek has beaten her, is openly and defiantly disobedient. Their relationship is sado-masochistic of long standing. Two years ago she had a miscarriage caused, she says, by father's ill-treatment. At present, living with Mr. X., a friendly, bucolic middle-aged bachelor, formerly in Regular Army. Since discharge, has been labourer and lorry driver. During treatment, Mother planned to marry this man if divorce was obtained. Mr. X. is also unable to manage Derek. The mother is determined to have the boy sent away, as she fears he will repeat his father's abnormal sexual behaviour.

Father: aged 31. A gardener. Discharged from the Army after 3 years' service, when Derek was 4, because of attacks he made on other soldiers. Described by mother as 'lean, skinny individual who frequently suffers from sores and styes'; 'sex mad'. Brutal, jealous, sexual behaviour abnormal, probably perverted. Ill-treated wife and child. After discharge from Army, he disappeared; wife obtained separation order on grounds of cruelty. Until Derek was 4, father saw him only when on leave. Derek idolized him, even though father preferred younger sister. Treatment of children severe; Derek caned and shaken for masturbation. In father's family, history of epilepsy, mental defect, and insanity.

Sibling: a girl, aged 4, who is terrified of Derek, and towards

248

whom he is aggressive and destructive, swearing he hates her. Health poor. Cruelly treated by father, yet is nice, good child; mother perplexed why, with similar treatment, two children are so different in behaviour. She has, however, observed sex-play between the two children; frequently finds them in bed together despite reproofs.

There have been frequent changes of home; for periods the family lived with both maternal and paternal grandparents, and once in a condemned, rural cottage. The mother now lives with Mr. X. and a relative of his in a labourer's cottage where she has one room for herself, her children and all their things.

History: Pregnancy normal except for ill-treatment by father. Birth was Caesarian. While mother was in hospital, another girl in the district became pregnant by father. This child now lives nearby and is disturbed like Derek. Derek breast-fed for 2 months; weaning difficult. No response to habit-training, never became dry or clean, and faecal incontinence continues. At 3, began to talk with stutter, which still persists. Because he was so difficult, sent to a foster-home by a child guidance clinic, but was so troublesome that he was returned home. At 4, began wandering and ran away from home. He interfered with his small sister, and at 5 achieved sexual intercourse with her which, the mother says, has been repeated 4 or 5 times. Openly masturbates during day and night. Set fire to things several times, killed 2 cats by stamping on them. Talks and walks in sleep, has night terrors. Health good.

School record and intelligence: at 4½ went to school but refused to learn, truanted; considerably knocked about by other children. Teachers say his mind seems far away. Unable to dress himself; is backward in all subjects, but adjustment better at school than at home.

His I.Q. assessed as 96. He was anxious and insecure, used only his left hand; unable to concentrate. Has a peculiar hand movement, and will interrupt conversation to relate incomprehensible fantasies or to play weird games. Wanted to take away toys from the clinic.

Personality and behaviour: mother describes him as never having wanted affection; kicked her away as a small boy; never shows feeling; is aggressive, yet bullied by other boys. Though restless, is slow and day-dreams. He was involved with other children in setting hostel beds alight and in pilfering. He likes drawing; is said to be devoted to animals but is also cruel to them.

Clinical summary: taken on for a long period of observation, and sent to a specialist for examination for epilepsy. The E.E.G. showed no likelihood of epilepsy. Later diagnosed as primary antisocial conduct, and taken on for treatment. Subsequently charged in the juvenile court on account of uncontrollable and aggressive behaviour and stealing. In the clinic, when he acted out aggressive fantasies and weird stories, he seemed to have some difficulty in differentiating between reality and fantasy. Established good relationship with therapist, but attendance was irregular. Home environment was too unsettled, over-crowded, and rejecting for treatment to be undertaken with any hope of cooperation. Derek then placed in a foster-home by the education authorities, and an attempt made to work with foster-mother and help her to gain insight and to relax her rigid standards. At first she praised the child, denying any difficulties, then rejected him after he stole food from her and wished him to be taken away. Thus only moderate success was achieved. After the court case, he was placed in the care of the education authorities until he is 18. His behaviour at school and in the remand home is satisfactory. Prolonged period of treatment away from home has been recommended, and was arranged. Prognosis is thought to be only fair, and the outcome of the case remains inconclusive.

Causative factors: father's bad family history and his personality; his violence to Derek in infancy; unstable home environment; parental discord; inconsistency and indecision in mother's handling, and her rejection because of his resemblance to father; early separation from home.

Case No. 4: Reginald. *Age:* 7 years, 2 months. I.Q. 103.

Reginald is a delicate-featured, rather 'pretty' boy, healthy, clean, and tidy, with a self-confident manner.

Referral: by maternal grandmother and probation officer on account of aggressive, uncontrolled behaviour at home and at school, truanting, stealing, enuresis, encopresis, and feeding disturbances.

Family background: illegitimate; parents never married. Mother poses as widow; she and children live with grandmother.

Mother: aged 31. Childish, impulsive Irish woman, whose good looks are marred by a facial disfigurement. One of 6 children; mother reports that she was rough and destructive as a child, suffered from nerves. At 19, left home and worked as children's maid in family of middle-aged ex-Army officer. Became pregnant by her employer, who was upset and wanted pregnancy interrupted. Because of this, wife denounced them, left him and her two children, made a scandal, and as a consequence, he lost his job. Wife refused to divorce him. At first mother was fond of father; later he was cruel, and she had to defend the boy. Mother has always been religious; is a spiritualist. She is disturbed, anxious, and guilty, and has suicidal thoughts. Felt her disfigurement to be a handicap, feared Reginald would inherit it.

Father: more than 20 years older than mother; a moody, difficult man. Only home at irregular intervals, and then tried to keep his children under rigid military discipline. Could not bear sight of Reginald, would beat him severely with army cane for disobedience. N.S.P.C.C. called in because of his cruelty to Reginald. Assists the family financially.

Reginald and his mother have had frequent changes of home and much financial stress. Mother has twice left father and taken Reginald and his young brother to her parents, who are unhappily married. Grandfather is drunken and quarrelsome, grandmother possessive and argumentative, and eventually left her husband after 30 years of marriage. Grandmother has shared control of Reginald, who is particularly insubordinate with her. At present Reginald lives with his grandmother (who takes in lodgers in summer), mother, a half-sister, and a younger brother aged 5. He has always been jealous of the other children.

251

History: Mother very unhappy during pregnancy, which was kept secret, and she had no medical care. Breast-fed for 3 weeks; mother became ill and anaemic, had to go to convalescent home. Father wanted baby adopted, mother refused, and sent him to foster-home for 1 year, where she and father visited him weekly. Reproaches herself for sending him there, as home was unsatisfactory. Because of his feeding difficulties and weak legs, she took him to a spiritualist healer, who continued to see him for 5 years. At 1 year, mother and father set up an irregular home together and the father's youngest daughter lived with them. There was quarrelling, physical violence, unhappiness, and insecurity, with recriminations from real wife and children and their grandmother. Reginald has been with mother ever since. Regularly wet bed, but mother says was frightened out of it at an early age. Habit-training difficult; still soils himself occasionally. Poor appetite, but can be bribed to do anything with sweets. At 2½ father went overseas; Reginald told he was dead. Reacted to father's reappearance, when he was 5½, with outbreaks of jealousy, soiling, wetting, and difficult behaviour. At present he never mentions him. For some time, suffered from chronic colds and catarrh; chickenpox and whooping-cough shortly after going to school. Now very healthy.

School record and intelligence: went to school in Ireland at 4; liked it at first, but soon began truanting. Became disobedient and dirty, would be found playing on beach during school hours, angry and resentful if questioned. Said to be intelligent, can concentrate when interested, making quite good progress. Dislikes arithmetic, good at reading. Teacher says he is interested only in reading, is always sullen and scowling and at war with the world. Constantly pilfering, aggressive towards others, is then bullied and attacked by them in return.

In the intelligence test, I.Q. 103; cooperative and responsive, enjoyed himself and talked with animation about games of cowboys and Red Indians at school. He is usually the biggest chief with the biggest gun and most weapons. Becomes expansive when praised.

Personality and behaviour: at home he is described as temperamental and demanding; enjoys only drawing, or fighting-games out of doors; steals small objects such as razor blades, paper clips, and nail clippers. Destructive, negative, careless, no respecter of property. Easily becomes angry and sullen; has a way of walking that suggests defiance. Tries to keep up the pretence that he has no emotional ties or concern for the consequences of his behaviour. Seems to possess no feeling that can be appealed to. Play stereotyped; no friends, usually associating with naughty boys of class.

Clinical summary: diagnosed as primary antisocial conduct disorder. He and mother taken on for treatment. After some time, mother became less rejecting and guilty over his illegitimacy; modified her handling. She also became more independent of her own mother, though remained fundamentally childish, impulsive, and erratic. Reginald continued to maintain his pretence of lack of feeling or guilt; this mechanism was interpreted, and his sibling jealousy difficulties discussed. Began to produce sado-masochistic fantasies, but retained defiant, pre-delinquent attitude. Before treatment had advanced very far, the case was withdrawn, as the family left the district. Prognosis thought to be poor without major environmental changes in which the mother is unwilling to cooperate. The follow-up showed that Reginald was still showing delinquent and regressive behaviour. He was then admitted to hostel for maladjusted children.

Causative factors: irregular and unsettled home background; inconsistency of handling; harsh, unsympathetic treatment from father and his prolonged absence; disturbed and immature personality of mother.

Case No. 5: Thomas. *Age:* 7 years, 8 months. I.Q. 115.

Thomas is small for his age, but well-built and sturdy, alert, and independent. Perky, cocky manner.

Referral: by school medical officer, on account of lying, pilfering, moodiness, and aggressive behaviour at school.

Family background: third child of large working-class family.

Mother: a tall, thin, anaemic, harassed-looking woman, one of a family of 16, 8 of whom died in infancy. Before marriage, was warned that her health was too poor for child-bearing. Rheumatic fever 2 years ago; now careworn and very run down. Throughout marriage, dependent on her own mother, says she could not have stuck it out without her help. Because of the children she remains with husband; fundamentally a good mother; carries a heavy load of responsibility, as father is said to show neither concern nor affection for children. Physical care for children is good, discipline lax and inconsistent. Makes a drudge of eldest girl, who accuses her of trading on ill-health. This girl brought up almost entirely by grandmother. Headmaster of school says mother is shiftless, always out dancing and drinking. She does part-time work in school canteen. N.S.P.C.C. officer regards children as neglected.

Father: a skilled labourer; said to have married beneath him. Irresponsible, alcoholic; beat mother in fits of temper, which ceased when grandmother stepped in and mother threatened separation. Before marriage, he had mental breakdown, ill for 11 months, but not certified. Frequently out of work; during these periods a Church fund pays for children's school meals. When working does not always give money to mother. Takes no share in upbringing of children beyond thrashing Thomas on account of his thefts. He and Thomas are openly jealous and antagonistic; boy's attitude towards him is brazen. Marital difficulties have so increased recently that separation is again considered. Mother blames father for all present trouble with child.

Siblings: there are 6 children between 12 months and 12 years; boy of 10 is on probation for stealing. Thomas gets on well with older children and the very small ones; intense quarrel relationship with brother, aged 6; rivalry in terms of toys and comparative strength. Thomas sometimes beaten by siblings, who consider he disgraces them at school. Oldest girl has been before juvenile court.

Family has a bad name in the village, where villagers and they dislike each other. The mother takes in two lodgers, one of whom is on probation. Material conditions fairly good; house dirty, garden neglected. Financial difficulties when father out of work.

History: pregnancy and confinement normal; breast-fed for 10 months; weaning easy, but subsequent feeding difficulties. Habit-training slow and difficult, clean at 4, but still wets bed occasionally. At 2, shortly after birth of next baby, Thomas drank gargling fluid; three weeks in hospital with severely burnt mouth. Following this, was difficult to handle, particularly in feeding. Periods of severe diarrhoea. Beyond period in hospital, no separation from mother. Has had measles and chickenpox in infancy. Health and appetite good.

School record and intelligence: attends village school, is one year retarded; difficult to control, rude to teachers, intensely disliking one of them whom he declares to be domineering. Lazy, though good, even precocious in oral work. Almost daily lapses of stealing and lying, for which he is caned.

In intelligence test, I.Q. 115. Showed excellent memory, quick, accurate reasoning powers; perky in manner, talked a great deal, and liked praise. Outgoing and impulsive.

Personality and behaviour: According to headmaster, Thomas has no moral code, no sense of guilt, lies with cunning, is cruel to other children, uses bad language in class. Appears to lack affection and care, shows no misgivings at prospect of changing present home for another, has no possessions, steals for a definite purpose, is generous with stolen money. No response to ordinary methods of discipline. Mother describes him as quick tempered, at times sullen, discontented, and unwilling to share with other children, can be aggressive. Attacks older siblings. Sociable and forceful character. Mother says he is fond of her, is obedient to her because she knows how to handle him, nevertheless he is frequently beyond her control; probably most intelligent of family; regarded as 'black sheep' and 'like his father'. Belongs to scouts, sings in choir, interested in flowers, drawing, and painting. Fantasy life very real; vivid and plausible liar. 'A clever thief'.

Clinical summary: diagnosed as primary antisocial conduct disorder; taken on for period of observation in order to get clearer picture of school and family stresses, and in hope of discovering legitimate outlets for child's assertive tendencies. Made easy contact; with remedial education attainments began to improve and from this derived satisfaction. Treatment and progress satisfactory, until boy's attendance at clinic became irregular as mother found it impossible to attend. Recommended that he should be sent to a hostel, but before this was done, he was charged at the juvenile court with minor theft, sent to a remand home, and put on probation for 3 years. Prognosis thought to be fairly good, depending on stability of home situation, success of probation, and continued psychiatric supervision.

Causative factors: unstable home conditions; marital discord; irresponsible, alcoholic father; early separation from mother; inconsistency in discipline at home; mother's poor health; boy's deep antagonism towards father. A constitutionally assertive, aggressive child in a social problem family.

Case No. 6: Ernest. *Age:* 7 years, 10 month. I.Q. 105.

Ernest is a well-grown, pleasant-looking boy with over-active, excitable manner. Babyish; sucks thumb and lisps.

Referral: by head teacher, on account of fighting and aggressiveness in school, disobedience and difficult behaviour at home.

Family background: only child of separated parents. Lives with mother in employer's house.

Mother: disturbed, shy woman, unable to make contact easily. Suffers from headaches; weeps on receiving letter from husband. Lonely in her job as cook-housekeeper in isolated house; no friends. Ambivalent, over-emotional, and disturbed relationship with boy, who has long-established sado-masochistic relationship with her. Blames father for all difficulties.

Father: journalist who wanted to be an artist. Went abroad when Ernest was 6 months; mother and child supposed to follow. Letters continued to come from him until a year ago, and occasionally some money. Through a social agency, mother discovered he was living with another woman, so started divorce proceedings. Father showed no interest in Ernest; once or twice sent books, which the boy has treasured. Position not explained to Ernest; recently mother told him that they would not now be going abroad since father did not want them.

History: mother hints that Ernest was unwanted; some doubt as to legitimacy. Early years disturbed as mother was upset and depressed following departure of father. Mother has always worked, never had own home; child forced to keep quiet. Harsh habit-training, control achieved at 1 year; walked and talked at normal time. Takes long time to go to sleep, fears dark, calls out to mother in room he shares with her to stroke his head, rub his back, and play with him; this stimulation excites him; unable to sleep until she comes to bed. As baby, ate well, now has food fads. Sucks thumb and lips. Jealous if he sees mother with another child; seldom leaves her. Hangs round headmistress at school in way that disquiets her. Relationship with mother uninterrupted until he was 6, when he was in a Home for 3 months. Health good.

School record and intelligence: many schools because of mother's frequent changes of work. At present school, gets on well and work is satisfactory. Teacher here takes more interest in him than those at former schools.

In intelligence test, I.Q. was 105. No unusual features.

Personality and behaviour: mother describes him as cheeky, disobedient, and difficult to manage; sometimes affectionate, babyish, and wanting to be kissed. Blames himself for mother's headaches; apologetic if he has had fights at school; gets on well with employer's children, who go to better school; fights with village boys. Can be helpful in house. Talks a good deal about his father, greatly interested in geography. Takes care of toys; likes drawing and painting, and wants to be an artist like father. Likes indoor games; screamed with fright when mother wanted to take him to swimming-pool. Most evenings spent in talking to mother in bedroom; continues talking after she is in bed; would like to share her bed, but she forbids this.

Clinical summary: diagnosed as primary antisocial conduct disorder in very immature boy. Mother taken on for treatment, and boy for observation in playroom. Mother tried to establish sado-masochistic relationship with the therapist. After some time it was thought improbable that she could change her attitude without prolonged individual treatment; boy takes husband's place emotionally for her. Treatment for neither mother nor boy likely to succeed under present living conditions.

Ernest over-dependent upon mother; emotionally immature; disturbed in most social relationships. Mother tried to compensate for hostile feelings towards boy and husband by spoiling, which resulted in an intense and complicated relationship. Hostility and resentment towards people probably led her to choose a lonely life. She is angry and guilty towards Ernest, and brings all her conflicts into her relationship with him. The possibility of undertaking treatment under present conditions was pointed out, but the mother was unwilling to cooperate herself or to change the situation; consequently the case was closed with doubtful prognosis.

Causative factors: unstable home conditions; broken family life; desertion by father; mother's disturbed personality and sado-masochistic relationship with boy.

Case No. 7: Felix. Age: 7 years, 7 months. I.Q. 83.

A well-built, healthy boy, but so frightened at the clinic that he hardly dared react at all, and spoke in a hoarse, strained voice.

Referral: by school medical officer, at father's request, on account of uncontrollable behaviour at home, and sexual offences against little girls.

Family background: youngest in large working-class family. Mother has 5 children by first husband, who was killed in the war.

Mother: a hard-working, dour Scotswoman; shrewd, but with little warmth of feeling towards her children. Resentful about Felix's behaviour; rigid disciplinary ideas, frequently hits Felix and keeps him constantly under her supervision; warns neighbour's children about him. For many years, she did part-time job in an hotel, but stopped this when Felix became troublesome.

Father: elderly civil servant; over 25 years in Navy before retirement. A small, hard man, with rigid disciplinary ideas. Angry about Felix's behaviour; thrashes him unmercifully, sometimes for trivial offences.

Siblings: Felix is shunned by 5 older step-siblings, of whom youngest is 10, eldest 20. He is bullying and spiteful towards youngest girl; feels that others have more than he has.

Considerable financial difficulties in home; father's pension and pay cannot meet family needs. Eldest girl is married, and lives at home.

History: mother anaemic during pregnancy. Birth normal; bottle-fed; no feeding disturbances. Habit-training rigid; clean at early age, reliably dry at night since 3. Walked at $2\frac{1}{2}$, talked at $3–3\frac{1}{2}$. From 4, temper tantrums so severe that he hurt himself; periods of twitching in sleep. Mother always found him difficult. Sleep, appetite, and health are good. None of the usual childish complaints.

School record and intelligence: Felix is in class where average age is 5 yrs. 11 mths. Restless, difficult to handle, unable to concentrate, cannot yet sound his letters. Provokes other children, is bullied by them. Frequently absent; some truanting.

In intelligence test, I.Q. 83; mental age 6 yrs. 4 mths. He was easily confused, frightened, and wanted to speak in whispers.

Personality and behaviour: mother describes him as the scapegoat of the district, though there have been no complaints from school about his behaviour. Obstinate; can be led, not driven; temper at times uncontrollable. Although he seems hard and fearless, mother realizes this attitude is a cloak for timidity and fear. Gets on fairly well with other children; shows no emotional reaction to father's beatings; owns up to misdeeds. Particular about personal habits, fussy about clothes. Is said to be in the habit of misconducting himself with small boys and girls by mauling. Mother received reports about this from other residents on the estate, and from mothers of small girls. Punished him severely. In his play, Felix seemed to have few normal outlets even for a dull boy. Mother says, 'He's hard as nails'.

Clinical summary: diagnosed as a case of primary antisocial conduct disorder. Recommended that he should be admitted to a hostel for maladjusted children, since treatment was thought unlikely to succeed while he remained at home. This has been carried out, and the boy is making satisfactory progress.

Causative factors: poor mental endowment; disturbed relation with mother and father; special position amongst step-siblings; particular factors of inconsistency in the family were attitudes of prudishness, false modesty, righteous indignation for small offences, alternating with rigid discipline and thrashings.

Case No. 8: Frankie. *Age:* 8 years, 6 months. I.Q. 88.

Frankie is a serious boy, over-polite, who volunteered nothing spontaneously to the psychiatrist.

Referral: by School Medical Officer on account of pilfering food and money, sleeping and feeding disturbances, encopresis, and lying.

Family background: mother died in child-birth, father re-married. The boy now lives in a stable home with three half-sisters and the step-mother's illegitimate daughter whom the father adopted.

Step-mother: a warm-hearted woman, of a voluble, fairly shrewd working-class type. Health poor: neurotic, suffering from severe obsessional thoughts such as cutting children's throats. Early life irregular; 11 years ago had an illegitimate daughter whom she brought up according to rigid standards in a home for unmarried mothers. About 7 years ago she married Frankie's father, who, adopted her child. Tries to be conventional in outlook. Welcomed Frankie, but is guilty about her methods of handling him; feels that because she is his step-mother must not be too hard on him. Persistent in efforts with the boy; before coming to the Clinic kept most of her difficulties to herself.

Father: in the Forces for $3\frac{1}{2}$ years; demobilized this year and now a skilled artisan. Fond of Frankie, but worried and puzzled by his behaviour. Thrashes him for delinquencies, a fairly frequent occurrence.

Step-siblings: adopted sister, aged 11, who is bossy, tells tales on Frankie; three half-sisters, ages 7 and 5 years and 15 months.

The home conditions are good, no financial stress.

History: mother died during Frankie's (Caesarian) birth. At this time, father discovered that she had been stealing from her employers, found himself £300 in debt, and her mother admitted that she had been in a Home for 2 years on account of theft. Father described her as a kleptomaniac. After her death, grandmother looked after Frankie for 4 months. Bottle-fed; difficulties in feeding and habit-training from the beginning. At 4 months, step-mother took charge; difficulties continued in extreme form until 4 years. Late walking; at 18 months began to talk, but with a stutter. At 2 developed abnormal feeding habits and obsessions over food. Smacked for this; began to eat his faeces, and continued this until 4. When this habit was forcibly stopped, developed intense liking for some special and sometimes bizarre foods; began pilfering money. Without consulting anyone, the step-mother tried to deal with this by rigid methods. Has been encopretic and enuretic; walks and talks in sleep. Now eats enormously and greedily, and steals food. He had chicken-pox before going to school; measles, whooping-cough, mumps, and scarlet fever. since. A year ago in hospital because of poisoned finger. Now healthy; despite peculiar feeding habits has had no digestive disorders.

School record: generally backward; weak in reading. Constantly in trouble on account of pilfering, but in other respects behaviour in class and on playground said to be good. Gets on fairly well with other children, though no friends of his own.

In intelligence test, I.Q. 88. Reading age on Burt's Accuracy Test 6 years, 8 months; on Burt's Mental Arithmetic Test showed no spontaneity, enthusiasm, or initiative, was extremely retarded.

Personality and behaviour: is helpful and affectionate at home, but can be obstinate, disobedient, and stubborn; reacts only to loss of love; at times thrashings are without effect. Shy, inhibited, with some odd tendencies in his play; clean and tidy. Teases his sisters by urinating in front of them. Likes to pose as martyr; wistful and pathetic with neighbours who regard him with pity. Used to pick fingers constantly.

Clinical summary: diagnosed as primary antisocial conduct disorder, possibly with some constitutional basis. Frankie and stepmother taken on for weekly interviews over a long period. During this time, he could not establish a relationship or become aware of his problems; produced little material, played in stereotyped, inhibited fashion. Relationships with people tend to be disturbed, though well-adjusted at school. At first mother appeared to cooperate, but gave up when child showed no quick improvement; this partly due to her own neurotic symptoms, preoccupation with smaller children, poor health, and further pregnancy. It appeared that during his early period with grandmother, Frankie had been greatly spoilt. This was followed by more severe and rigid training by step-mother than she had at first admitted. Over a period of 18 months, Frankie failed to respond to individual treatment; sent for special residential treatment in a hostel for maladjusted children. Diagnosis remains doubtful. Outcome inconclusive.

Causative factors: loss of real mother; complete break in mother-relationship at early age; inconsistent handling; step-mother's disturbed, unhappy, and reserved personality, her greater interest in her own children; possibly some constitutional basis or heredity from unstable mother.

Case No. 9: Philip. *Age:* 8 years, 10 months. I.Q. 79.

A bright, friendly boy; healthy-looking, talkative, and responds immediately to sympathetic interest.

Referral: by Juvenile Court, for lying, stealing, truanting, enuresis, encopresis, sexual offences, and wandering from home. In Remand Hostel at present.

Family Background: illegitimate; little known of parentage. Adopted by present parents after death of first adoptive ones, who were friends of father.

Adoptive mother: prefers her own son, now aged 3, who was born after she had adopted Philip, towards whom she is resentful and rejecting; expects him to behave like an adult, and to help with younger child, a sullen, detached boy who shows no emotions and whom Philip teases. She alternates between emotional appeals to Philip and thrashings. Wants to be rid of him, as she considers him to be abnormal. She takes in lodgers, loves cooking, and is very house-proud.

Adoptive father: formerly in the Navy; has deserted the family. Wife's picture of him is vague; tried to hide the fact of his desertion, says he was restless, regarded Philip as backward until the age of 6.

Philip believes that he has had two fathers and two mothers, that his first adoptive parents were his real ones. Adoptive parents have expected impossible standards; mother now permits him few outlets. Mother and two boys live in poor working-class home.

History: little known of early years; second adoption when he was 4; appeared to be normal and well-developed, though dirty. Long history of delinquencies, mainly lying, pilfering, wandering, and truanting. Suffers from enuresis, frequency of micturition; occasionally encopresis. At 6, thought to be backward because of lack of response to training. Nailbiter; slight stammer, persistent nervous cough. Appetite good, sleeps soundly, though, in absence of father, begs to be allowed to sleep with mother and younger child. Mother often permits this. Badly frightened in an air-raid when 6 or 7. Health good; backward, forgetful, and dreamy.

School record and intelligence: began at 5; attainments always below average; attendance erratic; began truanting. Bullied by other boys. Can read only two-letter words; unable to recognize capital and script letters, does not know phonetic value of diphthongs. Reading at six-year level.

In intelligence test, I.Q. 79. Concentration variable, lacked sufficient confidence to try hard on reading tests. Results slightly better on practical tests.

Personality and behaviour: destructive with toys; temporarily sorry for misdeeds, but constantly repeats them. Easily excited; follows

263

mother about, worried when she leaves him. She says he cannot think for himself. Play at home very restricted; plays with younger children; refuses to fight, gives his things to other children, frequently complains that he has nothing to do. Likes travelling, wanders a good deal.

Clinical summary: diagnosed as primary antisocial conduct disorder; taken on for observation. Made good contact with therapist, enjoyed individual attention, but only attended four out of nine appointments. Truanting and pilfering increased; charged at Juvenile Court for theft. Moved to hostel for maladjusted children where he was sexually assaulted by master. Was then seen weekly for 3 months to help him over difficult period. Relationship with mother discussed, and attempt made to help him accept home situation. Parents encouraged to allow him better outlets. Sexual behaviour for which he was charged in Court was exhibiting himself to girls, and open, exaggerated masturbation. Sexual problems partially worked through with him in treatment. Brought material indicating strong feelings of insecurity, aggressive wishes, fears, and passive tendencies. Mother failed to cooperate, and Philip has remained at hostel where he has settled down; some symptoms have cleared up. Prognosis rather doubtful and dependent upon continuation of treatment.

Causative factors: personality of mother; unsatisfactory home background; secrecy about parentage; broken mother-child relationship; inconsistent handling in dull and passive boy.

Case No. 10: Ivor. *Age:* 8 years, 9 months. I.Q. 99.

A good-looking, solemn boy who talks in a monotone.

Referral: by probation officer on account of masturbation and being 'far away' following his being charged, with other boys, in the juvenile court for stealing articles from a shed. It is also said that he cannot differentiate between right and wrong, and that he is dirty.

Family background: large, poor, working-class family. Some instability on father's side.

Mother: aged 38: brought up in a Barnardo's Home, cannot read or write. Warm, good-natured, child-loving woman, has full charge and control of 6 children still at home. Good manager and mother, does her utmost for children, keeps their 8-roomed house and the garden well. Baffled by the trouble children have caused. Fears Ivor may take after father's family, because paternal aunt died in mental hospital a year ago.

Father: store labourer; tuberculosis suspect for many years; work-periods irregular; during illness, family on relief; only one hot meal a week. Been in regular work now for 2 years. Devoted to children; indulgent, unable to punish them, yet his passion for tidiness restricts their play and compels him to do much house-work.

Siblings: 5 brothers, 2 sisters, ranging from 2–20 yrs. 3 older brothers have been on probation for various offences; one is at an approved school because of stealing. Ivor particularly friendly with this brother. A younger sister is delicate.

History: a wanted baby, but always troublesome. Normal birth; bottle-fed. At 3 weeks, circumcised, apparently badly; mother had to give treatment for wound. At 2, had 2 bad fits in one day, seemed to be unconscious for 5 hours. Unexplained except that doctor thought it might be beginning of gastric flu. Walked at 1 year, talked at 2½. Habit-training marked by difficulty in urinary control; stopped soiling early. Wet bed until almost 5. Between 2 and 4 obstinate and self-willed, most difficult child of family. Only mother could deal with his screaming and bad temper. Between 18 months and 2 years refused to sleep in cot, slept with parents. Did not then wet bed, but this habit recurred when put back in cot. Health and appetite good.

School record and intelligence: began at 4½; disliked it and returned home at playtime. Teachers and children complained that he masturbated. Similar complaints received from second school where he went at 7. Continued to dislike school; took no interest in work; backward, especially in spelling, reading, and arithmetic. Dislikes teachers; feels things always go wrong with him.

Mother says he would truant were she not firm. Popular with other boys; mother thinks he is leader, but not bully.

In intelligence test, I.Q. 99. Looked unhappy and miserable. Cannot read. Tense and reserved.

Personality and behaviour: mother feels he is more demanding than other children, never seems satisfied; doesn't know what is in his mind. Can be so irritating, yet upset when punished, so she feels compelled to give in to him. Passion for bonfires; lies consistently, even when he knows he has been discovered doing wrong; gives in only after pressure. No response to beatings; more upset if sent to bed. Always occupied and with companions. Probation Officer who has care of Ivor and his brother finds them mischievous but not deceitful, especially Ivor. They undertake wild escapades. Ivor has stolen and stayed out late at night.

Clinical summary: diagnosed as primary antisocial conduct disorder; taken on for period of observation at clinic. Failed to make good relationship with therapist in individual interviews; brought evidence of disturbed relationship with mother. Was then seen in a group of boys, where he immediately established contact with the only delinquent boy, conspiring with him against the therapist. After some months, began to show some signs of conscience formation. Prognosis with continued probation was good. Follow-up shows that considerable improvement has been made in social relations, and that he is doing well.

Causative factors: crowded family life; inconsistent handling by parents due to their personalities; presence of several delinquent siblings; possible constitutional factors from father's family.

Case No. 11: Patrick. *Age:* 9 years, 1 month. I.Q. 116.

Patrick is a nice-looking, sturdy boy.

Referral: by Juvenile Court on account of stealing, tempers and screaming, smearing faeces, and being beyond control.

Family background: Patrick was deserted by his father when he was about 2 years old.

Mother: aged 26; an untidy, unstable, harassed woman, whose father was in police force. Intelligent; very tired, constantly yawning; scabies on hands. Upbringing strict; rebelled, became wild. At 16, became pregnant with Patrick; married the father, who deserted her after 2 years. Does housekeeping jobs, no support from husband during last 3 years. Patrick separated from her many times; fond of him, inconsistent in handling, considers he is like father and that they are 'both mental'. During war, had illegitimate child, whose father she now wishes to marry; husband refuses to divorce, and offers to adopt the child. Patrick has been strictly handled by the maternal grandparents with whom he has lived since father's desertion (while mother was working) and at various periods before this.

Father: aged 32; a psychopathic personality who is described as 'weak-kneed'; mother warned by his family against marrying him; after considerable marital discord, joined the Army as single man. Returned home when Patrick was 7; short, stable period while he was a sergeant. Deserted Army to avoid detention; long history of theft; took part in black-marketing and house-breaking activities; now in gaol. Nervous symptoms; frightened of dark; sleepwalks. Both Army and prison authorities consider he needs psychiatric treatment.

Patrick and his mother are at present living in the house where she does domestic work. Her employers are a crude businessman and his slatternly wife. The garden is unkempt, the house dirty, untidy and comfortless.

History: despite her youth, mother wanted baby. Pregnancy and confinement normal; breast-fed for 5 months; easily weaned. Before 2, outbursts of screaming and temper tantrums. Average progress. Strictly trained; clean and dry at 8 months. Following father's desertion, mother and child went to grandparents; grandmother took charge of Patrick, was stricter than mother. Patrick frightened of dark, disobedient, destructive and untruthful. Even when working, mother kept in touch with Patrick. Appetite fussy; difficult to get him to bed, needs nightlight. Openly masturbated despite threats of consequent illness. No sex information

267

given. Between 7 and 8, had habit of defaecating in paper and hiding it about the house. Stealing began in grandparents' house, and they charged him in Juvenile Court when he was 9. Health good except for bronchitis every winter.

School record and intelligence: began at 5; apart from truanting has got on well. Dislikes school, has truanted for as long as 6 weeks. First referred to Child Guidance Clinic for truanting when he was 7. Has attended three schools; not backward.

In intelligence test, I.Q. 116; poor vocabulary, marked practical bent. Results widely scattered.

Personality and Behaviour: mother describes Patrick as now being crafty and clever, yet talking foolishly. Destroys things, especially younger child's toys. Not upset when misdeeds discovered, even by policeman grandfather. Went through Court proceedings without sign of emotion. Rude to most adults; physically attacked Probation Officer. At times, anxious to please, to make good impression and gain affection. Sometimes nice to baby, declaring he is proud to have brother.

Clinical summary: diagnosed as primary antisocial conduct disorder; taken on for observation; established positive relationship at once on basis of needing help. Friendly, willing to talk about problems. Evidence emerged to show that there may be more compulsion basis to stealing than was at first recognized. Confused on sexual matters; hidden sado-masochistic fantasies. After consideration of long-standing antisocial conduct and relatively minor role of neurotic factors, it was decided that stable home background was, at present, most imperative need, for, without it, individual treatment impossible. As mother appeared to be too unstable to set up home by herself and father is in gaol, boy placed in hostel under psychiatric supervision, though this meant postponing treatment. Made good adjustment in hostel and considerable progress at school. Occasionally goes to see mother. Further problems about taking money, but in other respects, follow-up has been good during stay in hostel. Prognosis thought to be fairly good provided suitable psychiatric treatment can continue while at hostel.

Causative factors: unstable personality of mother; separations from her in infancy; dual control with marked change in behaviour standards between mother and grandmother; personality and absence of father; parental discord; confusion in sexual matters resulting from presence, without adequate explanation, of second father.

Case No. 12: Carl. *Age:* 9 years, 1 month. I.Q. 101.

A sturdy, likeable boy, grown-up and philosophic manner. Appeared to be mildly depressed; during first interview, frightened and stubborn, denied difficulties, kept conversation on reminiscent level.

Referral: by headmistress on account of thumb-sucking, encopresis, provocative and immature behaviour at school and at home.

Family background: eldest of 4 children in working-class home. Neither parent considers him a problem, regard him as high-spirited, intelligent and independent. Father's family known to be headstrong.

Mother: in her late 30's. Friendly, colourful and impulsive, with many grudges; often untidy, blowzily dressed. She and people in village dislike each other; criticizes old-fashioned ways of village, is excluded from activities there. Fond of children, anxious to do her best for them, but not intelligent; reiterates her husband's criticisms of teachers, nurses, doctor. Her discipline is lax, accepts difficulties as deriving from father's family.

Father: 4 years abroad when Carl was 4–8 years. Demobilized a year ago; works locally as tractor-driver. Good-looking, talkative and intelligent with strong personality. Blames community for poor conditions under which family lives, critical of village people and conservative land-owners. In Services, some contact with psychology, laughs at it. Quick-tempered, thrashed Carl with belt when he first returned home. Spends much time with Carl, would like to treat him as a grown-up; loses temper when Carl is demanding or naughty, and thrashes him. Family pattern appears to be aggressive.

The family has lived for 6½ years in a condemned cottage in a rural village. Though crowded, the house is tidy and the furniture good. Carl sleeps in one bedroom with his parents and 2 months old brother; two girls, 8 and 5, sleep in the other. Both girls are aggressive; one is a thumbsucker, a large, impudent redhead; shouts rudely at mother, and at school is regarded as another Carl. Relationships between the children are aggressive, but they enjoy playing together.

History: mother says Carl was a nice baby, bright from birth. Bottle-fed for 9 months without difficulty. Walked at 10 months; talked distinctly at 3 years. Until 1 year, had dummy which he bit to pieces; when removed, he sucked his thumb; mother did best to stop this, but the habit continues. Between 2 and 3, sucking very intense. Periods of intense nail-biting. Wet bed until 3; mother treated this leniently. At 4, father went to Germany. Since 5, when he went to school, has soiled his knickers 2 or 3 times a week there; ashamed, tries to hide them. Mother has thrashed him for this. At 7, aggressive towards other children, frequently hurt by them. Appetite good, no sleep disturbances. Health good except for 3 weeks in hospital at 3½ on account of suspected illness about which mother is vague. Not difficult to manage either in hospital or on return home. Has stayed with paternal grandmother for periods during births of siblings, and for periods as long as 2 months at Christmas. No reports of difficulties after these separations; contact between him and mother unbroken.

School record and intelligence: infant teacher says Carl is most difficult child in her experience. On first day, refused to sit down or follow routine, aggressive towards other children, quietened only by stories being read, when he sat sucking his thumb. Retarded in arithmetic, defeated by difficulties. Written work below 5-year level despite being kept in infants' class for 2 years. Reads well; chooses to read poetry in free periods; likes acting, practical work good. While in infants' class, threatened teacher; at attempts to control him, temper tantrums. Gets on better with present teacher, says he likes school, although bullied by others and comes home dirty and dishevelled.

FIFTY DELINQUENT CHILDREN

In intelligence test, I.Q. 101; detached, sucked fingers; pre-occupied, day-dreamed and unable to concentrate for long. Backward in arithmetic, reads fairly well.

Personality and behaviour: at home, no bother if occupied all the time; affectionate, helpful. Parents deny finding him irritating. Helpful at school, but noisy, clumsy, and a disturbing element in class; incapable of sustained effort. Tries to monopolize teacher's time, stubborn if frustrated, easily discouraged, impulsively anti-social; always demanding books to read. At home likes practical things; can help father mend lorry.

Clinical summary: diagnosed as primary antisocial conduct dis-order; taken on for treatment. Response to individual treatment poor; tried to establish quarrel relationship with psychotherapist; no response to interpretations. Revealed little capacity for genuine feelings. It was decided he should then have group treat-ment. Parents' attitude towards clinic unsatisfactory; psycho-therapeutic treatment thought to be unsuitable for this case. Carl's character trends were antisocial, thought to be fixated upon sado-masochistic level within framework of an aggressive problem family. Prognosis considered doubtful; follow-up showed that his difficulties at school were less, but his symptoms remain unchanged.

Causative factors: possibly constitutional, allied to an aggressive family pattern; laxity of concern by parents for child's training; aggressive, grudging and resentful personalities in parents; absence of father; crowded and unsatisfactory home conditions.

Case No. 13: Paddy. *Age:* 9 years, 3 months. I.Q. 137.

A small, nice-looking boy. In his relationship with adults, so suspicious and guarded that he is unable to reveal his thoughts, answers in monosyllables as though afraid he might give some-thing away.

Referral: by juvenile court on account of stealing, running away, tempers and disobedience.

Family background: elder of 2 children, the other a girl, whose parents were dead at time of referral. At that time, lived with step-mother and her 2 illegitimate children.

Mother: killed in an air-raid on factory when Paddy was 7. Apparently unmoved by her death as he had not seen her for some time; off-hand when he refers to her. Paternal grandmother reports that she neglected the children.

Step-mother: slovenly woman in her 30's; intelligent; some understanding, little affection for Paddy who has lived with her for 3 months. Concerned about his behaviour and long history of stealing.

Father: artisan until joining R.A.F. where he served for 7 years. Shortly after discharge, fall necessitated his going to hospital. Said to have had violent tempers and been difficult; evidence that relationship with Paddy's mother was disturbed. Married 3 times: first to Paddy's step-mother, whom he divorced; second Paddy's mother; on her death, remarried his first wife, knowing he was suffering from an incurable disease. Saw little of Paddy during war. After continual rows and physical fights, he and Paddy's mother separated. Children then looked after by friends while mother worked in factory. Paddy unconcerned about father's death; seems to have been afraid of him.

Siblings: Paddy and sister, aged 7, are very attached. She is difficult; pilfers and tells lies. Step-mother's illegitimate children are a girl, aged 12, a boy aged 2. The family live in a council house on a large estate. Conditions are clean and orderly.

History: little known of Paddy's early years. Birth normal. Until 4, lived in atmosphere of quarrelling. Mother had no home of her own. Parents separated when Paddy was 4, and mother and 2 children lived for long periods in lodgings. At one time, Paddy shared single furnished room with mother while she was on night work in factory. Frequently climbed out of window, ran away, stole, and was brought back by police. He and sister then placed in foster-home for a short time. At 4½, Paddy placed in a residential school, sister sent to another foster-home. At 7, mother killed. Paddy remained in residential school until father was demobilized when child was 9. Father re-married and later died leaving children with step-mother. Since 4, Paddy has been known to wander away, steals, is difficult to control. Since father's death, step-mother unable to control him and feels living arrangements have been unsuccessful.

School record and intelligence: attendance irregular; for long stretches did not attend at all. Has stolen a great deal, particularly other boys' bicycles; punished for lighting fires that led to considerable damage. Work careless; backward in arithmetic and spelling.

In intelligence test, I.Q. 137. Superior intelligence. Reading favourite lesson; wants to be an engineer. In spare time reads fairy tales and books about open-air life.

Personality and behaviour: step-mother says that at times he can be charming, at other times is callous. Passion for matches; tends to wander; has sat under a tree until 10 p.m. in heavy rain. First court appearance was on charge of stealing bicycle and money; has stolen many bicycles in one day. Placed on probation; during last 3 months has repeatedly run away from school and stolen. Attachment to sister so strong that at times he has taken the blame for her misdeeds. Reads voraciously. Step-mother, who fears he will be a criminal, tried hitting him with her hand. He laughed, told her he would make her a stick with knots and things in the ends, and if hit with *this* he would stop doing these things. Kept on talking about this stick, even to neighbours. Step-mother alarmed; talk of this stick her main reason for feeling unable to handle him, and fear that he would force her to do this and other thing she would not like. He ultimately owns up to his delinquencies.

Clinical summary: diagnosed as primary antisocial conduct disorder; taken on for treatment. Made strong, friendly relationship with psychiatrist, gave impression that every contact with an adult must be kept up, as though trying to collect those who are, or whom he imagines to be, fond of him. Attempt made to provide him with stable home background so that he could attend clinic. This was partially achieved by sending him to an overseas Farm School, where he remained for 3 months and then absconded three times. Placed in remand home during treatment. An attempt made to discover whether his stealing (of bicycles in particular) and frequent wandering had a compulsive element; not clear whether or not this was related to a specific fantasy. Various other attempts made to find him a suitable foster-home, but each time his delinquencies continued and, in accordance with his own wishes, he was sent to a hostel for maladjusted children with the idea of working for a scholarship to grammar school. The follow-up shows he has not absconded again, is making satisfactory progress. Prognosis good if psychiatric recommendations can be carried out.

Causative factors: largely environmental, in particular the unsatisfactory and frequently interrupted mother-child relationship; absence of father; early death of mother; changes of parent substitutes, and gross insecurity of early years.

Case No. 14: Keith. *Age:* 9 years, 6 months. I.Q. 88.

A quiet, well-behaved boy who is so small that he looks about 5. Appears timid and frightened.

Referral: by a police officer on account of lying, running away from home, and 'romancing'.

Family background: an orphan. As a baby, boarded out by public assistance committee; all trace of early foster-home is lost. It is known that he was not in any of his many foster-homes for more than short periods until 5½, when he came to live with present foster-parents.

Foster-mother: large, blowzy, middle-aged woman; ignorant, unintelligent and crude, but seems kindly and maternal towards Keith. A registered foster-mother, but refused to come to the clinic or cooperate in Keith's treatment. When visited, was unable to supply many details about him; complained that he was unhappy, did not like to play like a normal child. Appears to be out of touch with his activities; neither she nor her husband has formed a good relationship with Keith.

Foster-father: a middle-aged farm-labourer, hard working, little time to spare for Keith.

Home conditions are of poor working-class level.

History: when Keith came to present foster-mother at 5, he was enuretic, and has been until a few months ago, when mother lost patience and thrashed him for it. Extremely passive, is usually no trouble except that he is sly and tells lies. Ran away from home several times, refusing to admit where he had been. On last occasion, found by police sergeant, who thought he looked miserable, and brought him to the clinic for advice.

School record and intelligence: dislikes school; retarded in all subjects. Very passive in work and play; teachers thought him defective. They are puzzled by his behaviour, lack of effort or desire to learn; have been unable to teach him the elements of reading and arithmetic.

In intelligence test, I.Q. 88; dull in manner and intelligence; quiet, obstinate, and uncommunicative. Very inhibited.

Personality and behaviour: at home, is willing and obedient, generally seeking to avoid attention or trouble. Does not play, reads only comics; seems to have no interests. Inhibited with adults; not afraid when questioned by the policeman. Inclined to be more lively when alone with children.

Clinical summary: diagnosed as primary antisocial conduct disorder in a dull, deprived child. Personality make-up shows typical impoverishment and apathy often found in institution-reared children, or children who have had numerous changes of home in early years. Play is that of a dull child; no evidence of emotional conflict or other disturbance. Taken on for observation at the clinic, where he was mistrustful, and unable to establish relationship with therapist. Regarded adults merely from viewpoint of what material advantages they could offer, or whether they were dangerous and punishing. Prognosis considered to be poor, since foster-mother was unintelligent and uncooperative, although she wished to keep Keith as a foster-child.

Causative factors: gross deprivation at all psychological levels in early life; loss of parents, complete absence of strong, enduring substitute mother- or father-relationship; many changes of home; general neglect; haphazard upbringing.

Case No. 15: Donald. *Age:* 9 years, 7 months. I.Q. 111.

A tall, handsome boy, grown-up in manner.

Referral: by probation officer of juvenile court on account of stealing at home, staying out at night, disobedience and temper tantrums.

Family background: eldest of 5 children in working-class home, where father has been away for long periods in the Services.

Mother: aged 34; a depressed woman who, at the time of bringing Donald to the clinic, was desperately worried about the illness of her 5-month baby, and unable to give much attention to the boy's problems. Thin, miserable-looking; held the baby, who was thin and tiny, in her arms all the time. Appears to be a good personality and busy mother; overworked, confused by court proceedings and does not know what to do about it. Handling of Donald inconsistent and impulsive. Standards lax; has allowed stealing to go on without complaint since he was 4. Appears to have spoiled Donald at first; lost interest in him now, preferring younger children.

Father: tough-looking, unshaven, but likes nursing the baby and handles him well. Until a year ago, a Naval commando; talks much about his travels. Now a labourer on shift work, so sees little of Donald; wants to go back to sea. Originally went off for 6 months the day after his wedding. Minimized Donald's difficulties; appears to be unworried, ignores the probation officer, says that all Donald needs is a man's firm hand. Donald no better with him than with mother; disobedience has increased since father's return. No real contact between them. Father thrashed boy after theft; pleased with his method, yet denies concern about Donald's behaviour, blames other boys and says he himself truanted as a boy. Both parents appear to be superficially friendly towards the boy; in reality, not greatly interested.

Siblings: Donald quarrels a great deal with his 7-year-old sister, who has also stolen considerably. His small brother is enuretic. Donald's favourite is the baby.

The family lives in a poor-class labourer's house; the home is casual and over-crowded, reasonably clean and fairly well furnished. No room for Donald to put his things away out of reach of smaller children.

History: Pregnancy and birth normal; no feeding difficulties; habit-training easy. Temper tantrums and disobedience at 2, after birth of sister and removal of family from London because of air-raids. Between 2 and 4, father overseas; mother and children lived in several billets; mother quarrelled with people with whom they shared houses. At 4, Donald and another boy, aged 9, stole hand grenades; warned by police. Some weeks later, they broke into house, rifled gas meter. Between 4 and 6, often ran away in blackout and, as mother could not follow him, stayed out late. Several changes of home before father returned when Donald was 8. Health good; had usual childish ailments, none seriously.

School record and intelligence: reports always reasonably good; popular with staff and boys; bright, friendly, disobedient. Master considers him sly; suspicions are aroused when Donald is elaborately friendly and chatty. Stole stamps from another boy, then very upset, truanted after discovery of theft, persuaded another boy to go with him. Likes school; average progress.

In intelligence test, I.Q. 111; showed good verbal ability. Nervous but friendly. Wide scatter in results; some practical bent.

Personality and behaviour: mother describes him as never contented with anything; disobedient and cheeky to her, never helps her with other children, resents time she spends with them. Brags to school companions that he is going to join the Navy like his father. Not short of toys; plays football, learns the piano, has weekly pocket money though wants more than mother can give him. Steals things he wants when unable to buy them. Likes nature study; belongs to local library, reads animal and bird books in spare time. Likes to go to cinema. Yet mother described him as uninterested in things and seemed unable to give good picture of boy.

Clinical summary: diagnosed as primary antisocial conduct disorder; seen at clinic during period of observation with group of boys. For first interviews, kept up adult attitude, then became disturbing influence, fighting with another boy, provoking the therapist. Play a mixture of aggressive behaviour and superficial defences of a nonchalant type. Basically Donald was thought to be quite a good personality; delinquent conduct related to lack of good social standards in the home. Recommendations made for the probation officer to work with the boy. Prognosis considered doubtful, depending upon outcome of probation.

Causative factors: largely environmental, particularly absence of father, presence of large number of siblings; inconsistent handling by parents; lack of concern over delinquencies; constantly repeated disappointments and jealousies, and mother's withdrawal of original strong interest in favour of younger children.

Case No. 16: Jonathan. *Age:* 9 years, 8 months. I.Q. 98.

A tall, pale, odd-looking boy, with penetrating grey eyes. Neatly dressed; appears to be very nervous. Babyish manner.

Referral: by school medical officer on account of temper tantrums, jealousy at school, childish behaviour, inability to make contact with boys of his own age.

Family background: only child of elderly parents.

Mother: aged 58; curious-looking, eccentric woman; children's nurse until at 46 she married the groom on the estate where she worked. Small, fussy, deaf, regarded by neighbours as peculiar. Emotional, over-anxious, entirely devoted to Jonathan with whom she has intense relationship of sado-masochistic type. He baffles her as no child has done. Jonathan argues and criticizes, is disrespectful to her. She is a woman of the old servant type; now does domestic work to supplement family income.

Father: groom and handyman; can do only light work, as he suffers from bladder, leg and spine trouble; cannot support family. Passive, pink-faced and podgy old man, moves and talks slowly and ponderously. Jonathan quarrels with him, provokes and plays up to him, cries if he cannot get his own way. Father unable to manage boy when mother was ill. He is inconsistent in handling of him; never hits him, though mother smacks him repeatedly. Mother says boy treats father more like an older brother.

At time of referral, family lived in a small flat over the stables of a house in an isolated rural area; had lived there for 13 months; boy had to share bedroom with mother. During treatment, returned to live in seaside town in cottage of good working-class standard.

History: much wanted child, though mother would have preferred a girl. Being elderly and suffering from a tumour during pregnancy, mother had difficult time carrying baby. Birth was Caesarian; breast-fed with difficulty for 5 months. Easy baby, but from birth had poor appetite; still has food fads. Walked at 17 months, talked at 1 year. At 18 months had period of nightmares, which recurred after he started school. Mother unable to remember details about toilet-training, but said she was not rigid about it, and was not unduly concerned when he had period of enuresis before 5. Whooping cough when he was 2, after which mother sent him to paternal aunt for fortnight; this was followed by difficult behaviour, tempers and crying at home. Measles severely at 4, then chickenpox, tonsil trouble and nasal catarrh. Occasional earache now. Mother noticed he masturbated considerably as a baby; dealt with this by giving him toys to play with. At 3, talked to him about this, and at 6 made a point of giving him sexual information. Stressed that when he asked how the baby got out of her, she told him that first of all she was cut open. Disappointed that he refused to discuss the subject again. Thinks he still masturbates. At 5, sent for holiday with mother's sister for month; nightmares, talked in sleep. At 6, mother took him to nerve specialist because of nightmares, nervous and irritating behaviour.

School record and intelligence: at 3½ went to private school where he remained until 5. No complaints, got on well. At 5, went to council school; difficulties reported after 3 months. Constantly came home in tears, complained that other boys hit him. Has attended 3 other schools; in each was backward, did not get on with other boys. 1 year retarded in arithmetic and writing; reading of average standard. Reported that he teases, provokes and attacks other children, and is bullied by them.

In intelligence test, I.Q. 98; nervous and ill-at-ease; results showed wide scatter. Excellent memory for digits, poor in mental arithmetic; says he dislikes school on account of other boys' behaviour towards him. They call him 'daft'.

Personality and behaviour: mother describes him as very cantankerous; on one hand babyish and unhelpful, on other, adopts lordly air and knows everything. Honest; aggressive and vindictive towards other boys; shows cruelty, has tortured birds. Behaviour is irritating and attention seeking; at times is whiny and miserable. Goes to Cubs and to swimming; has only one friend to whom he is faithful. Interested in reading, enjoys pirate and adventure stories. General knowledge good; likes drawing but not good at it.

Clinical summary: diagnosed as an early and mild case of primary antisocial conduct disorder; taken on for treatment. Mother also seen regularly, and has made good response. She expressed marked ambivalent relationship with Jonathan in line with her sado-masochistic tendencies in all social relationships. Established very positive relationship with psychiatric social worker, was able to gain considerable information about the boy, and some insight concerning her handling of him. Produced some bizarre fantasies, one of which was concerned with kidnapping little girls whom she saw on the beach. Jonathan established good relationship; from the beginning was willing to talk. Play revealed elaborate defences against feelings of inferiority, a sado-masochistic relationship to his mother, and pronounced sexual preoccupation. Treatment consisted of an attempt to analyse these defences and help in finding a better way to deal with conflicts. It was possible to discuss some reasons for his provocative behaviour towards other boys, and the silly behaviour that disguised his fears and inferiority feelings. Has compensatory fantasies of being magical, a superman; basis of these worked over, as were his failure in school work and the significance of stealing food. Sexual curiosity dealt with by mother aided by the clinic. Boy's behaviour improved in all directions. Remains preoccupied with sado-masochistic fantasies, passive and easily led. Behaviour at home and relationship to parents greatly improved. Treatment was followed with attendance at holiday camp for 3 months. Follow-up shows improvement maintained. Recommendation of sending him to boarding school proved impracticable.

Causative factors: unwise and inconsistent handling by elderly eccentric parents; crowded living conditions accentuating his sexual interest; sado-masochistic relationship with both parents; constant parental bickering and father's failure to support family; mother's aggressiveness towards boy; several periods away from home.

Case No. 17: Monty. *Age:* 9 years, 4 months. I.Q. 100.

A dark-haired, neatly-dressed boy who appeared to be depressed, hostile and suspicious.

Referral: by school medical officer on account of lying, stealing, destructiveness, disobedience, educational backwardness, failure to mix with other boys, sleeping and feeding difficulties.

Family background: adopted child; adoptive father dead; adoptive mother borderline psychotic.

Parents: little known about them. Father was unskilled labourer who had been in and out of prison for various offences, and then joined the Merchant Navy. Adoptive mother describes him as a rotter. Mother is an irresponsible girl, very young when Monty was born. Now lives in the district, is fond of Monty's 11-year-old brother who lived for a time with Monty's adoptive mother, but has now returned to his mother.

Adoptive mother: aged 52. A big, red-haired woman, who looks eccentric and ill. Trained nurse, widowed in her twenties; intelligent and capable, but self-opinionated and quarrelsome, full of paranoid ideas. Devoted to Monty, but has little insight; is over-protective, unable to tolerate his boyish behaviour; punishes any sign of aggression. When he produced nervous symptoms, kept him away from school for long periods. Relationship with him is of an intense sado-masochistic type; all her emotions centre round him; cannot bear to be parted from him. Her mother died of senility in a mental hospital. For years had a small children's home, was in good financial circumstances when she adopted Monty. Later, threats of a libel action were brought against her on account of the death of a baby in her care. Makes accusations and hints about people working against her. Gave up home, took various residential posts as a matron in schools, taking Monty with her.

History: Monty was a sickly baby whose real mother was cared for and fed by adoptive mother during pregnancy. Adopted at 2 weeks, given devoted nursing. Suffered from pyloric stenosis with severe vomiting; too delicate for operation. Feeding difficulties severe; diet rigidly controlled, and still is. Excessively clean; upbringing very rigid, with much nagging. Until 2½, tied in cot and forbidden to walk; talked and played skilfully when released, walked immediately. Mother worried constantly about health, deafness, and stealing food. At 4, mother brought court case against N.S.P.C.C., which was quashed; says it was started by someone out of spitefulness. Monty forbidden to mix with other children by whom he was bullied. Involved in sex episodes with older boys, Before 2½, had pneumonia, measles and bronchial trouble; then constant temperatures; allergic to milk; has had urticaria, chickenpox, German measles, whooping-cough. Said to be healthy now.

School record and intelligence: began at 5, disliked it from start; knocked about by other children. Constant trouble with teacher because mother kept him away for trivial reasons. Attended 5 or 6 schools irregularly; is now backward in all subjects. Rude and disobedient to master, provokes other boys; mother calls for him, accuses boys of bullying him. Headmaster says Monty most difficult child he has had to deal with in 30 years.

In intelligence test, I.Q. 100. Attractive boy, suspicious and inattentive. Some ability in drawing.

Personality and behaviour: an affectionate, demonstrative child, very dependent on mother. Well-mannered with strangers, but disobedient and difficult at home. Untruthful and spiteful to other boys; invariably manages to get his own way. At home and school is demanding, thoughtless and untidy. Looks after his toys, destroys those of others. Over-protected at home, solitary at school. Draws well; likes to read children's newspapers and schoolboy books; prefers aggressive games.

Clinical summary: diagnosed as primary antisocial conduct disorder; taken on for long-term individual treatment. Made fairly satisfactory progress, but was charged in court for theft and sent to hostel for maladjusted children. Behaviour improved; mother cooperated well until court sent him away from home. Case terminated owing to lack of cooperation from probation officer.

Causative factors: abnormal and grossly unsettled home; total absence of father; elderly and disturbed personality of adoptive mother; inconsistent discipline and abnormal rearing methods.

Case No. 18: Percy. *Age:* 10 years. I.Q. 92. See *Case No. 34.*

Case No 19: Leonard. *Age:* 10 years, 10 months. I.Q. 125.

Leonard is pale and apprehensive-looking, fearful of the toys in the psychiatrist's room.

Referral: by parents and P.S.W. of mental hospital for stealing, lying, destructiveness, and cruelty.

Family background: second child in a family of four children in working-class home which has been broken by father's long absence, infidelity and marital difficulties.

Mother: aged 32; over-anxious and intense. Married at 16, first baby at 17. Long periods of instability, so treats the children inconsistently; admits that during father's absence has little control over them. Intense sado-masochistic relationship with Leonard, who is everything to her. Defends him from consequences of his

283

delinquencies; condones and covers up his misdeeds. Discusses domestic discord with children.

Father: aged 36; in the Army for 6 years; only short leaves at home; repeatedly unfaithful to wife. Now works long hours in small shop. Intelligent; severely disturbed relationship with wife; spends little time with children; excessively strict. Children dislike him, possibly as a result of mother's influence. Father unknown to Leonard during early years.

Siblings: aged 13 and 6 years, and 6 months. There was an induced miscarriage after third child. Leonard and his two sisters are spiteful and jealous of each other.

Standards of the home are low; financial circumstances poor; parent lenient about money-stealing.

History: mother's pregnancy normal, though she was anxious. Instrumental birth. Breast-fed for 3 months; milk lost when father announced that he was in love with another woman. Leonard was a stubborn baby, yelled when frustrated. Said a few words at 6 months; walked at 16 months. Cleanliness-training slow but not difficult; never dry at night, still enuretic. Sleep good. From 3–3½ stayed with grandparents; frequently thrashed, then spoilt. Developed fears, began taking things, for which he was thrashed. Mother saw him daily. Until 6, took things from mother, would swop lipstick and powder for articles he wanted. After 6, stole money, wandered, truanted and was destructive. Mother sent him to grandparents again, where he stayed until 9, when the father returned and grandmother died. While with grandparents, both were ill. Grandmother often collapsed, Leonard would send for help. Grandfather had gastric ulcers. Both disliked mother, who declares they turned the children against her, Leonard disturbed by grandmother's death. Slight whooping cough as baby, measles at 3, mastoid operation at 5, which disturbed him considerably. As well as stealing, long history of truanting, lying, cruelty, attempts to interfere with sister.

School record and intelligence: began at 4½; difficulties from the beginning. Considered clever; did well at first, now unable to concentrate; bad reports. Many friends, tends to be a leader.

In intelligence test, I.Q. 125; was cheerful and cooperative. and made attempts to hide underlying anxiety.

Personality and behaviour: at home he is willing and active; enjoys helping. Plucky; likes to appear tough, but cries easily, becomes defiant if deprived or frustrated. Good at sport, learned to swim easily. Likes getting dirty and digging on the beach for worms for fishing.

Clinical summary: diagnosed as primary antisocial conduct disorder. As it was considered impossible to treat Leonard in present environment, efforts were made for him to be suitably placed away from home. Parents left the district before this could be arranged, and he was transferred to another Child Guidance Clinic. It was recommended for this intelligent boy in a disturbed family that he should be sent to a boarding school which had some understanding of his problems. This has been arranged and the follow-up shows that he is making satisfactory progress.

Causative factors: mother's unstable personality; psychologically broken home; mother's disturbed relationship with the boy; inconsistent handling between mother and grandmother; father's prolonged absence.

Case No. 20: Ian. *Age:* 10 years, 6 months. I.Q. 90.

Ian is healthy and strong, but looks suspicious and unhappy. He talks in undertones; is quiet, controlled and altogether unchildlike in manner and speech; has slight squint.

Referral: by probation officer, for stealing, truancy, wandering, lying, dirty habits, destructive behaviour, cruelty to other children.

Family background: illegitimate; adopted at 11 months after adoptive mother's miscarriage of twins, when she believed further child-bearing impossible. Nine years later more twins were born, then a third child. Adoptive father's army duties caused frequent family moves. There are no financial difficulties.

Adoptive mother: a well-built but tense and haggard woman in her thirties; capable and confident; has rigid standards. A twin, youngest of a large family; childhood hard; father died when she was 8; was made responsible for nephews and nieces, which displeased her. Preoccupied with her own children with whom she is affectionate and patient, though strict. Openly rejected Ian, threatening to leave her husband unless he was sent away. Her relationship with Ian is sado-masochistic.

Adoptive father: Army officer with over 20 years' service; intelligent, handsome, and successful, if rather priggish, demanding a high standard of his family; is at home only at week-ends. Is fond of and interested in his children, anxious for their success, yet deliberately intimidates Ian. Took the initiative over Ian's adoption; unconfirmed evidence that he is real father.

Mother: promiscuous; has several illegitimate children. Husband refused to accept Ian, severed relations with her on his birth.

History: before adoption at 11 months, had 9 foster mothers. At 11 months weighed 17 lb., was covered with sores and bruises, dressed in rags and so repellant that mother gave him a trial only to please her husband. At first, slow and stubborn during feeding. Walked at 14 months, backward in talking. Between 2 and 3, had temper tantrums to which mother responded by throwing water in his face. Habit-training difficult; dry at 3, clean at $3\frac{1}{2}$. Smeared faeces, but harsh punishment made him excessively clean. Until 5, played with his urine, and reverted to this on birth of third child, when the twins shared his bedroom. At 3, a Service doctor was consulted about his obstinacy and naughtiness, and advised thrashing, which the mother inflicted. Between 3 and 5, set things on fire. At 5, was told of his adoption. While appearing to take this information easily, even boasting of it to other children, he urinated on the furniture, despite severe smackings. For about a year, had nightmares; once walked in his sleep. Health good except during early infancy. Mastoid operation in hospital at $2\frac{1}{2}$; recently a cut in the leg which required stitches.

School record and intelligence: has attended 9 schools and been in trouble at all. Frequently truanted; reports bad. Owing to mother's pregnancies and father's absence, attendance has been irregular. In class he is idle and indifferent, though not badly behaved. He prefers practical work and mechanical things or looking after animals to school work. Reading fair, arithmetic poor; well-mannered towards teachers, but aggressive towards children with whom he seems nervous and ill-at-ease.

In intelligence test, I.Q. 90; showed no sign of affect. Did not talk spontaneously, kept an immobile face. Results widely scattered.

Personality and behaviour: Mother describes him as a bully, attempting to dominate others but running away from bigger boys. At one time started a gang armed with sticks to beat other boys. Is polite, but sulky and plausible; tells lies and prevaricates; is unreliable on errands, has tantrums. Since 7, has stolen from mother, especially food. Involved in sexual play with little girls. Openly masturbates, picks at his clothes and himself, and sucks his hand until it is sore, then picks the skin. Was a severe nail-biter, now bites his lips until swollen. Greedy for punishment, and provokes his parents to get attention or rebuke. After punishment, seems satisfied, becomes cheerful, and bears no malice. Reading confined to comics.

Clinical summary: diagnosed as primary antisocial conduct disorder; taken on for observation for 3 months. He established with the therapist a friendly, if superficial, relationship from which he sought to derive material gain, openly demanding gifts and assistance. Lied convincingly, showing no guilt or shame. On discovering that his desires did not coincide with the aims of treatment, started to play truant from the clinic and, the parents failing to cooperate in the treatment, he continued to do so. In his fantasies, he invariably pictured himself as strong and a tough fighter. He is aggressive; threatens other children, including the twins. Recommended for a hostel for maladjusted children, or an approved school. Prognosis thought to be poor without prolonged period of environmental treatment. May become hardened delinquent, or later a psychopathic personality.

Causative factors: unhappy babyhood; lack of relationship with mother; harsh, inconsistent handling; rejection on birth of twins; doubt and secrecy about true parents; constitutional factors.

287

Case No. 21: Bobbie. *Age:* 11 years, 8 months. I.Q. 100.

Bobbie is a good-looking, friendly boy, who seemed to be worried and rather depressed.

Referral: by the juvenile court, on account of stealing, truanting and running away from home. He appeared to be beyond the control of his step-father, had spent several nights away from home, sleeping on doorsteps, engaging in minor delinquencies.

Family background: illegitimate, mother dead; has never had a stable home for more than 2 years nor known secure family life and affection.

Mother: married to Mr. X. for 3 years before he went abroad. During his absence, lived with Mr. Y., who became Bobbie's father. Little known of him; he is a grocer, an old friend of the mother's and was Mr. X's rival. Bobbie is supposed not to have heard of him and to regard Mr. X. as his real father. When Bobbie was a year old, Mr. X. returned, set up house with his wife and regarded Bobbie as his own child. The mother died, when Bobbie was 2, in giving birth to her husband's child, a girl now aged 8.

Step-father: A bar-tender; pleasant, casual, weak; fond of Bobbie; unauthoritative in his attitude; has little interest in what becomes of the boy, though anxious for him not to be considered a rogue; treats him as an adult, unprepared to consider the needs of a boy of 11.

Maternal grandfather: simulated blindness, stole money from a Blind Society. Charged with attempted suicide.

After his mother's death, Bobbie and the baby were looked after by a maternal aunt for 3 years. Father seldom saw them. When Bobbie was 5, father re-married, took the children to live with him and his wife and her children. The marriage was not successful, and Mr. X. deserted his wife. He and the children have lived with his mistress for 3 years, and she is known as 'Mrs. X.' Bobbie is supposed to believe this Mrs. X. is his mother, but he never refers to her, or to any woman who has looked after him, as mother.

'*Mrs. X.*': a good-looking girl; talks freely, is shrewd and observant. Fond of Bobbie, looked after him well for 3 years, but is now more interested in her own child. The household consists of Mr. and 'Mrs.' X., her parents, her 18-month child, Bobbie, and his sister. Because of trouble caused by Bobbie's delinquencies, he is no longer wanted in the household.

History: Bobbie's behaviour difficulties have only been outspoken during the last year. The second Mrs. X. reported that while Mr. X. was living with her, Bobbie took a ring from her and things from Woolworth's, but Mr. X. dismissed this as part of his wife's trouble-making. After the birth of the baby, Bobbie stole money from third 'Mrs. X'; owned up and was thrashed by Mr. X. Bobbie showed no concern; spent the money on food. Stole money on two further occasions; no tensions in the household over the incidents. Some time ago, Bobbie was kept home from school to look after the baby who was ill. After this, systematically truanted for 3 weeks, always giving plausible excuses; spent time in parks. A week later, failed to return from school; found at midnight, asleep in a doorway, in possession of 6 bicycle lamps, pencil sharpeners, books and a lady's bicycle. Thrashed for this, which he did not resent. Although kept under close watch before court proceedings, ran away, stole money, food and father's watch. Charged in court for all these offences, remanded for 2 weeks, then put on probation. After further theft, again brought before court, and remanded for psychological investigation. During all this, Bobbie was unresentful and the family casual. He has never shown sleeping or feeding difficulties; health excellent except for an accident a year after baby was born, when he bumped into a wall, was in hospital for 8 days when his head was stitched.

School record and intelligence: Headmaster reported Bobbie was one of the best-liked and brightest boys; despite frequent absences, work was good and up to scholarship standard. Bobbie says he was bored in junior school, now likes senior school, but has no friends.

In intelligence test, I.Q. 100; is well-adjusted at school, friendly but nervous and insecure. Weak reasoning power, unself-critical, good vocabulary.

Personality and behaviour: described by Mr. X as a lonely boy without friends. Helpful at home, liked by the whole family. Reads newspapers and comics; regarded as being intelligent and adult. 'Mrs. X' says she has never seen him play, will have little to do with sister. At 9 complained of boys at school hitting him; never cries now. Undemonstrative, never affectionate to anyone, frequently answers 'I don't mind'. Probation officer has impression Bobbie was not happy at home; Bobbie loyally says he is. Belongs to Cubs; plays in Salvation Army Band.

Clinical summary: diagnosed as primary antisocial conduct disorder; appeared to have only relatively minor emotional disturbances. Personality was in some ways similar to that of deprived institutional child. Made good relationship with the psychiatrist, responded quickly to encouragement and trust; showed clear indications of progress in conscience development during treatment. In view of his basically stable personality and impossibility of his developing satisfactorily until he was placed in a home environment which made genuine re-education possible, and in accordance with the boy's wishes, he was recommended for an overseas Farm School. Was accepted; sent to Australia from where he writes friendly and enthusiastic letters to the psychiatrist; has obtained good report for school work and personality. Latest report referred to his honesty. Outcome considered satisfactory and prognosis good.

Causative factors: lack of genuine father and mother relationship; frequent changes of mother-substitute; broken and insecure home life; fundamental indifference and rejection by Mr. X. and 'Mrs. X', emphasized by the birth of their own child.

Case No. 22: Clive. *Age:* 11 years, 3 months. I.Q. 111.

Clive is a tall, slim, good-looking boy, awkward and ill-at-ease. He is one of the tallest boys in school.

Referral: by Head Teacher, who refuses to have him at school because of aggressive and unmanageable behaviour.

Family background: younger of two boys whose parents have been separated since the war. The boys now live with their mother.

Mother: a tall, plaintive woman, affected in manner, and on the defensive. Intelligent, but neurotic, over-emotional and up against people. Suffers from neuralgia; adopts a self-sacrificing attitude; rationalizes her failure to maintain a happy family. Full of theories about right and wrong. Does not admit Clive's difficulties, shields him from consequences of his delinquencies and blames school. Handling of boys is ineffective; relationship with them ambivalent; violent quarrels followed by lectures, petting and fussing. Regards Clive's behaviour at school as tomboyish. Superficially, she wished to cooperate in treatment; showed no insight; after short time, terminated treatment. Formerly worked in National Fire Service, now in business of her own.

Father: held commissioned rank in Services during war; now a businessman. When Clive was a few months old, father was flirting with another woman; mother stopped this. He had a serious affair when Clive was 18 months on account of which mother wished to divorce him, but he refused. Came home temporarily, but deserted again for several periods of 18 months to 2 years. Clive has not seen him for 4 years. He neither writes nor takes any interest in the boys; mother receives regular allowance for them. Clive is supposed not to know of the separation, but elder boy does.

Sibling: brother, aged 17; studious, bright boy, at present at High School. Enuretic from infancy until two years ago. Periods of rages; jealous because Clive is mother's favourite; Clive is loyal, admiring and generous towards him.

Mother and boys lived with maternal grandparents during war years, following damage to their house and so that grandmother could look after boys while mother worked. Mother and boys not permanently together until 3½ years ago. They now live in a small flat of middle-class standards and are rather cramped.

History: pregnancy and delivery good; large baby; breast-fed for a few months. Mother rigid in her methods; habit-training easy.

Feeding difficulties began at early age. Talked between 9 and 10 months, walked at 10 months. At 3, in hospital for minor operation. At 5 or 6, periods of pilfering; was aggressive and bullying towards other children. At present, is a clean, healthy boy; some degree of flat feet and a weak knee, for which he attends private doctor. Suffers from nose-bleeding attacks.

School record and intelligence: several changes of school coinciding with mother's moves. Does not fit in well; aggressive towards teachers and pupils; cannot concentrate. Described as one teacher's work. Is in the retarded class, ranks as E grade in class of thirty-five. Good at general knowledge, likes reading and oral work best; written work and arithmetic far below standard. Wants to go to High School, but Head Teacher is doubtful if he will gain a scholarship. He is noticeably superior in dress to other boys; mother ambitious for him. Head teacher has tried every method of dealing with him.

In intelligence test, I.Q. 111. Boasted about achievements, which were not as good as either he or his mother says. Best on verbal tests; good on tests of spatial relationships. Superficially cooperative; denied all difficulties to the psychologist.

Personality and behaviour: mother says he refuses to admit anxiety or problems. Happy-natured child, has many friends, mostly a year younger than himself. Worries when mother and brother have petty quarrels. Likes sport, especially football, cycling and boxing; enjoys reading and children's cinema shows.

Clinical summary: diagnosed as primary antisocial conduct disorder of long standing with possible minor neurotic tendencies. Mother and boy taken on for treatment. Mother's cooperation soon failed, and her attitudes partly adopted by the boy. She maintained that Clive would be all right if only he could go to a better school. Clive took up defensive attitude at the clinic; was aggressive, rough, untruthful, restless and dishonest. Showed fair amount of sex curiosity and ambivalent relationship with mother. Behaviour at school improved, and progress in treatment was considered satisfactory, but treatment was incomplete. Mother terminated treatment as soon as the school situation was made easier. Prognosis thought to be poor; Clive continues to be aggressive and antisocial in outlook.

Causative factors: mother's personality and insincerity; her ambivalent relationship; inconsistent handling; the older brother's jealousy contributing to the unstable emotional environment; absence and indifference of father.

Case No. 23: Martin. *Age:* 12 years, 0 months. I.Q. 134.

Martin is a serious-looking boy who stared constantly at the psychiatrist, and was disconcerted when asked questions about family relationships. Response was quick, slightly aggressive, with a ready sense of humour, and a matter-of-factness beyond his years.

Referral: by the Headmaster of his High School for stealing, truanting, school failure and sleep disturbance.

Family background: younger of two children of a broken marriage. For the children's sake, the parents live together, but the children hear much quarrelling.

Mother: aged 35. Irresponsible, hysterical and uncontrolled. Makes noisy scenes before the children. For 4 years during the war, when the children were evacuated, she worked on country buses, earning as much as her husband. Now works part-time, does little housework, contributes little towards general expenses, spending money on drink and superficial things. Flaunts her many men friends to her husband, whom she recently sued for maintenance, and lost her case. Suffers from headaches and nervous eyestrain. Four years ago, refused to sleep with her husband, since when Martin shares her bed. Relationship with Martin is intense and disturbed; undermines the father's authority, shields the boy from the consequences of his delinquencies. Makes constant threats and promises, which she fails to keep.

Father: aged 36. A neat, quiet, painstaking man, formerly a skilled craftsman, now a civil servant. Has done the housekeeping, looking after children's clothes, regulating of pocket money, for several years because of wife's irresponsibility. Goes his own way, lets wife go hers. Over-conscientious and rigid with children; prefers the girl, so house is divided between mother and boy on one side, father and girl on other. He has thrashed Martin for delinquencies.

Sibling: older sister; enuretic, poor scholar. Martin jealous of her, resents father's preference and affection for her, and dislikes them both.

The family live in a house that was partly burnt down during the war and has not been repaired; there are still many household shortages. Constant financial difficulties and quarrels about ownership of furniture, insurance, etc. Home conditions are of poor, working-class level.

History: pregnancy and confinement normal; parents delighted to have boy. Bottle-fed; progress normal. Health good; no sleeping or feeding disturbances in early years. At 5, evacuated to country; stayed with childless, elderly foster-mother. Settled down well. Parents rarely visited him. Troubles began when he returned home at 9; reluctant to do homework, truanted from school; difficult at home, made no friends, began to steal.

School record and intelligence: began school while he was evacuated; made good progress. At 11, won scholarship and now attends local High School where he is twenty-fifth in class of thirty-two. Best subjects mathematics, geography, history, and writing. Says he likes school; mixes well on a superficial level. Frequently late, has no wish to work hard, achievements have steadily fallen below standard. Latest ambition is to go to university, of which father approves; Martin not prepared to undertake extra work necessary for this.

In intelligence test, I.Q. 134. Results excellent in mathematical reasoning; weaker on verbal tests.

Personality and behaviour: Martin belongs to Sea Scouts. Sells primroses in spring and does other odd jobs to earn pocket money. Reads a great deal, usually boys' books, books on swimming, and comics. For long time, ambition was to go on stage.

Clinical summary: diagnosed as primary antisocial conduct disorder. School failure, in spite of high intelligence, was thought to be due

294

to a mild emotional disturbance associated with adolescence since the development of which his level of school work has dropped considerably. Placement away from home was recommended, but parents refused this; attempt made to treat him while at home. For a period, attended with a group of adolescent boys, but mother's cooperation was withheld; after a few months, Martin came before the Juvenile Court for stealing. On the advice of the Clinic, he was placed as a boarder in a carefully selected grammar school. Follow-up reports have been satisfactory, and the prognosis, if he is given a long period of re-educational treatment and continued psychiatric supervision, is considered good.

Causative factors: mother's disturbed personality, allied with passive and inadequate father; inconsistent handling of boy by both parents; disturbed parental relationships; open disharmony and uncontrolled quarrelling; separation from family during evacuation at 5–9 years; very unhappy and unstable home.

Case No. 24: David. *Age:* 12 years, 3 months. I.Q. 97.

David is a lean, healthy type of boy, with a pleasant face; over-polite and anxious to be liked.

Referral: originally by his choir-master, when the case was investigated, a report sent, and the case then closed. Later, the boy came to the Clinic of his own accord with problems of stealing, truanting and disobedience.

Family background: adopted child in a stable home. Problems worse since the discovery of his adoption at 11.

Adoptive mother: middle-aged; pale and tight-lipped, looks tired; tries to impress with her respectability. Suffers from kidney trouble. First child, a boy, died in infancy. Imagining that further pregnancy was impossible, adopted David; when he was 3, an adoptive brother was born. Since then, David has been openly rejected by her, and he is jealous of the second child, now 9. Mother grudges David money and clothes, wants to force him to do things, considers father is too lenient with him. Justifies this

attitude by saying it is because of his delinquencies, but it has obviously persisted over many years. Wishes to send him into the
Navy to get firm discipline. She goes to work in mornings.

Adoptive father: large, burly, well-meaning man, in skilled trade.
Was 3½ years in service; discharged a year ago on account of poor
health and bad feet. Puzzled by David's behaviour, anxious to do
his best for him. Reiterates that he treats both boys alike, but
clearly younger one is his favourite. Disapproves of what he calls
David's bad habits and bad companions.

The conditions of the home are of comfortable, working-class
level situated in a respectable neighbourhood.

History: adopted at 21 months from an Adoption Society. Nothing known of real parents. Mother says that he was pale, with
flabby flesh and no muscle, and still fed from a bottle. Early development slow; at 2 years could make only isolated sounds. Nervous; frightened of crowds and large buildings. Until 3, was clean,
but after birth of adoptive brother became dirty, had screaming
attacks, and later became exceptionally difficult. Apathetic, unable to amuse himself, so sent to school at 4. Continued soiling
until 5, wetting until 6; played with faeces, for which mother
smacked him. After 6, became over-clean, is now most particular
about personal habits. Always anxious and fearful. Appetite enormous; sleep occasionally restless. Reacted strongly on discovery
of adoption, used bad language, for which he was thrashed. Told
mother he could now do what he liked; later told psychologist he
had heard of his adoption 3 years earlier from his cousin. Health
good except for usual childish complaints. Slightly defective
vision; mild degree of flat feet which causes no disability.

School record and intelligence: has always been difficult; likes to go
to school but is unhappy there. Talks and romances a lot; has
truanted and stolen from school. Sat three times for scholarship,
but failed because very backward in arithmetic, though above
average in reading. Is now a year older than average age of class.
Head teacher says he is weak, but a lovable, wayward lad, adventurous and romantic. No inherent vicious traits, owns up, is
penitent and takes punishment. Influenced by older boys; when a

leader himself, is aggressive; willing and good worker, but unstable.

In intelligence test, I.Q. 97; not fluent verbally, weak in rote memory; did better in practical tasks.

Personality and behaviour: mother says he is sunny-tempered and highly strung. Shares things with brother, can be kind and willing, bears no malice; undemonstrative, does not cry easily; sometimes cheeky; has tempers and is then disobedient and obstinate; penitent feelings, if any, are hidden from her. Ambitious to join Navy and go abroad; father reluctant to give permission, and so far, defective eyesight has prevented acceptance in Navy. David hates being indoors; likes animals; is good boxer. Dismissed from church choir for cheekiness and unsettled behaviour. Easily distracted. Earns pocket money doing paper round and errand job, which he likes; quarrels with mother about what he does with this money. Likes to go to cinemas, whereas mother makes him do much housework, especially when she is not well.

Clinical summary: diagnosed as primary antisocial conduct disorder; came to Clinic of his own accord for once-weekly treatment. Established good relationship with therapist, but became demanding for material things and for practical help for various projects that he fancied, such as going to Naval School, or art classes, and having typing lessons. Delinquencies and feelings of rejection at home were discussed with him; helped to deal in more effective way with jealousy of adoptive brother, and his reaction on discovering that he was adopted. Placed for a time in a Naval School, but rejected again on account of eyesight; this time was able to stand the disappointment without reverting to delinquencies. Arrangements then made, on his request, to place him in hostel for maladjusted children which he had visited. Follow-up shows that he has made good adjustment and still has hopes of going to sea when he is 15. Prognosis thought to be very good if period of re-educational treatment can be carried out.

Causative factors: insecure babyhood period; lack of early mother-relationship; parents' concealment of adoption and his reaction to the discovery of this; inconsistent and unwise handling by mother; jealousy of adoptive brother; rejection by mother.

Case No. 25: John. *Age:* 12 years, 10 months. I.Q. 132.

John is an undersized boy, very brown and healthy, suspicious in manner.

Referral: by Headmaster on account of school difficulties and backwardness, truancy and lying.

Family background: illegitimate child of an unstable, middle-class woman now married to an eccentric, elderly man who has legally adopted the boy.

Mother: about 40; active, odd-looking, dresses in eccentric manner. Difficult childhood; parents went abroad, leaving her in England. Has had rheumatism, heart-trouble, and has a small goitre; married when John was 6; now lives open-air, carefree life, and looks healthy. Father is wealthy professional man, twice married and now lives overseas. Maternal grandfather distinguished clergyman who has rejected her. Her sister, 6 years older, has also had an unhappy life. She is a strange personality, devoted to John; has not provided a suitable home environment, makes no complaint about his behaviour, blaming school.

Step-father: aged 74; very odd-looking, oddly dressed; speaks in hearty, bluff manner; lower social class than mother, who is his second wife. Formerly a salesman. Health poor. Joins wife in denying difficulty with John, and in blaming school. Anxious for boy to do well, is good to him but lacks insight. Mother maintains that John has never asked about real father, and that from the beginning he and step-father got on well.

History: pregnancy and confinement normal; breast-fed for 3 months. Father saw him often until he was 9 months old; mother's maternity order against father failed, since when there has been no contact. Until John was 18 months, mother lived with friend, Mrs. X., who had small son. Rigid training; clean by 1 year, dry by 2. No difficulties; good sleep and appetite. At 18 months, mother went to work, leaving John in charge of Mrs. X. who cared for him almost entirely until he was 6. Mrs. X. was sexually promiscuous; no ill-treatment of John, but he was frequently left on his own or with Mrs. X.'s boy. Saw and heard things disturb-ing to a child. At 6, mother married, and they moved into present house. John began bed-wetting, which continued until 9. At 7, tried to run away. Severe measles with delirium soon afterwards. At 11, jaundice; 6 months later, severe attack of 'flu, again deli-rious. Health now good.

School record and intelligence: difficulties began after he moved to a free place in grammar school 2 years ago. Has had poor reports from the beginning, made no progress, and is not considered worthy of special place. Chronically absent; cries so easily that he is treated leniently. Likes only French; backward in mathematics. Does not mix with other boys; unable to stand up for himself without encouragement.

In intelligence test, I.Q. 132; found to have superior intelligence with mental age 16: 10.

Personality and behaviour: very sensitive, especially upset if anyone is ill. Highly distractable, rarely settles to anything for long; likes to read, mainly thrillers. Domesticated, cooks family breakfast and Sunday lunch (in this follows step-father who does cooking and housework). Step-father says he is a liar, but makes passionate and convincing denials. Has many enemies amongst other boys; truants easily. Isolated from other children during holidays. On the whole, shares parents' interest in their garden and poultry. Collects stamps; wants to study science and work on railway.

Clinical summary: diagnosed as primary antisocial conduct dis-order; taken on for group treatment in order to help him make a better social adjustment. School difficulties, in spite of high ability, thought to be due to conflicts centred upon his relationship to people in authority. Recommended that he should attend the group over a long period, and be transferred to a more suitable school. Parents disinterested and failed to cooperate, and treat-ment was not carried through. Follow-up shows that school transfer was successful and that John has made some response. Prognosis without treatment is poor. Case closed as unsatisfactory, but it was hoped that it would be reopened when a new clinic nearer to the boy's home was opened, since distance was one fac-tor in the parents' refusal to continue treatment.

Causative factors: irregular upbringing with a change of mother-figure at 18 months; extreme inconsistency in handling by the two women. Unusual background, boy's failure to adapt satisfactorily to his elderly step-father and secrecy about his own father have reinforced his tendency to take the easy way out of difficulties by running away from them.

Case No. 26: Christopher. *Age:* 13 years, 2 months. I.Q. 111.

Christopher is a good-looking, polite boy with a bright and charming manner.

Referral: by his father, with a history of lying and pilfering, inability to concentrate and difficulties in school.

Family background: only child of separated parents; lives with paternal grandparents.

Mother: Frenchwoman whom father married before the war while working abroad; now middle-aged; intelligent and sincere, but nervous and highly emotional. Her mother committed suicide, her sister is in an institution. Early years of marriage satisfactory, though father admits sex life always disturbed. Mother discontented with English life. In 1935, father joined Regular Army and family moved to Singapore. During evacuation of that area, mother and boy went to Malaya and she had a good job with the American authorities. On arrival of Japanese, sent to internment camp, later released. Mother and boy separated for several periods; mother faced charges of espionage. On liberation was sent to camp for 3 months, where boy was ill and undernourished. Then both sent to America, and mother received salary for 5-year war period. American experiences increased feelings of dissatisfaction with England. She took him home, but father felt unable to cope with him because of delinquencies that had occurred during stay in America, so approached a Child Guidance Clinic for advice. Mother has no interest in Christopher's future; her handling of him is impulsive and inconsistent.

Father: superficially friendly and understanding, with little insight. Although always with the boy during early years, has had no real contact for 7 years. On demobilization has applied for civil service job; wants to settle in England and re-marry.

The standards of the home are comfortable, middle-class level. *Paternal grandparents:* both over 70; devoted to the boy. Mother visits them since she is in England, but finds them too cold and unemotional and is unhappy at their home.

History: pregnancy and birth normal. First 3 years in England uneventful. At 3, went to Singapore, looked after by an ayah; no difficulties; mother's relationship preserved. At 7, family came to England on leave; returned to Singapore for 2 years before evacuation to Malaya. During first separation from mother, truanting from school and stealing began. Between 9 and 12, lived in various camps; separated from mother, but when with her, she nagged or spoilt him, and left him to his own devices. Truanting and stealing continued, despite severe punishment, during separation from mother in Malaya and later when separated from her in the U.S.A. and Canada. Lies plausibly and cleverly. Health now good, but for 4 years in prison camps suffered from malnutrition, dysentery and considerable privations.

School record and intelligence: changed school eleven times in America; travelled with mother for a year, and in school for only a few months. Writing and spelling weak, but not as far below average as might be expected.

In intelligence test, I.Q. 111; results showed exceptionally wide scatter, poor memory, good vocabulary. Rushed breathlessly into tests, despite reassurance. Talks in adult fashion.

Personality and behaviour: lives considerably in the past and in world of fantasy; unable to concentrate. Proud to have killed a pigeon with a rock. Lacks persistence in what does not appeal to him. Rude to adults; difficult to handle. Uses stolen money to treat other boys, but never tells mother how he spends it. Never admits thefts, impervious to punishment. Likes gadgets, ambitious to be radio technician. Talks like an American; interested in radio and books; likes arithmetic and is not backward in it. Father wants him to go to good school and to study in field of humanities. Much conflict in family values and ambitions for boy.

Clinical summary: diagnosed as primary antisocial conduct disorder, taken on for observation while the father was helped to find a satisfactory environment for the boy. After some interviews father decided definitely to separate from wife, and was able to discuss the situation with the boy. Chris was less emotionally disturbed than at first appeared, and towards the end of the observation period had already become interested in and ambitious about his school work; was willing to go to boarding school. The prognosis was thought to be good; follow-up shows that the boy has settled down well, but attitudes and character remain rather self-centred and antisocial in outlook.

Causative factors: lack of stable home life; incompatibility and disturbed relationship of parents; various separations from both mother and father; inconsistent discipline from a temperamental mother; some encouragement to steal in internment camp; long series of gross environmental disturbances.

Case No. 27: Jeremy. *Age:* 13 years, 7 months. I.Q. 87

A well-grown boy, with a round face and pink cheeks. Ears prominent. Easily becomes wilful or evasive, and is withdrawn.

Referral: by mental health visitor, on account of running away from home, and being beyond control.

Family background: eldest of 3 children; father in India.

Mother: a thin, tense and anxious woman; rigid Roman Catholic. Has difficulty in all social relationships, probably mildly paranoid. Marital relations disturbed in early years; worse since husband started to drink heavily. At present, is in England in order to place children in boarding schools. She is hostile and resentful towards Jeremy; appears to reject his father in him. Is alternately strict and lacking in insight, and impulsive, which provokes his aggression; she feels hopeless because he rejects religion. He provokes her, flouts her control, then asks if she loves him. She has had little care of the children as they lived for some time with grandmother in Singapore. The mother is impatient and irresponsible towards them.

302

Father: an engineer. Harsh and impatient; drinks heavily, knocks his wife about; she is frightened of him, resists him, and has several times broken off relations with him. He shows no interest in Jeremy, and their relationship has always been difficult.

Siblings: one sister and one brother. Mother prefers the girl to Jeremy, who is spiteful towards his sister and attacks her. She is satisfactorily settled in a boarding convent. The younger boy, aged 2, will return to India with the mother.

The family has had frequent changes of home; spent 2½ years in a concentration camp, all living together in one room.

History: born in India; healthy baby, bottle-fed. No difficulties until birth of sister at 1 year; refused solid foods, for which mother smacked him. Wet at night until after 2; smacked for this, and wetting ceased. Walked at 14 months, talked a little later. Periods of restless sleep since before stay in internment camp. Always evasive and uncommunicative; tells lies. From 10–12½, when he was in camp, he must have gained extensive sex knowledge, as youngest child was born there. Present symptoms have developed since coming to England. He has absconded from four schools; forged a cheque with his mother's signature; kicks and attacks mother and sister.

School Record and Intelligence: Began at five in Singapore; some irregular schooling in internment camp. Unable to fit in with routine in either boarding or day school in England; does not get on with other boys; feels he is unwanted and disliked. Not abnormally backward, and progress should be good with steady work.

In intelligence test, I.Q. 87; poor verbal ability; answers scattered and uncertain. Easily gives up.

Personality and Behaviour: Mother says that earlier he was a happy and ambitious boy, and still likes, occasionally, to be childish and affectionate. On the other hand, he is stubborn and resentful, and has a don't care attitude. Careless and untidy in appearance, tells many lies, refuses to go to church or to the priest, and is generally disobedient and defiant. Says he wants to be an engineer. He is good with engines, can drive a car. Interested in designing aeroplanes and in scientific experiments, geography and mathematics; would like to discover a new gas. Denies his school difficulties. Likes to spend his time racing around on a bicycle.

Clinical summary: Diagnosed as primary antisocial conduct disorder; taken on for short term of treatment in order to improve the situation at home until a suitable school could be found which could keep Jeremy for the holidays. Mother is uncooperative towards treatment, and intolerant and rejecting towards the boy. She expressed much hostility towards him, used interviews to complain about him, but clearly provoked many of the scenes at home by her own attitude. In treatment hours, Jeremy maintained his defence that everything was going well both at home and at school, and he was unable to discuss his difficulties. He expressed a number of fantasies and daydreams, showing his inability to accept his own limitations and his deep resentment of what he feels to be his parents' rejection. Treatment was terminated suddenly by the mother's impulsive decision to take Jeremy back to India. Prognosis remains doubtful and Jeremy might easily become a hardened delinquent and rebel.

Causative factors: Unhappy parental relationship; his parents' rejection of the boy; mother's inconsistent handling; disturbed home life; effects of concentration camp during puberty; very free life led in India contrasted with strictness of English schools.

Case No. 28: Steven. *Age:* 13 years, 7 months. I.Q. 106.

Steven is a bright, talkative boy, with a rather jaunty air.

Referral: by the probation officer on account of feeding disturbance, disobedience and defiance, stealing and temper tantrums.

Family background: only child whose mother is a chronic invalid. The father is devoted to her and excludes Steven.

Stable working-class home. Maternal grandparents live in same street.

Mother: aged 40; a helpless cripple who has suffered from rheumatoid arthritis since she was 17. She is frail and patient, but manages to look pretty and happy. Youngest of 7 children, always dependent upon her mother. Spends her time in reading. Her relationship with Steven has been uninterrupted; worries about his food fads. She has good insight into his difficulties, and into his clash with his father. She secretly wanted to have a girl.

Father: aged 42. Irritable, highly strung and severe, quick-tempered and nervy. Graded C3 in Services; advised to give up heavy work; cannot bear monotonous, indoor work; has been furniture remover, painter and decorator; is now a labourer, working irregular hours. Does all the housework; vents irritability on Steven, gets angry, makes threats and whips him. Always sharp and impatient with him, resents his playing with toys and soldiers instead of reading books. Fussy about cleanliness. Openly disappointed not to have had a daughter. Mother says he has been jealous since birth of Steven.

History: pregnancy and birth normal; refused to feed at breast; screamed and lost weight, put on bottle. Feeding difficulties and screaming continued until 13 months. Mother blames overfeeding by grandmother, who also carried out toilet-training. Scolded and slapped until he was dry at 11 months, clean at 13 months. Suffered from disturbed sleep and head-banging when cross. At two had pneumonia, and bronchitis and catarrh before seven. At nine, mumps and measles, chickenpox, chest trouble and broken arm in quick succession. Ran away from hospital when left there with broken arm. Always been afraid of doctors. Until seven or eight, played with and fondled dolls. Later he injured them with chemicals, then bandaged and treated them. At 10½, when mother was ill, truanted with gang of toughs; was involved in stealing and malicious damage. Placed on probation for two years. Feeding difficulties and destructiveness have persisted.

School record and intelligence: started at five. Happy until he was moved to senior school at 11. Truanted, played only with younger, less rough boys and girls. Best subjects are reading, writing, composition and nature study. Mental arithmetic worst subject. He is in the top group in his class.

In intelligence test, I.Q. 106. Response very quick and cooperative; easily satisfied and inclined to insist that everything was all right.

Personality and behaviour: Mother says he hides his delinquencies at home. Afraid of his father's anger, threatened to run away when father was cross. Irritable and highly strung, has to be coaxed in everything. Never shown fear, except of father and doctors. Affectionate towards mother, but takes advantage of her illness and father's late hours to carry out misdeeds. Helps mother in house; likes getting dirty. When with younger children or girls, likes to be boss; is easily led and drawn into bad company. Fond of reading, mainly comics and thrillers; likes cinemas and music. Joined the junior brigade of the Salvation Army. Determined to be a painter.

Clinical summary: diagnosed as primary antisocial conduct disorder; taken on for treatment with a group of boys. Parents were seen at home, and helped to gain some insight into the boy's difficulties and need for firmer control. Steven made good progress in the group, left school, and remained in the care of the probation officer, who reports satisfactory progress, and good adjustment in his first job.

Causative factors: difficult home environment, especially the illness of his mother; disturbed relationship with father; father's difficult personality; inconsistency in discipline in early years at the hands of mother and grandmother.

Case No. 29: Alfred. *Age:* 16 years, 3 months. I.Q. 114.

Alfred is a tall, healthy boy, with an off-hand manner.

Referral: by Probation Officer after being charged in Court with larceny and running away from home. He had absconded from the Remand Home. At 13 was on probation, having been charged with other boys with stealing books from a salvage depot during a vacation. Probation passed without incident.

Family background: eldest of four children of a stable, working-class family.

Mother: aged 37; clean, tidy, pleasant-faced woman who gives the impression of being a good, capable mother. She is friendly, sensible, of average intelligence, reasonable and practical towards

306

Alfred's difficulties, possibly hiding her worry. She is the third of four children whose father was killed; went into service at 14 to help her mother support the family. One brother is restless and unsettled. She has done domestic and factory work during most of her married life, but gave this up on birth of third child.

Father: aged 42; lorry-driver for business firm; away from home from 6.30 a.m. until 6 p.m. daily. Worked away from home during most of the war. Easy-going, likes to spend free time at home. Eldest of a large, highly respected family. He is annoyed and displeased at the disgrace and loss of time Alfred's troubles have cost.

Siblings: girl, aged 13; two brothers, aged 4 and 2½. The family is a happy one, though without strong bonds. Health good, no apparent nervous disorders. Normal pleasures and outings.

History: pregnancy and birth normal. No difficulties in feeding, weaning or training, bottle-fed. Walked and talked at normal age; appetite good. Usual childish ailments, but mildly. Had periods of nose-bleeding which have recently recurred. Nailbiter. At 4 or 5, woke up in the night screaming and saying there were things in the room.

School record and intelligence: remained at first school until he was 9; made average progress, only problem was arithmetic. At 9, evacuated to the country; attended four schools; remained at one for 2 years while living with a miner, his wife and son. Happy and well-adjusted there, but missed his family. On vacation at this time, got into trouble with other boys and was put on probation. During this period away from home, a brother was born; 4 weeks after he returned home, another child was born. Alfred never settled down under these changed home conditions. Normal adolescent difficulties were increased by jealousy of siblings. Left school at 14; final school report said he had limited capacity allied to poor effort; elusive, not dependable; boyish scrapes, but no vice.

In intelligence test, I.Q. 114; intellectual performance very scattered with a tendency to give up and not to set himself a very high standard.

Since leaving school, he has held three jobs; at present works in jobbing company, is well-spoken of by employers, but finds the job monotonous and it gives him headaches.

Personality and behaviour: at home, Alfred is sharp-tempered and moody; secretive, full of flights of fancy. He is restless and cannot let himself join in family life. Wants to join the Navy or Army and to travel. Bad mixer, has few friends. Sometimes he spends evenings at home, at other times stays out until late at night. Used to belong to Sea Cadets, now belongs to no youth organization; has no hobbies.

He was referred to Court following several attempts to run away from home and stealing father's fountain pen and 30s.; tried to join Army and Navy; rejected because he was too young; hid in woods, brought home by the police, but refused to stay, so spent night at police station. He was sent to a Remand Home, absconded next morning. Broke into a house, appeared before the Court.

Clinical summary: diagnosed as primary antisocial conduct disorder exaggerated by adolescent difficulties. Seen by psychiatrist over this difficult period. Recommended that he should be helped to leave home, but to remain in contact with it. It was thought that he would benefit from a period of hostel supervision, and that, with a stable re-educational environment, the prognosis was good. Parents and boy agreed, and he was sent to a hostel where there has been no further delinquency. Follow-up reports show that he is getting on well, has made new friends and interests, and is more confident and contented.

Causative factors: long period of evacuation during pre-puberty; return home to find a new family in which he felt himself a stranger. Difficulties in establishing independence at adolescence in this crowded home were exaggerated and experiences in his earlier childhood and schooldays had prepared him for taking the line of least resistance.

Case No. 30: Paul. *Age:* 16 years, 9 months. I.Q. 131.

Paul looks more than 16. He is tall, well-built, healthy; faulty sight in one eye.

Referral: by the out-patient department of the local hospital on account of his having embezzled money during the past ten months.

Family background: eldest of three children from good, working-class family.

Mother: aged 39; reserved, uncomplaining; worked as domestic servant throughout married life. Her relationship with Paul is intense and disturbed, and no longer close.

Father: formerly a manservant, now an ambulance worker and away from home a good deal, especially at night. He is impatient and difficult; relationship with wife has been unhappy for some years. Strict with children, who do not confide in him; little in common with Paul. Did not punish him for embezzlement offence.

Siblings: two sisters, aged 15 and 6 years; Paul is on good terms with them, though jealous because the elder earns more than he.

Until Paul was 15, the family lived in a small cottage on the estate where parents were employed. A year ago, family went to mother's relatives in nearby village; Paul was pleased because he enjoyed membership of local youth club. Some months ago, family moved to more isolated village where there is no youth club. The conditions of the home are of respectable working-class level.

History: a wanted baby. Breast-fed for nine months; lively and forward. No difficulties until at 20 months, sister was born, and Paul was sent to relatives for two weeks. On return home, refused to have anything to do with mother, appeared not to know her. Obstinate, always wanted his own way; no apparent hostility to baby; period of night terrors. Habit-training easy; clean during infancy, but breakdown between three and five; spells of wetting until 12. Thumb-sucking after he started school, continued this until three to four years ago. No feeding difficulties, no serious illness, no early delinquencies. Mother says that during childhood he invariably hurt himself more severely than most children when he fell over.

L

School and post-school record and intelligence: good reports for work and conduct. Gained scholarship to technical school, spent two terms there with friends; was well-liked. Left school to join Navy; failed because of eyesight, and was very disappointed. Got job as office-boy at £1 per week; began taking insurance money each week for 10 months—£50 in all; spent it on friends and impressing girls. Father paid back most of the £50; Paul dismissed from job.

In intelligence test, I.Q. 131. He showed superior intelligence, and clearly present work is unsatisfying.

Personality and behaviour: mother says he has been moody, irritable, and withdrawn during past months. Recently he has taken things belonging to his father. Always passive, never facing difficulties directly. Likes smoking, dancing, football, cinemas, and going to youth clubs. He has a girl friend. Likes reading, especially cowboy yarns and murder stories.

Clinical summary: diagnosed as adolescent disturbance with delinquent trends; taken on for observation to determine whether or not treatment was necessary. After a short period it was felt that he would probably remain stable if he now succeeded in getting the post he wanted in the R.A.F., and a strong recommendation was sent in support of this. If this plan failed, longer observation at the clinic and possible treatment was advised. Prognosis thought to be good. The outcome was satisfactory. Paul was admitted to the R.A.F. Follow-up shows that he has settled down and is enjoying his new life.

Causative factors: unsatisfactory job with low salary, and strong desire to be adult and able to treat his friends. Paul is passive, effeminate type who reacts to disappointment by taking easiest way out without considering consequences. He has fundamental feelings of inferiority amongst his equals which he tries to combat by appearing to be the great man before his friends. Sister earning more than he did was particularly irksome. Intense and disturbed relationships with mother, dating from time of early separation from her, unhappy marital relationship of parents, poor relationship with father have increased his desire to be grown up and to get away from home.

Case No. 31: Alice. *Age:* 6 years, 5 months. I.Q. 101.

An attractive, sturdy girl with a slight squint. Her air of self-possession and independence hides feelings of insecurity and inferiority.

Referral: by the Psychiatric Department of a Mental Hospital on account of pilfering, lying, inability to mix and behaviour difficulties.

Family background: youngest of three children from broken home; she has had several foster-mothers.

Mother: intelligent and capable, with little fondness for children. She rejects Alice, feels guilty, but makes plausible and hypocritical excuses. Works in an office and is the main wage-earner of the family.

Father: works only irregularly. Bad-tempered, odd, possibly psychopath. Suffers from arthritis deriving from leg injury; finicky, worries over trifles, is upset by dirt. Unreasonable with children, takes his meals apart. Mother fears he will beat Alice unmercifully. Alice has seen little of him.

Siblings: sister, aged 16, brought up by grandmother, a shy girl who stammers. Brother, aged 9; nervous, intelligent, jealous of Alice and fights with her.

The family has never lived together. Mother has now bought a house and hopes to unite them.

History: 2 weeks after birth, was taken by foster mother, Mrs. X., an intelligent, middle-class woman with a son of 14. Alice was bottle-fed, greedy, suffered from acidosis. Rigidly trained; reliable toilet habits at 11 months. Until 2, was sickly; severe reaction to vaccination; had whooping-cough. At 5½, Mrs. X. had to give up caring for Alice on account of poor health and advancing years. Spent 2 weeks with mother, then went to second foster-mother, Mrs. Y., a rough, working-class woman in a poor-type home. Alice slept with two boys; learnt sex-play and bad language. A third foster-mother, Miss Z., is elderly, frail and nagging. Alice is at present with her, but she finds the child too difficult and wants to get rid of her.

School record and intelligence: started school at 3½; Head Teacher says she was naughty, spiteful and difficult. Alice had been to three schools before 6, including a private school, from which her removal was requested because of rough and rude behaviour. She cannot read, writes fairly well, can sound her letters. Concentration is poor, and she is easily distracted.

In intelligence test, I.Q. 101; she was insecure and needed encouragement.

Personality and behaviour: behaviour with other children is difficult; takes their things, hits them, spits at them; has pilfered since 3; has a mania for pens. She has tempers, swears and grimaces, openly masturbates, picks her nose, scratches her head, wriggles. Lies with fantasy stories. Because of severity of behaviour disorder she was taken for examination to a Mental Hospital. At the Clinic, she tried to be tough, sought adult attention; dissatisfied with herself; disliked by children and cannot give and take in play. She shows no response to punishment, but tells Miss Z. that she does not smack her hard enough.

Clinical summary: diagnosed as primary antisocial conduct disorder; it was agreed to take her on for treatment. The mother, however, refused this, failed to bring her for her appointment or to acknowledge letters. It was heard from Mrs. Y., the second foster-mother who is fond of the child, that Alice has returned to live with her parents, where she is unhappy and badly treated. She seems to have settled down, however, and no further stealing is reported. The prognosis is doubtful; with unsuitable treatment Alice may become a hardened delinquent.

Causative factors: chiefly environmental; total lack of normal family life or secure home. Four changes of mother-substitute in 6 years, and now does not make genuine relationship with any of them. Rejection by her parents who are unsatisfactory and difficult personalities; their marital difficulties and unsettled life; choice of unsuitable foster-homes have all added together a chain of adverse influences to which Alice has reacted with defiance and dissocial behaviour.

312

Case No. 32: Freda *Age:* 6 years, 8 months. I.Q. 93.

A vivacious, active child, small for her age, thin and wiry. Friendly and self-possessed at interviews; talkative.

Referral: by school medical officer, on account of stealing (with her twin sister) and uncontrollable behaviour.

Family background: Freda and her twin, Peggy (who is not identical), are eldest in unstable, irregular family in which there are five children. Parents are separated; father, who lives with his mother, is seeking a divorce. Mother has the twins and one younger girl, aged five of this father. She has also had four illegitimate children, including deceased twins, by an American soldier who has now returned home. The two surviving babies are 7 and 16 months old.

Household consists of maternal grandparents, maternal uncle and aunt, mother and her five children, an old lady lodger, and three maternal uncles who come on leave at intervals.

Mother: a stocky, well-built, pleasant woman. Low intelligence; easy-going, irresponsible and ineffectual. Has had seven children in seven years, is now harassed with care of two babies; perplexed by inability to control twins and five-year-old girl. Discipline inconsistent, content to leave discipline to grandmother who has had care of twins at frequent intervals.

Father: a builder; was in Navy during the war, now demobilized; was a juvenile delinquent; since marriage has served sentence for stealing.While in Navy, went about with other women, drank heavily; now defaults with maintenance money. Mother says he kicked her, causing breast abscess for which she had to go to hospital. Irresponsible towards children; twins are uncertain as to who is their father.

Family has had frequent moves and lived in overcrowded conditions, yet maintained reasonably good home conditions of poor, working-class standard.

History: mother hints that twins were conceived before marriage and were unwanted. Bottle-fed; normal progress. Peggy is duller, sturdier, and more stable; still wets bed occasionally. Freda is

313

more intelligent, emotionally less stable. Habit-training satisfactory, health and appetite good. Twins share room, sleep well, but sometimes have to be locked in before settling down to sleep.

School record and intelligence: both below average in fundamental subjects. Freda knows a few letters, cannot read; poor vocabulary, talks incessantly. According to her teacher, she is inattentive and unable to concentrate. Steals, incites others to mischief.

In intelligence test, I.Q. 93 (twin sister 83). Response was impulsive and easily confused; concentration poor.

Personality and behaviour: twins are attached to each other, but quarrel; jealous of younger children, aggressive towards babies. Mother finds Freda, who resembles mother's family, easier to handle than Peggy, who resembles the father's family. Freda is full of vitality and daring, never nervous, defiantly untruthful, easily upset, and then cannot be persuaded to talk. Mother thinks that Peggy plans, and Freda carries out the delinquencies. They steal separately and together. They have no friends, bribe children to play with them. Both have a mania for money, and drinking water. Both will drink anything obtainable, including disinfectant and indigestion remedies. Freda is volatile, facile, suggestible and over-active. She quarrels and is spiteful with other children; loves attention and makes scenes. Likes drawing and writing better than playing with toys; likes to go to the cinema.

Clinical summary: diagnosed as primary antisocial conduct disorder; prognosis without prolonged re-educational treatment thought to be poor. Placement advised in foster-home where she and her sister could have individual care and re-education over a long period. This proved impracticable; recommendation made that the twins should be sent to a hostel for maladjusted children. Outcome inconclusive.

Causative factors: weak and unstable personality of mother; father's antisocial personality and rejection of children; disturbed and broken marital relationship; early interrupted mother-child relationship; inconsistent and divided discipline; broken family and irregular home background since early years. Constitutional inadequacy may also play some part in Freda's disturbance.

314

Case No. 33: Petula. *Age:* 7 years, 0 months. I.Q. 93.

Petula is a sturdy, pleasant-faced child who seems to be with-drawn and self-conscious, and unable to talk spontaneously.

Referral: by School Medical Officer, on account of pilfering, dis-obedience and sulky behaviour.

Family background: eldest of three children of unhappy marriage. During the war, the home was broken up. After father's demobi-lization, second child was very ill, parents then made up their differences for children's sake, but without success. Petula now lives with parents and maternal grandparents.

Mother: aged 34; a large, tearful, neurotic woman, depressed and miserable, with hysterical symptoms. Embittered, and anxious to discuss her disturbed relationship with husband; probably in need of treatment. She feels superior to her husband, is preoccupied in mourning the loss of her American lover, a married man who has returned home. She wants to believe the youngest child is his and does not want to accept husband's children. Relationship with Petula is ambivalent; feels her to be like she herself was; less fond of her than of the others. Nine months ago, made suicidal attempt in front of her.

Father: Artisan; joined Forces soon after marriage; unhappy with wife and lived with a married woman. Seldom at home until after demobilization. Less intelligent than his wife, and there is a marked difference in their tastes. Has few interests, takes no in-terest in his home, and openly dislikes the children.

Maternal grandmother: shared in children's upbringing, as family lived with her for a long time. She says mother is too lenient with them, and now threatens to turn her out of the house unless she is more firm.

The family has moved frequently; now lives in fairly comfort-able flat.

History: born in coastal town during air-raids. Breech birth. Parents' marriage already unhappy. At 4 months, mother went to live with grandmother and worked in a factory. Grandmother cared for the child, who lived in a nagging, restrictive atmosphere. Habit-training strict. At 2½, feeding difficulties. Mother then returned to husband; family lived in one room, but Petula's night-screaming forced them to leave. At 3, second child born; Petula had severe facial burn necessitating long treatment. At 3½, mother returned to grandmother, where she remained until a year ago. At 5, Petula was sulky, unhappy and disobedient. Feeding difficulties continued. Mother then expecting third child, and Petula would wander into other children's homes. She regarded her mother's American lover as her father.

School record and intelligence: started school at 5; likes it and works hard; good progress in all subjects. Friends are mainly older children, especially girls who swear. Twice Petula took other children's lunches. She is not regarded as a problem in school.

In intelligence test, I.Q. 93; she was self-possessed and grown-up; silent and showed no feeling.

Personality and behaviour: present problem includes pilfering flowers, food and jewellery, disobedience and sulky behaviour. She takes money from grandmother, spends shopping change. Whines and cries easily; undemonstrative; imaginative and tells lies. Usually shows aggression by silent, sullen behaviour.

Clinical summary: diagnosed as primary antisocial conduct disorder with minor neurotic tendencies; taken on for treatment. Made excellent progress; neurotic element in behaviour cleared up and she began to express herself in many achievements. Became more girlish, less defiant and difficult. Relationship to mother improved, and stealing ceased. Mother's attitude was changed, and she was able to modify her handling of the girl. Improvement has been maintained over some time. Prognosis good for normal character development, provided the home remains stable.

Causative factors: broken and unhappy home; unsettled environmental conditions during early years; disturbed marital relationship; rejection by the mother on account of the latter's hysterical disturbance; prolonged absence of father; inconsistency in

316

handling, with changing standards between mother and grand-mother.

Case No. 34: Ellen. *Age:* 8 years, 9 months. I.Q. 86.
and *Case No. 18:* Percy. *Age:* 10 years, 0 months. I.Q. 92.
    Ellen is pretty, wild, and defiant, and looks older than her years. Percy is good-looking, shy, and timid.

Referral: by probation officer. Percy, on account of breach of probation and breaking a glass window after having been remanded on probation for larceny and house-breaking; Ellen on account of being unmanageable and beyond control. Each has a long history of delinquent behaviour. In Percy's case this includes stealing, destructiveness, disobedience, truanting, staying out late at night, lying, house-breaking, and sexual games; in Ellen's, temper, tantrums, disobedience, screaming attacks, stealing, sexual offences, and staying out at night.

Family background: Ellen and Percy are the eldest of six children, each of whom is a social problem. The home background has always been unsatisfactory.

Mother: at 21, married a man many years her senior; husband reported impotent. After three years, lived with her cousin, Mr. X. Percy and Ellen were born before her marriage to Mr. X. Mrs. X. is quiet, washed-out looking, nervy, easily exasperated and tearful; unreliable in clinic attendances, and looked dirty and ill. She is overwhelmed by the children, inconsistent in handling them, continuously nagging. She has little to give them emotionally, intellectually, or materially. Particularly irritated by Ellen, whom she thrashes but cannot control; relationship is sado-masochistic and ambivalent. She prefers Percy, can handle him when he is not with Ellen. Does not give children pocket money; horrified when asked if Percy had received sex information at time of sexual offences and curiosity. Observed no masturbation, and says she would thrash if she did.

Father: works as a jobbing painter or as a porter in a public house. Was in the Army for $5\frac{1}{2}$ years, three of these abroad. Six months ago, as a result of a court order, obtained compassionate discharge because mother was unable to control the children. Discharged as medically unfit; operation before returning home. Dull intelligence, easy-going. Children are better when he is at home; his idea of discipline is to give periodic thrashings. Has little interest in children; neither Percy nor Ellen is fond of him.

Siblings: Sheila, aged seven, a bed-wetter, uncontrollable by mother; Paul, aged five, enuretic, screaming attacks at night; Simon, aged three; and a baby born during period when mother attended clinic. Percy and Ellen are very irresponsible with younger children.

Family originally lived for three years with mother's parents; during father's absence abroad, lived in another house, also overcrowded. Mother's brother lived with them; children know him better than father. At present live in council house, poorly furnished, dirty and smelly. Mother is a poor manager, children run wild. The family is notorious in the district.

History: (Percy). Unwanted baby, but mother consoled herself that he would supply evidence for divorce. Forceps delivery; breast-fed for three weeks. Handed over to grandmother who cared for him until he was two, by which time he was walking, talking and very clean. On return to mother, threw stone at Ellen, then a new baby. Sleeps alone; mother emphasizes need to separate girls and boys, but denies having seen sexual play between Percy and sisters. Healthy; appetite and sleep good. Never stolen from home. At nine, placed on probation after court appearance on charge of stealing and attempting to sell razor and watch. Unmoved by court proceedings; difficult while under supervision by probation officer. Six months later, he was charged with larceny of bicycle and indecent assault on girl of five. Charge dismissed because of insufficient evidence. Other offences, one with Ellen, included lighting a bonfire, wasting £5 worth of paraffin, joining other boys in smashing a butcher's shop.

History: (Ellen): also illegitimate. As baby was always crying. Breast-fed for one year because she kept crying for the breast. At
318

one year, was in hospital for three weeks, was weaned there. Toilet- and habit-training difficult, for which mother smacked her. Clean at three. When three, spread new baby's clothes on bed and urinated on them. Health good; sleeps well, but wakes early and fights with Percy. Slept in parents' bed until two years ago, now has her own bed in younger sister's room. Good appetite. No sex information given, thrashed for sexual games when younger.

Personality and behaviour: (Percy): mother protects him, makes excuses for his misdeeds yet thrashes him, and is furious because he does not mind. He delays owning up, unmoved by threats from police; says he will run away when father threatens to thrash him. He is disobedient and defiant at home, refuses to help; never plays but constantly fights with Ellen. Likes to read, but Ellen stops him, then they quarrel, but she wins. Complains that other boys fight him; never sticks up for himself. He is not reluctant to leave home.

Personality and behaviour: (Ellen): quick and impulsive; defiant, hard, with defensive veneer that makes her humourless. Talkative to family, indiscriminately so to strangers; provokes quarrels with younger children, spiteful to them, bites, hits and tyrannizes over them. Denies mischief until it is beyond proof; impervious to punishment. Mother is inconsistent with her. Ellen's attitude is one of defiance and fear; she has no genuine play activities or toys; likes needlework and handwork. At school, seeks limelight, bullies other children and demands show of affection. She was seen by the probation officer in the park with her face made up, rushing up to soldiers, and throwing herself on men lying in the sun; this led to one of them slapping her. Stole child's tricycle; grabs anything she wants. Temper tantrums when thwarted. Mother says she doesn't know right from wrong. Both parents are anxious for her to go away. Ellen is clearly a greater problem in the home and contributes considerably to Percy's disturbance.

School record and intelligence: the children go willingly to school and get on relatively well. Ellen's reports are fairly good, though the teachers say that she needs constant attention and is the ringleader in any trouble in class.

In intelligence test, *Ellen's* I.Q. was 86. Inadequate vocabulary. Reasoning powers specially poor. Says she dislikes school.

Percy's I.Q. was 92. Adequate vocabulary, good manner, some common sense. Slow in response, on the defensive, did not smile.

Clinical summary: (Percy): diagnosed as primary antisocial conduct. Since he has a strong relationship with his mother, the first recommendation was that he should attend the clinic whilst staying at home, and the sister should be sent away. This proved unsuccessful; the home environment deteriorated; boy was summoned for breach of probation when he absconded from remand home, and later truanted from school. Percy became more openly delinquent, failed to keep appointments at clinic. Placement in 'Q' camp or approved school then recommended. Observation of play at clinic revealed mild neurotic tendencies superimposed on a pronounced antisocial character. Preoccupied with sado-masochistic fantasies; submissive to authority; poor control of aggression; considerably dominated by delinquent sister. Percy is unable to act out his aggression in a socially accepted way; allows himself to be bullied for long time, then finds outlet in impulsive, aggressive act. Special difficulties in boy's character disturbance, especially his inability to voice grievances, necessitate environment where special care is taken not to mistake his submissiveness for obedience and social behaviour. Does well under very strict discipline, but character remains unchanged, and will be delinquent again if discipline is relaxed. Outcome inconclusive.

Clinical summary: (Ellen): diagnosed as primary antisocial conduct, and thought to have personality of prospective prostitute. Immediate placement in hostel recommended, but could not be carried out at once; treatment during intervening period advised. Ellen kept all appointments; quickly established good relationship to therapist; strong exhibitionistic tendencies became paramount. In time, strong sexual fantasies expressed; aggressive feeling towards mother, and positive feelings for father became conscious. During treatment, behaviour at home improved, but owing to circumstances beyond control of the clinic, she was sent to unsuitable hostel where she behaved violently, did malicious damage; said to be uncontrollable; returned after two months. Stayed at home for six months; now in hostel for maladjusted children. Outcome inconclusive, but case is being followed up. Prognosis thought to be doubtful, and definitely bad if hostel treatment is unsuitable.

Causative factors: (Ellen): largely environmental, allied to girl's personality. In particular, mother's weak personality, and her interrupted and sado-masochistic relationship with the girl; inconsistent handling; low standards of the home; presence of four younger siblings; father's prolonged absence from home when the situation became too much for the weak, over-burdened and ill mother.

Causative factors: (Percy): an unwanted child; disturbed relations with weak and neurotic mother; inconsistent and capricious handling from birth; low standards in crowded home; father's absence and ineffectual performance of role as parent.

Case No. 35: Maryann. *Age:* 8 years, 7 months. I.Q. 101.

Maryann is awkward and shy, and unwilling to talk about herself. Avoids personal contact, turns head away.

Referral: by R.A.F. Association welfare officer and by her grandmother on account of uncontrollable behaviour at home and at school, cruelty and spitefulness to other children and temper tantrums.

Family background: child of divorced parents. Mother remarried, and is about to divorce again. Child now lives with maternal grandmother.

Mother: aged 30; attractive actress and singer who has many men friends. Impulsive, unpredictable; quarrelsome, bad-tempered and fault-finding. As a child, she was difficult and uncontrollable. At 21, married Maryann's father after two weeks' acquaintance; he was 20 years her senior. Went to Burma. Divorced shortly after child's birth. When Maryann was five, married Mr. X., who is five years her junior; he is in the Army, and is being invalided out because of hysterical conversion symptoms. Mother scorns his low rank, refuses to live with him. He is the father of her two-year-old son, towards whom Maryann has behaved violently. Mother gives music lessons; refuses to have Maryann in her second home, a dreary, undecorated flat amongst ruined houses in a poor area of the city.

Father: Army officer, previously divorced; alcoholic, drug-addict. Unfaithful to wife during her pregnancy; uninterested in mother and child.

History: pregnancy and birth normal; bottle-fed. Rigidly trained by Norland nurse who tied the child's hands down at six weeks to prevent face-scratching. Before five, was intermittently with mother, father and grandmother, an aunt, foster-mothers, and at several boarding schools; two years in children's home; then with mother's second in-laws. Difficult baby, greedy and faddy about food; at two, aggressive, temper tantrums. At four, expelled from boarding school because of spitefulness, cruelty and violent behaviour towards other children. Between four and eight expelled from four schools for similar reasons. Longest period of adjustment is two years. At five, reacted to mother's second marriage by becoming coarse and playing with faeces and urine. Sleeps well but makes scenes about going to bed; appetite still greedy. Health good except for discharging ear at five; sent to hospital which she feared and hated. Now lives with grandmother and aunt; established extreme degree of quarrel relationship; rages are uncontrollable. She is physically violent, her manners are terrible; swears and provokes scenes. Grandmother thinks she is sexually abnormal.

School record and intelligence: despite frequent changes of school, progress good; likes school and is not backward.

In intelligence test, I.Q. 101; reserved and revealed little about herself. Scattered results. Rapport difficult.

Personality and behaviour: although grandmother and mother were frequently advised by numerous child guidance clinics over several years to send Maryann to a special school for maladjusted children, they refused to do so. Maryann is now exhibitionistic, attention demanding; afraid of other children and refuses to play with them. She is violent, uses rough language, shouts and kicks when thwarted. Likes to help at home, keeps her room tidy; is affectionate, but grandmother says this is cupboard love. Likes dancing and gymnastics and singing; reads a great deal. Maryann can be good as long as she has constant admiration.

Clinical summary: diagnosed as primary antisocial conduct disorder; thought to be a child who has been constantly mishandled over eight years. Taken on for observation; made good relationship at once; immediately gave evidence of her most pressing problems, which were largely sexual. Suitable placement away from home was recommended as the first step in treatment. An attempt was made to give grandmother insight enough to deal with the present situation until a suitable placement could be found; plans were made for Maryann to go to foster-home after period of psychiatric treatment. Grandmother was unable to cooperate on account of her own considerable disturbance, and broke off treatment and sent the child to a mental hospital. Prognosis is poor unless permanent placement can be found.

Causative factors: possibly constitutional, since both parents are unstable; complete absence of secure home life; failure to form a mother-relationship with any of the many people who cared for her; inconsistent handling; rejection by both parents; mother's marital difficulties; intense sado-masochistic relationship with mother and grandmother.

Case No. 36: Florence. *Age:* 9 years, 10 months. I.Q. 122.

A pale, sensitive child, silent and intense. Volunteered no spontaneous remarks; matter-of-fact in manner. Her mask-like expression and controlled voice indicated rigid control of anxiety. She wanted to be told what to do, and denied worries.

Referral: by Headmistress of school on account of stealing and lying and having been found searching other girls' things.

Family background: parents abroad, having left two daughters in hastily chosen boarding school a year ago. Family consists of a boy of 18 by mother's first husband, the father and two girls of mother's second marriage.

Mother: elderly; appears over-anxious; little security in her own life; self-deprecatory, says she has periods of uncertainty; believes that she has been too lenient and indulgent towards the girls, both of whom are fond of her. Well educated. At the Clinic, Florence expressed disappointment in mother, and showed much insecurity and uncertainty about parents' movements. Mother left girls in boarding school, and neither visited nor told them of her departure. On return, was a week in England before visiting them.

Father: many years abroad, and has seen little of Florence since she was 3. Unable to settle in England. Widely travelled.

Sibling: sister, also untruthful; Florence is jealous of her, believing that Pat had more as a child than she had. Pat is less disturbed than Florence. All the family are musical.

History: as a baby, Florence was with her mother. Made normal progress; no difficulties. Before 4, evacuated to grandmother's because of air-raids; mother visited her every fortnight. Florence was bewildered and frightened by evacuation and separation from mother; worried if mother failed to come. Grandparents elderly and restrictive. Father had returned to London when Florence was 3, but she went back to her mother only after father had gone abroad again. Health good; no sleeping or feeding disturbances. Family has had little security or home life; future is uncertain.

The children have not been abroad.

School record and intelligence: from an early age, Florence has had bad reports. First she went to village school; did not get on with other children. A year ago, went to boarding school; is bottom of class, knows she is backward, and expects to do badly. Daydreams; has history of purposeless lying; steals food for which she has no need; is envious.

In intelligence test, I.Q. 122. No unusual features.

Personality and behaviour: quiet, tense; popular at school; tells ghost stories, but unable to talk to therapist about them. Likes singing, plays piano and 'cello; rides and likes animals; dislikes French and arithmetic. Upset at having no letters from parents for 3 months during political crises overseas, and was preoccupied with fantasies. Has no special friends, feels left out of things and prefers to play with little ones. Likes strenuous games. Her matter-of-fact attitude towards all activities suggests that none of them is important to her. Shows great interest in talking about early memories.

Clinical summary: diagnosed as primary antisocial conduct disorder; taken on for individual treatment; made good emotional contact with therapist and responded well. Progress very satisfactory. Treatment continues.

Causative factors: lack of security in home background; generally unsettled living conditions; absence of parents; Florence's long periods away from home; mother's casual handling and possible neglect; frequent interruptions in mother-child relationship.

Case No. 37: Caroline. *Age:* 10 years, 4 months. I.Q. 90.

A plump, friendly girl, active and self-assured, and decided in whatever she does. Finger-nails severely bitten.

Referral: by Juvenile Court on account of truanting, stealing, running away from home and school retardation.

Family background: fourth child in Irish working-class family of eight children.

Mother: pretty, feckless Irishwoman who uses charm to escape responsibilities. Lives for the moment, is impulsive, unstable, casual, unreliable and ignorant. Probably of poor intelligence. Vague about details of lives of children, who have been given much sexual misinformation largely because of mother's denials and undue secrecy about the births of her children. Mother has poor health. She is too much occupied with younger children to give Caroline needed supervision, so Caroline goes her own way. Mother threatens, but never carries out punishment. After periods away from home, child reacted with difficult behaviour. Mother dismisses this, says all the children have been away, only Caroline gave trouble. Parents are resentful and ashamed about the disgrace Court proceedings have brought on family. Caroline punished for this disgrace. Mother is unconcerned about sending her away again.

Father: aged 37; artisan. Came from Ireland 10 years ago. Healthy, easy-going; not over-concerned about children. Sometimes knocks mother about, and mother in turn has treated older children harshly.

Siblings: four younger children are 6, 5 and 2 years and 2 months; Caroline good with them. Fifth child was born when Caroline was 4, and usurped her place in the home. She is hostile and jealous towards three older children, who knock her about.

Family have frequently been dispersed. They now live in crowded working-class home in poor street. House very clean.

History: pregnancy and birth normal; breast-fed while mother was in bed, then abruptly changed to bottle. Easily trained; good health and progress until 5, when evacuated to country. Lived there for a year with grandmother, several aunts and cousins. At 8, returned to grandmother for 4 months when seventh child was born (so far as mother can remember). Grandmother fond of Caroline, would have liked to keep her permanently. Caroline then had 7 months in a convent, a period in an institution and another in a children's home, and has been away from home more than any of the children. First stealing episode involved taking money from aunt during family quarrel; aunt took revenge by charging Caroline in Court with theft. For over 2 years, Caroline has been pilfering, lying, and for a year, running away from home. No evidence of neurotic difficulties beyond occasional night fears.

School record and intelligence: many absences from school; much below average in all subjects; has reached 7-year level in reading and spelling. Except for pilfering, behaviour in class and playground satisfactory; has definite practical bent.

In intelligence test, I.Q. 90. Some glibness and verbal facility; impatient; poor concentration. No special gifts.

Personality and behaviour: mother says Caroline is the most demanding of all the children; more resentful of punishment and

326

threats than the others. She feels neglected; is bewildered by her own dishonest, impulsive and wilful behaviour. When not in trouble, is friendly and talkative; when in difficulties, is silent, resentful of correction, and reacts to criticism or rejection by outbreaks of wandering. Looks after baby reliably, and does household tasks. Likes dolls and jewellery; is anxious for attention. Since Court case, other children have avoided her; feels ostracized at school. Has to be cornered before owning up to truanting and stealing.

Clinical summary: diagnosed as primary antisocial conduct disorder with mild neurotic trends; taken on for treatment. Made good relationship to therapist, showed some degree of progress, but mother was casual and failed to keep appointments. Case had to be closed when Caroline was sent by Juvenile Court to an Approved School. She settled well in a Remand Home, and says she prefers to be away from home, but is reported to be one of the most difficult 10-year-olds ever to have been in the home. She is disobedient, lies, scribbles on walls, and is precocious. Cried every night during first week because she slept alone. Prognosis thought to be fair if school handling is sympathetic, and if re-education away from home can be carried on over long period. Follow-up shows that she has now settled down happily in the approved school, has an understanding Mother Superior, and her school work has begun to improve satisfactorily.

Causative factors: frequently interrupted and disturbed mother-child relationship; position in the family in relation to her overburdened and weak mother; rejection by parents and older siblings; inconsistent discipline over many years; insecurity about her rightful home background.

Case No. 38: Susan. *Age:* 11 years, 7 months. I.Q. 81.

Susan is a tall, pale-faced girl, neatly dressed, but clumsy and awkward. Rather overgrown.

Referral: by probation officer on account of stealing and unmanageable behaviour at home

Family background: only surviving child of working-class parents separated six months before referral. Susan lives with her mother.

Mother: aged 37; excitable, attractive, hysterical. Looks stern and has hostile, anxious, and truculent manner. Came to clinic dressed in heavy mourning for her son, aged 9, who had died of tuberculosis 2 years previously. She idolized this boy, makes an exaggerated show of putting flowers on his grave; practised strict economies to save £50 for tombstone. She has extreme quarrel relation with Susan, resentful that she is left with girl instead of with father and son. Blames Susan for all domestic troubles, is openly hostile and rejecting, and always deriding her. Despite quarrels, Susan and she dependent upon each other. Discipline inconsistent; has beaten her until neighbours called in N.S.P.C.C.; at other times indulges her. Mother and child rival each other for father's attention, and for food, money and clothes. Mother's family has history of tuberculosis and childhood fits.

Father: aged 36; invalided out of Army, now unskilled labourer. Difficult and miserly. Suffers from rheumatism and backache; alcoholic. Did not want Susan, and has no affection for or interest in her; nags and hits her. Father's family has history of temperamental instability.

History: mother badly treated by father during pregnancy. Baby breast-fed for two weeks; greedy. At one month, mother developed breast fever, went to hospital; Susan cared for by maternal aunt until three months. Cried a great deal; greedy, lazy. Habit-training rigid, rapidly became over-clean, and early disgust of messing became pronounced. Active, tomboyish child. Sleep restless, some sleep-walking. Eats ravenously, never satisfied, yet daily quarrels when mother forces her to eat what she does not like. Mother washes her. While not robust, no serious illnesses; week in hospital recently for removal of birthmark from top of head.

School record and intelligence: began school at 4½; attended four schools, which she liked. Retarded in all subjects; now in class for backward children. She creates disturbances, is excitable and quarrelsome with other girls, cannot be trusted, is demanding and discontented. Makes quarrel relation with one particular teacher. Dislikes holidays. Achievements are sketchy.

In intelligence test, I.Q. 81. Thought processes rather primitive, mainly associative links; uncritical, with poor memory. Likes first-aid classes, and wants to be a nurse. Unworried by failure.

Personality and behaviour: Mother says she never shows affection, is always demanding money and food, angry when refused. Accuses mother of hurting her, is aggressive and cheeky; makes scenes; begs mother to beat her. Is good and helpful with strangers, likes to visit; at home is greedy, provocative and unmanageable; has stolen food and money from home, and once from neighbour. Is a girl guide; likes going to socials where she gives recitations. Likes films. Dislikes going to church, which mother compels her to do three times every Sunday as well as visiting brother's grave.

Clinical summary: diagnosed as primary antisocial conduct disorder; taken on for treatment at clinic for 10 months. At first, nervous and apprehensive; later became defiant and provocative, tried to quarrel with the therapist. Talked a great deal about ill-treatment she had received from her father, vowed that she was worse off than other girls. Did not want to stay in present home because, she said, she would not grow right. After some treatment, her adjustment improved. With much persuasion, mother agreed to let her go to an approved school as a voluntary scholar. Made good progress for two terms with the support of a cooperative probation officer. Mother failed to cooperate, demanded her return because she herself was lonely. Family situation had deteriorated. Follow-up is being continued, but case is regarded as unsatisfactory owing to mother's failure to continue with clinic's recommendations.

Causative factors: Mother's aggressive disturbed personality and rejection of girl whom she unconsciously identifies with her own hated sister; difficult, alcoholic father; loveless home and disturbed family relationships; inconsistent discipline; sado-masochistic relation between parents and between mother and girl.

Case No. 39: Rita. *Age:* 11 years, 9 months. I.Q. 132.

Rita is a well-grown girl; has marked facial disfigurement. Very tense manner of speaking covers up anxiety; walks with exaggerated swaying of the hips. Nails badly bitten.

Referral: by her mother on account of stealing, lying, dirtiness and disobedient and defiant behaviour.

Family background: elder of two girls who resemble each other like twins, from stable but unhappy home.

Mother: short, thick-set woman with affected manner. Her upbringing was strict. She is intelligent, and is highly trained accountant; carried on full-time work while Rita was a baby. Since birth of second child, gave this up, now does part-time work, but wishes to resume career. Is preoccupied with her own health; talks to Rita about past illnesses, about an internal growth she thought to be cancerous, and threatens Rita with imagined 'future paralysed condition'. Has quarrel relation with her own family; identifies Rita with her young sister, with whom she has seriously quarrelled. She dislikes Rita, sees no good in her; denies her pocket money, beats and slaps her during quarrels, and is disgusted with her dirty habits. She denies the girl's obvious facial disfigurement and opposes treatment for it. Mother feels that whole relationship with Rita went wrong at birth; made bad beginning; the child was cared for by a housekeeper in early months, then had many changes of nannie.

Father: a salesman; was in Services for four years, and abroad for 18 months. From six to ten, Rita saw him only when he was home on leave. He now travels daily to London. Rita and he are fond of each other; he is strict, threatens to cane her, but usually only shouts and makes scenes. More patient than mother, but supports what she says. Dislikes Rita's dirty habits. The girl tells the parents they do not love her, and that no other children are expected to do so much housework. Discipline is old-fashioned and restrictive; bread and water for a week after quarrels.

Sibling: sister aged five, who resembles Rita. She is sunny-natured, affectionate, and mother's favourite. Although Rita is jealous of her, she prefers her to anyone else.

The family live in a comfortable, clean home of lower-middle-class standards.

History: mother's pregnancy difficult because she continued working. Birth normal; rejected immediately by mother because of poor, thin appearance; breast-fed for two weeks. Mother then returned to business, baby bottle-fed and cared for by house-keeper. At three months, severe gastric illness; at 15 months, whooping cough; measles, chickenpox and German measles before three. During first year, had three nannies, one of whom had nervous breakdown. Excessive frustrations of infancy led to feeding difficulties; habit-training strict; reliably clean at nine months; relapsed at 15 months during whooping cough; after struggle, clean at two. Walked and talked early. Sleep good, though occasionally talks. At three, visited maternal grandmother for three months; standards greatly relaxed; grandfather gave the child the pocket money the mother had denied her. At nearly four, severe facial burn during London blitz (detailed circumstances as to how this occurred are unknown). Bandaged for five months. At 4½, meningitis; three months in bed, a further three months' convalescence. At five, 12 days in hospital with tonsillectomy. At eight, occasional wetting and soiling, which were promptly and harshly dealt with. Since going to school has had mumps and recurrence of measles and chickenpox. During last two years, ear and mastoid trouble, further operation probable. A hair wart on her face was medically treated. Rita worries greatly about her mother's health, and is preoccupied about the permanent paralysis which the latter threatens.

School record and intelligence: started school at 4½, but many absences because of illness. Went to convent boarding school at time of sister's birth, and to three other schools. Attainments average; teachers think highly of her, but say she has periods of looking dense.

In intelligence test, I.Q. 132; matter-of-fact and impersonal; examiner found her too reserved to make a real contact. Responses quick and accurate, showed a wide scatter from nine years to superior adult level on verbal tests.

Personality and behaviour: since six to seven, Rita has been defiant and disobedient; since eight to nine, has been stealing. Fierce nail-biter; episodes of wetting and soiling during last three years.

DELINQUENT AND NEUROTIC CHILDREN

Mother describes her as sulky, defiant, self-pitying; does not value things; is out to please outsiders. She is untidy, lazy, and has tempers; her habits are dirty, and she refuses to wash. Obstinate, but always lies in such a way that she is found out. Not aggressive towards other children, but prefers younger ones. Has no special friends or real interests. Hates housework, likes only swimming and cooking and collecting stamps. She is a girl guide and wants to be a domestic science teacher.

Clinical summary: diagnosed as primary antisocial conduct disorder; she and mother were offered treatment. Some adjustment made in mother-child relationship but mother showed little insight, failed to cooperate, and treatment was discontinued when both said they wished to stop. Both partners unwilling to give up their intense quarrel relationship. Prognosis under these family circumstances is poor, but Rita will probably be helped to some extent by her move to high school, where she will have better opportunities for her good abilities. Outcome inconclusive.

Causative factors: primarily mother's complete rejection; general neglect of child's psychological needs throughout babyhood; lack of enduring mother-relationship, with frequent and haphazard changes of nannies and others caring for her; girl's severe illnesses in early years and resultant need for special care; disturbed relationship between mother and child which has resulted from mother's dissatisfaction with her role as a woman, and refusal to play part of mother; father's long absences; harsh and unsympathetic methods of discipline used by both parents.

Case No. 40: Minnie. *Age:* 11 years, 10 months. I.Q. 84.

Minnie is small, attractive and friendly, though subdued and fearful. She talks with a slight lisp.

Referral: by head teacher on account of stealing, lying, soiling her bed, nail-biting, feeding difficulties and defiant, obstinate behaviour.

Family background: adopted at 2½ by a couple because they could not have children of their own. They wanted a boy, but because both they and Minnie were Roman Catholics, she was given to them.

Adoptive mother: middle-aged, untidy woman, unstable and strong-natured. Ambivalent towards Minnie, frequently threatening to send her away. Strict but inconsistent, and makes wild threats. Takes holiday lodgers, and has many domestic problems. Looks after a boy cousin, with whom Minnie is unfavourably compared. He is three classes above Minnie at school; she is antagonistic towards him, and has stolen his watch.

Adoptive father: a waiter. Cold, thin-lipped, middle-aged man of Italian extraction. Hard, impatient and strict towards Minnie, without feeling for her. Openly declares he wants her sent away. Much vacillation between him and wife about Minnie's upbringing, and quarrelling over whether or not she is to be kept. There are many restrictions and little affection in the home.

The family live in moderately comfortable circumstances.

History: shortly after birth, Minnie was abandoned on doorstep of a church. For first 20 months, lived in a charitable Institution. First foster-home was unsuccessful; moved from one social institution to another until she was adopted. On arrival at new home, was passive and fearful, undersized and badly nourished. Had walked since 18 months, but knew only the word 'sit'. Toilet habits reasonably well established at time of adoption; then some expected lapses, which were dealt with fairly tolerantly. Sleep and appetite good. Except for colds and sore throats, health good. Snores and mouth-breathes; removal of adenoids recommended by school doctor. As a child, cried easily. Apparently unmoved by air-raids. At nine, because of local gossip, was told of adoption; received information calmly, but imagined there was no longer any need to obey her mother. First period of stealing began shortly after starting school, second after she was nine, and continues. History of feeding difficulties, nail-biting, picking and pulling at herself.

School record and intelligence: first school was in a city; she disliked it and quarrelled with other children. Then went to convent school for two years; poor reports; unable to concentrate, talked to herself. At present school, does badly; reading very elementary; average age of class is 10, and her work is below the average of the class in all subjects. Requires constant individual attention. In intelligence test, I.Q. 84; basal age seven, results showed long and irregular scatter. Failed all reasoning tests.

Personality and behaviour: Minnie is tomboyish and lively; picks dull friends. Gets on better with girls than boys, but lives largely in world of her own; acts and talks to herself while walking in street. Lies pointlessly and arrogantly, brazen about stealing. Spiteful and aggressive with other children, mischievous in school, disobedient to mother. Reacts to insecurity with arrogance and aggression. Prefers to play out-of-doors, and is devoted to her dog and kitten. She has regular pocket-money.

Clinical summary: diagnosed as primary antisocial conduct disorder; she and mother taken on for treatment. Mother continued to vacillate a good deal about sending Minnie to an institution. Over a long period, however, it was possible to modify her attitude and to show her something of how both parents were rejecting and ambivalent towards the child. Minnie responded quickly, whereupon the mother refused to send her for further treatment, saying that Minnie had become more amiable and her personality had 'mellowed'. Follow-up showed one further episode of stealing, with which the school had dealt satisfactorily, but Minnie's behaviour is basically unchanged. Case was closed as incomplete and unsatisfactory, and prognosis without prolonged re-educational treatment remains poor.

Causative factors: insecure babyhood in institutions; lack of early mother-relationship; adoption by unsuitable and unstable parents; inconsistent discipline; parents' ambivalent and rejecting handling; disturbed relationship between parents and their unsatisfactory relationship to the girl. The stealing episodes were found to be related to her jealousy of the preferred boy cousin in the home.

Case No. 41: Maureen. *Age:* 12 years, 2 months. I.Q. 120.

A pretty, friendly girl who makes an easy superficial contact. Active, alert, and interested, but talkativeness may cover anxiety.

Referral: by head teacher and parents on account of stealing, truanting, temper tantrums, social maladjustment, and gossiping.

Family background: illegitimate child, adopted by mother two years after marriage, 4½ years ago. No stable home until she was 10. Now lives with mother, adoptive father and mother's three legitimate children who are all under three years.

Mother: an attractive but hard-faced, emotional woman. Suffers from high blood pressure and is said to have temper tantrums. Maureen's real father deserted mother before child was born. Mother is exasperated by Maureen's gossiping about her illegitimacy, which mother has tried to conceal, and refuses to discuss with the girl. She has no insight into the girl's difficulties; handles her with extreme severity, restricts all activities unnecessarily, and allows her little responsibility. She feels the girl is an intolerable burden and that she is becoming like her father. In her anxiety about this, has beaten Maureen with a dog leash, for which she was reported to the N.S.P.C.C. Much unconscious hostility to the girl, and has rejected her over a number of years, but more openly since the birth of her three babies.

Father: wealthy, spoilt only son, who has made no contribution towards keeping the mother or child. Mother describes him as a rotter. Maureen remembers nothing of him, but recalls her change of name. While talking of him to the therapist, made a model of mongrel dog, said it was like her father and sobbed broken-heartedly. She believes he is dead.

Adoptive father: large, friendly, thoughtful man. Was in business before the war. Boyhood ambition was to be a tramp; became successful officer in the Army for five years. Likes military routine and order, which he would like to bring into home life. Stable influence on mother, excuses her rejection of Maureen as nerves and war strain. During treatment showed greater insight than mother, but was prevented from genuine cooperation by her uncompromising attitude. He tries to treat Maureen as he treats his own children, but admits he prefers them. Blames mother for Maureen's gossiping, but is equally adamant about refusing to discuss the true position with the girl, who shows no attachment to him.

The family now live in stable home in comfortable circumstances.

History: Maureen lived in three foster-homes between four months and 10 years in addition to being evacuated at five years. During and following pregnancy, mother in great financial difficulties. Birth normal; breast-fed for two months before going to first foster-home at four months. Satisfactory home; mother visited her weekly. In third year, second foster-home where there were six older children. Feeding difficulties developed before this removal and continued. Habit-training not achieved. Until three, sucked piece of blanket while sleeping; sleep much disturbed by walking, talking and head-banging. Appetite slow. At five, evacuated to home of elderly couple in country who were devoted to her, anxious she should have perfect manners. Mother's visits infrequent. Because elderly couple became ill, child removed to third foster-home where there was a large rough and tumble crowd of children, and, unlike previous home, Maureen had to do everything for herself, but adapted herself and responded well to change. Although mother married at this time, Maureen remained in foster-home, as mother could not find a house. At 10, returned to mother who now had eight-months baby; two more children quickly followed. Shared mother's room at first during father's absences, but head-banging disturbed mother, so slept in baby's room. Now likes to share adoptive father's bed. Not yet menstruating. Masturbated after birth of second baby; shows great interest in sex matters; mother unable to discuss these or pre-menstrual fears with her. Six months ago mother, in anger, told her adoptive father was not real father. Maureen's behaviour then changed, feeding difficulties returned, number of fears developed, began stealing food, especially baby food, at home.

At five, tonsils and adenoids operation, otherwise health good.

School record and intelligence: started school at four; liked it at once, but naughty and attention-seeking. Through evacuation, missed much; backward on return, but has now caught up and is making good progress; working hard for matriculation. Wants to be a nurse, an ambition she has had since seven. Best subjects art, needlework, and handwork.

In intelligence test, I.Q. 120. Quick in responses, independent, able to evaluate her performance. Excitable. Insecure.

Personality and behaviour: mother complains of her jealous, quarrelsome nature; lacks standards about her person and clothes, behaves like the nobody she feels herself to be. Good in the house, likes to look after babies, but if allowed authority takes too much. Lacks staying-power. Makes scenes at home; chooses undesirable, older girl-friends; over-dramatizes herself and slanders her mother to neighbouring women.

Clinical summary: diagnosed as a case of primary antisocial conduct disorder; taken on for treatment. Made good progress in which she played out aggressive fantasies towards siblings and parents; certain neurotic tendencies were revealed as subsidiary to her dissocial conduct. She became aware that her mother's rejection was because of her illegitimacy; her own difficult personality and feelings of inadequacy were somewhat overcome and her school work improved. An attempt was made to modify the mother's attitude and to persuade her to deal more satisfactorily with the 'gossip', but she was uncooperative, failed to keep appointments, refused to accept help or explanations for Maureen's behaviour. Rejection of Maureen remains unchanged. Boarding school placement recommended and case is being followed carefully. Prognosis remains doubtful.

Causative factors: in the girl's 'slandering' these were directly related to the deliberate and clumsy deception about her true parentage, and failure of mother to overcome her own guilt about it and accept Maureen. Factors underlying the faulty character development were thought to be insecurity of early years, unsettled home throughout childhood; lack of enduring mother-relationship; rejection by mother; complete absence of father until 10. Homecoming to find parents preoccupied with new babies intensified jealousy and feelings of inadequacy. Mother's pregnancies and reticence about sexual and family

337

matters important to the child exaggerated her pre-pubertal, sexual curiosity, led to her stealing, gossiping, and other dis-social behaviour.

Case No. 42: Meg. *Age:* 13 years, 3 months. I.Q. 109.
   Tall, red-haired girl, rather odd-looking; wears glasses. Tense and unsmiling in initial interview, looked unhappy.

Referral: by School Medical Officer on account of telling lies, being 'light-fingered', unhelpful in the house. This has been a problem for six months. She makes up stories and tells purposeless lies, mainly about things she has not done, or people she has not met. Stole money and pilfered food from larder.

Family background: illegitimate child of sailor who lived with mother while father was overseas in the Navy. Mother died of pneumonia when Meg was 3. Child now lives with her aunt, Mrs. X., with whom she and the other children and 'Gran', their guardian, came to live after the house was bombed. Because Meg resembles her mother, father and aunt are particularly fond of her.

Father: aged 46; solid, taciturn. Kept in touch with family all through separations; anxious to have all children together and have housekeeper to care for them. Demobilized 2 years ago, now works as rural labourer. Does his best for children, but lacks sympathy and imagination; adopts harsh and ignorant attitude to Meg's romancing which he wishes to deal with by repressive measures. Expects Meg to do much domestic work, but is fond of her.

Aunt: an ignorant old lady, untidy and unkempt. Well-intentioned; gossips freely; fond of the children. Places great emphasis upon saving money, expects children to work for her. Maintains strict discipline, forbids friends to come to the house and children to join in youth clubs or inter-school activities. Deals with Meg's lying by frightening her with stories about God hearing her and going to prison. Talked freely about Meg in the child's presence, ignored the child's sobs.

Siblings: two older step-brothers who work on nearby farms; one sister, aged 11, is prettier than Meg, who gets on well with all siblings except older boy.

The family lives in half of a broken-down cottage in an isolated rural area.

History: little known of Meg's early history. After her birth, father came home, forgave wife and accepted Meg. He was overseas when mother died. Children were cared for by elderly guardian, who found difficulty in dealing with four young children; she disliked Meg, favouring the others. Despite protests from relatives, guardian refused to leave her home in coastal town during 'blitz' until house was bombed, when Meg was 6. After this, children were nervous of the dark and aeroplanes, but settled down in new surroundings; did not mind guardian leaving them after 3 months. Though shy, with some feeding difficulties, Meg was no more difficult than other children. Always greedy; pilfered food from larder. Not really difficult until 6 months ago. Menstruated 3 months ago; no information given about this.

School record and intelligence: makes average progress. Teacher feels home discipline is too restricting. Meg likes school, but has no friends; is regarded as bossy by other children.

In intelligence test, I.Q. 109. Good vocabulary.

Clinical summary: diagnosed as showing a mild primary antisocial conduct disorder; not thought to be very disturbed. Recommended that she should be taken on for observation in order to find out more about the story-telling, which seemed to be connected with her doubts about her father and her wish to please her aunt who she felt was the only person to whom she belonged, and whom she feared leaving. Father refused to co-operate, however; insisted on the girl's return to him and would not permit further attendance at the Clinic. Treatment remains inconclusive, but the case is being followed up.

Case No. 43: Peggy. *Age:* 13 years, 6 months. I.Q. 124.

A pretty, self-possessed girl, on the defensive and withdrawn. Healthy-looking, well dressed.

Referral: by School Medical Officer for lying, stealing, temper outbursts, wandering, staying out at night and destructiveness.

Family background: illegitimate; deserted by mother at 14 months; boarded out by Public Assistance Committee to various homes until Mr. and Mrs. X. took her from hospital when she was almost 2. They considered adopting her, but as parental history was unknown, did not do so.

Foster-mother: hard-faced, bad-tempered-looking woman; anxious and disturbed. Attitude towards Peggy is selfish, neurotic and emotional. Plays on child's feelings, keeping her in state of insecurity and dependence, and is demanding. Professes affection, yet torments her; takes sadistic satisfaction in girl's tears and unhappiness. Lacks sympathy, insight and understanding of her needs; out of touch with her activities. Denies anything is wrong, yet made accusations publicly. Told school that Peggy had been in approved school. Keeps her with her as constant companion. Declares that real mother was of no account, that she has it on good authority mother was well known to police. Her own unhealthy, emotionally seductive attitude to the girl and her instability have contributed to the girl's difficulties.

Foster-father: Artisan; not in Services. Quiet, placid. Peggy is shy but fond of him. He fails to understand her needs; does not carry out his threats; dislikes punishing her.

Family lives in well-kept flat of good standard.

History: nothing known of early history. Apparently sleep has always been restless; appetite ravenous. When she steals food, leaves tiny portion behind. Has attended two other clinics because of severe nail-biting, destructiveness, cruelty towards cats and dogs, lying and pilfering, and not mixing with other children. Fantasy companions younger than she is. Has wandered for a number of years; on several occasions spent night out of doors, because she 'just had to'. First of these incidents occurred following discovery from Sunday School companions that foster-mother was not real mother. Other such incidents followed scenes with foster-mother. Health good, though slightly pigeon-chested. Measles three times between 5 and 8; whooping cough at 6. Later it was found that Mrs. X. had at first considered legally adopting the child, but, on discovering that she was illegitimate, had cancelled the arrangement, and she was returned to the Public Assistance Committee. She has also been returned to the children's home for a month or so when Mrs. X. was ill. When questioned, the girl was polite and apologetic for the trouble she had caused, and wanted to return to Mrs. X.

School record and intelligence: regarded as a problem child; when younger, did not play with other children. Now goes to secondary modern school; progress fairly good, but failed in scholarship examination because arithmetic was below standard. Teachers describe her as polite but restless, with poor concentration; year older than class average. Foster-mother forbids her taking part in school social activities.

In intelligence test, I.Q. 124. Quick reaction, facile, adaptable and vivacious. High verbal fluency, but restless and insecure.

Personality and behaviour: as a young child, was destructive; did not mix with other children, screamed and kicked when they came near her. Now described as a nice personality, well-mannered, but inhibited and still does not mix with others. Good imagination, speaks well, good sense of humour. Some dramatic ability. Erratic and temperamental, sometimes childish. Her strong tendency to romancing makes her difficult in social situations. No liking for sewing, reading or writing; occasionally watches sport. Fond of animals, but has no established or sustained interests.

Clinical summary: diagnosed as a case of primary antisocial conduct; taken on for observation with group of girls. Adjustment in foster-home thought to be unsatisfactory, with insufficient scope for her abilities; boarding school recommended, and attempts made to find place for her. In the group, she was shy and inhibited at first, but confidence increased, relationships improved. Liked to promote activities, showed pleasure in them. Individual interviews revealed material indicating that disturbance is only partially resolved, and long period of re-education away from home

M

DELINQUENT AND NEUROTIC CHILDREN

required. But considerable progress has been made, and prognosis thought to be good. Mrs. X. pleased with progress, but reluctant to let her go to boarding school; has permitted her to join Youth Club and another club. Follow-up shows improvement maintained over long period; girl now enjoys life more. Various possibilities for a career were opened up.

Causative factors: unhappy babyhood with desertion of mother and failure to form satisfactory mother-relationship; disturbed personality of foster-mother with inconsistent, ambivalent and sadistic treatment; lack of adequate father-relationship; general insecurity of home background.

Case No. 44: Doreen. *Age:* 13 years, 11 months. I.Q. 94.

A healthy-looking, nicely-dressed girl; wears glasses. Voice is high-pitched and monotonous. Appears to be fairly mature, but attitude is defiant.

Referral: by school medical officer for stealing, lying, not mixing well, difficult behaviour at school and home.

Family background: younger of two children; father died when she was three and brother 12, since when family has had much financial stress. Standards of home maintained at good working-class level.

Mother: childishly dressed, harassed-looking woman; readily becomes nagging and complaining; unreliable in her reports. Fond of Doreen, but impatient; ambivalent and inconsistent. At clinic, insisted child was abnormal, blaming head injuries for delinquency. Deals with situation by exhorting promises to be good, but constantly finds fault. Later refused treatment for child, despite continued complaints, saying she could not spare her. Since father's death, mother and child sleep together.

Father: builder; invalided out of Army with T.B. Family highly strung. Doreen hardly remembers him, believes he died from pneumonia.

Sibling: older brother; served in Army during war. He and

342

Doreen used to e good friends; now he is strict and critical, and she is less fond of him. He was difficult as a boy; enuretic until 14. *History:* miserable baby. Bottle-fed; feeding difficulties from birth; difficult to handle; temper and breath-holding attacks; screamed when thwarted. Nervous as a child; bed-wetting until five or six, though almost dry at three; relapsed after father's death when family lived with younger brother of father. Periods of screaming in sleep; difficult to get to bed at night, refused to get up in morning. Frightened of birds and of jokes played on her by brother. Mother says she is spoilt by uncle, a confectioner, unmarried, who has poor health and is deaf. Though generally giving in to her, occasionally the uncle becomes strict. Suffered from usual childish illnesses. At 12, tonsils and adenoids removed; at 11, away from school for 10 months as T.B. suspect. As baby, fell off chair; at three, stood on uncle's tennis racket, fell and was knocked out; between four and five, fell downstairs and had concussion; at five, several falls, hurting head each time. Knocked over by dog; fell off bicycle at six; at 13, accident to arm. Thumb has slight disability following an injury.

School record and intelligence: described as restless and lackadaisical, with much attention-seeking and babyish behaviour. Reports poor; is careless and clumsy, bad at games and P.T. Head teacher describes her as wild and uncontrollable, not amenable to school discipline; wilful, does not mix well, has to buy her friends, and is said to have sadistic tendencies towards other children.

In intelligence test, I.Q. 94. Attitude was submissive, anxious, deferential and apologetic for failures. Good verbal facility.

Personality and behaviour: mother says Doreen is cruel to animals and small children; is provocative, makes scenes; impatient and destructive; quickly flares into temper; demanding from mother; throws things on floor when requests refused; dirty and untidy; careless about personal hygiene; cannot save money; must have what she wants at once. Unwilling to help mother; likes to play mother and uncle off against each other. Well developed; has started menstruating. No friends; likes to play with younger children, whom she either torments or plays with as one of themselves. Few interests. Wants to be waitress or nurse. Happiest when she can have sweets and go to cinemas. Likes music; has fine singing voice.

At the clinic, she was lifeless, without energy, uninterested in interviews or intelligence tests.

Clinical summary: diagnosed as case of primary antisocial conduct disorder; recommended that she attend clinic with group of adolescent girls. In group, was at first blushing and unsure of herself which she counteracted by exhibitionistic behaviour. Gradually paired off with child of stronger character, but in many ways demonstrated poor ego-development and inhibition of imagination and action. Made conscious of dependence and inability to stand competition, which brought out obsessional traits as defences. Continued to show off and bluff, talked much rubbish to confuse therapist. This and other defences were interpreted; reacted with histrionic behaviour, noisiness, copying of other girls and sadistic behaviour. Discussed her feelings about examinations at school, delight in dressing up and acting. Then became quieter; strong transference to therapist developed. Behaviour at home improved; at this point, mother declined further treatment with insincere excuses, saying girl was now no trouble. Prognosis thought to be only fair; danger that girl will become confirmed delinquent.

Causative factors: disturbed and sado-masochistic relationship with mother; mother's ambivalent and inconsistent handling; early loss of father; failure to form good relationship with either brother or uncle, which might have helped her.

Case No. 45 : Bertha. *Age:* 13 years, 11 months. I.Q. 110.

An attractive, plump girl with friendly manner; mature for her age. Expression was solemn and sulky when she came to Clinic.

Referral: by mother for stealing, lying, 'wolfing' her food, nail-biting, staying out late at night with men. She has a history of being uncontrollable since infancy.

Family background: only child of parents who have been legally separated for the past 2 years.

344

Mother: aged 40; has petulant, sullen expression, slight defect in one eye; smartly dressed. Intelligent, but highly emotional; quickly dissolves into tears. Unsympathetic towards Bertha, expressing open hostility. Much animosity towards husband whose faults she sees in Bertha. Restrictive and rejecting in handling the girl, soon gives up in exasperation. Very tied to her own parents with whom she and Bertha have lived for many years. Several changes of home which is now shared with many outsiders and relatives.

Father: a skilled artisan, never in Forces. Work has necessitated absence from home. For some years, has been living with another woman by whom he has a child. This affair went on for 3 years unknown to wife; other affairs previously. Mother says marriage was unsuccessful from beginning; Bertha blamed for much parental discord. Father maintains mother and child, sends gifts at Christmas. Mother used to threaten child with father, while he undermined her discipline by reversing her decisions. Bertha threatens to go to father.

Grandparents: autocratic, possessive; ill-disposed towards father. Bertha is only grandchild.

History: birth normal; breast-fed for 6 days until mother developed peritonitis and appendicitis; in nursing home for 4 weeks, and Bertha sent to maternity home. For next 6-8 months, cared for by maternal grandmother. Mother vague about early history; baby protested about weaning. Habit-training rigid; periods of wetting if upset until 8-9 years. Until 4, father home only at weekends. Unmanageable since early years; screaming fits and temper tantrums from 2-8; later nail-biting and wolfing of food. Appetite always enormous, though faddy about food. At 4, whooping-cough; at 5, chicken-pox; measles at 6. Health then good. A year ago, in hospital for two hammer-toes; said to have been a trial.

School record and intelligence: five changes of school. Failed scholarship examination at 11; now in third year at secondary modern school; thirtieth in class of thirty-one. Regarded as difficult problem, since more mature than other girls, making difficulties.

Behaviour is sullen, temperamental and unreliable. Teacher describes her as an excitable, play-acting type.

In intelligence test, I.Q. 110; mental age 15. No unusual features.

Personality and behaviour: mother describes Bertha as disobedient and argumentative; dominates other children; cannot keep friends; constantly enthusiastic about people, then tires of them. Uncontrolled; mother fears sexual precocity; likes male company, has boy friends whom she meets with group of girls. Good at games and needlework; likes animals, wants to work in kennels. Likes to work out of doors. Wants to leave home. Declares she gets on better with her own friends than with mother.

Clinical summary: diagnosed as a case of primary antisocial conduct disorder with mild neurotic trends in an adolescent girl with a provoking and unsympathetic mother. Taken on for treatment and some remedial education. Has not yet worked up to the level of her intelligence, but otherwise has done well despite unsatisfactory home environment. Improved relations with her teachers. Recommended that she go to boarding school. Follow-up satisfactory.

Causative factors: rejection by parents at early age; parental and grandparental discord; prolonged absence and desertion of father; inconsistent and divided discipline from parents and grandparents; mother's own maladjustment to adult life.

Case No. 46: Joyce. *Age:* 14 years, 6 months. I.Q. 104.

A healthy, well-built but pale girl; slightly deaf.

Referral: by Juvenile Court with a long history of larceny and difficult behaviour at school.

Family background: sixth child in family of ten children.

Mother: a smartly dressed, plausible, highly emotional woman; was a nursemaid. Aggrieved and antisocial in attitude to society. Probation officer reports that she is a pub-crawler and shop-lifter. Fond of her family, seems to have strong, affectionate relationship with all of them; spoils them, though frequently leaves younger ones alone. Denies Joyce is difficult at home. Family very united.

Father: works as rural labourer; reported to be unstable; dominated by mother.

Siblings: eldest brother killed in war. One sister has been on probation for larceny, is defiant and rebellious, has now returned home with her child after unsatisfactory marriage. Older brother fined for larceny. Married sister, on probation, is reported to have been concerned with mother in shop-lifting.

Family has a bad reputation with court officials; standards of conduct in the home are unusually low. They are housed in a modern council house, which is crowded and neglected.

History: easily handled baby; bottle-fed; good appetite; health good except for usual childish complaints; has adenoids and ear infection. Difficult to get to bed; talks in sleep. Development entirely normal.

School record and intelligence: likes school, and gets on well, but there are continual complaints about her behaviour. Wants to leave. Thought to have slight disability in learning owing to ear infection.

In intelligence test, I.Q. 104; no unusual features beyond some weakness in verbal comprehension owing to slight deafness.

Personality and behaviour: willing and helpful at home; gets on well with siblings, especially the boys; looks after younger children when mother is out. Long history of pilfering; twice on probation for larceny. Told court fantastic tales in unconcerned manner. Plans to leave school and take job looking after children. Belongs to Girl Guides and Christian Science Club. Earns money delivering newspapers.

Clinical summary: diagnosed as case of primary antisocial conduct disorder in a problem family. Child sees nothing wrong in stealing since the family standards are low, doing only what mother and sister do. Mother not annoyed with her except when she is found out. Only long period of re-education in special surroundings thought to be helpful; sent to an Approved School. Outcome inconclusive.

Causative factors: 'vicious home' in which she learned delinquent conduct without guilt feelings, just as she has adopted other attitudes; unstable personality of mother and weakness of father thought to be chief cause of poor quality of the home.

Case No. 47: Sarah. *Age:* 14 years, 6 months. I.Q. *81.*

A tall, fair girl with bright colouring; childish-looking. Has slight tics.

Referral: by school medical officer for tempers, destructive and violent behaviour, uncontrollable at home.

Family background: elder of 2 children of separated parents. Lives with mother, 13-year-old brother and aged great-uncle and great-aunt.

Mother: smartly dressed, grey-haired woman, who adopts a self-righteous attitude in talking of the good home which Sarah has and fails to appreciate. Odd manner suggests rigidly suppressed emotion underlying hypocritically pleasant manners. Easily irritated, quick-tempered. Has long-established sado-masochistic relationship with Sarah, and no love for her. She and Sarah constantly struggle for domination. Sarah has been sent to a convent, a mental hospital, a children's home and public hospital. Mother now reluctant to have her home. Prefers son; Sarah accuses her of loving him most and that he has not been sent away. Mother found to be an unreliable informant, with little feeling for the girl; was two-faced, failed to cooperate in giving the girl a fair trial to settle down at home during treatment period.

Father: skilled labourer in civilian life; voluntarily remained in Army. According to mother, is drunken, wasteful, squandering. Rarely home on leave. Matrimonial difficulties and disturbances from the beginning; associates with other women; has been known to spend entire pay on drink, sell furniture, and waste proceeds. Irresponsible, unreliable and untruthful. Mother says

348

Sarah is fond of him, but seldom sees him. He contributes nothing towards maintenance of children. Mother welcomes his remaining in Army in order to get regular allowances.

Sibling: younger brother; according to mother, he is no trouble. Sarah is jealous of him, teases him; interferes until he becomes aggressive, then there are open fights. Once knives were thrown.

Great-uncle and Great-aunt: both nag. Sarah quarrels with and provokes them. They cannot stand noise or wild behaviour and have exaggerated Sarah's temper outbursts.

History: early childhood uneventful; bottle-fed; no feeding difficulties; no habit-training or sleeping difficulties. As baby, considerable bronchitis; between 7 and 8, severe measles followed by series of attacks of bronchitis and colds. At 9, had chorea, since then enuretic. Residual choreiform movements involving the head, shoulders, lips, eyelids, and a repeated nervous cough which have now developed into habits of which she is not fully aware, such as blinking, fidgeting, fumbling, tongue movements and grimacing. Temper tantrums and scenes followed recovery from chorea together with periods of shouting, swearing and destructiveness. Developed fears of dark, became clumsy. For a period, was under observation in mental hospital, given modified course of insulin treatment, which was a failure. Discharged as unsuitable for mental hospital. Sarah says she supposes her mother wanted to get rid of her because she quarrelled with her brother.

School record and intelligence: began school at 5. Liked first school, where reports were good. At convent, where the standards were strict, Sarah failed to fit in; repeatedly sent away. Performance fairly good considering limited mental capacity.

In intelligence test, I.Q. 74. On a re-test some time later, I.Q. 81, and on the Raven Progressive Matrices, she made a score of 21, Group E. Her intelligence is therefore low but not defective, and she has some verbal facility.

Personality and behaviour: friendly, easily liked by friends, but soon takes advantage of them and is troublesome. Mother says she kicks and shouts if wishes not immediately granted. Shows off, needs attention; is babyish in some ways; plays only with small girls or dolls. Helpful domestically, trustworthy on errands. During quiet periods, can be affectionate and helpful. Likes films and film stars, to whom she writes. Has now left school; is assistant waitress. Would like to learn typing.

Clinical summary: diagnosed as a case of primary antisocial conduct disorder in a dull, unstable adolescent. Taken on for treatment as it was felt that, although she has a constitutionally unstable temperament, this has been aggravated by constant mishandling and her infantile regression of enuresis, tantrums and destructiveness was largely reactive to a bad, rejecting home environment. Began to respond well to psychotherapy, made good relationship with therapist on basis of needing help in a situation in which she feels rejected and defeated. Brought much material related to her quarrel relationship to mother and brother, her menstrual fears and fears of attack. Behaviour at home improved, but mother failed to cooperate, prevented child from attending for her sessions, broke off treatment on the grounds that no attempt was being made to find a place where the child could be sent away. The prognosis is thought to be poor, and Sarah may become a confirmed delinquent, or possibly develop psychotic tendencies.

Causative factors: constitutional inadequacy, but this was exaggerated by gross mishandling and unsatisfactory home environment; disturbed mother-child relationship and frequent interruptions and rejections brought about by the mother; the absence and desertion of the father; the preference of the mother, as well as of the great-aunt and uncle, for the boy; their combined rejection of the girl from the home.

Case No. 48: Monica. *Age:* 14 years, 11 months. I.Q. 97.

A spotty-faced, adolescent girl with unformed features and greasy hair. Talks freely in a giggling way, takes no responsibility for her actions.

Referral: by probation officer on account of stealing, lying, truanting, destructiveness, temper tantrums, sexual offences and swearing.

Family background: only child of parents who were divorced when she was a year old. Mother remarried when Monica was 4, and son of this marriage is now 7. Mother separated from second husband.

Mother: aged 36; a heavily made-up woman who seems older than her years. Hard and unmotherly; calls herself a smart business-woman; works as waitress in an hotel. Nervous, impatient, bad-tempered in dealing with Monica, who resembles her in appearance. Bitter and vindictive about Monica's delinquent behaviour, condemns her, lacks understanding and is rejecting. Relationship of mother and daughter, according to grandmother, has always been antagonistic, but is worse since birth of step-brother. In frequent rows, Monica generally wins. Mother has no patience with girl's sloppiness and slowness, feels that she should also work hard, and that she does her no credit.

Father: aged 34; Scotsman. Divorced by wife on discovery that he was living with another woman. Lives in same town as Monica and mother; pays no alimony. Monica supposed to know nothing of him.

Step-father: nervous man, unable to settle down. Prisoner-of-war for 5 years; on return, was difficult, rejected Monica, whom he previously spoilt, having preferred her to his own son. After a succession of violent quarrels, deserted wife. Unknown to her mother, Monica meets him.

History: pregnancy and confinement normal; a wanted girl, 4½lb. at birth. Bottle-fed; constant feeding difficulties until 6 months. Mother went to live with grandmother because of marital disharmony; remained there until after divorce. Mother then went out to work; Monica alternately handled by mother, grandmother, and aunt. Habit-training easy; talked early; developed enormous appetite. Sleep poor; always wanted night-light. When 4, mother re-married; continued working until Monica was 8, when step-brother was born. Soon afterwards, Monica was evacuated, lived in two foster-homes, where she was difficult; jealous of other children. Menstruated early; has been interested in boys for some time. Diurnal and nocturnal enuresis from 7–11. At 8, began stealing, which coincided with birth of step-brother and evacuation. At this time, grandmother was ill, mother ceased to work; family forced to move to poorer neighbourhood. Monica's health irregular. At 5, doctor advised operation for tonsils and adenoids; this was postponed owing to suspected diabetes which is said to have disappeared without treatment at 7. Scarlet fever and diphtheria before 9.

School record, intelligence, and post-school work: started school at 5, attended 2 schools when evacuated. On return, at 11, was in 'C' stream of secondary school, later in 'B' stream. No outstanding abilities or disabilities; not educationally backward. She caused trouble, was defiant and unmanageable, until last summer. Headmistress refused to keep her. After conference between Headmistress, probation officer and mother, she was found a job in a children's home. This was regarded as satisfactory as she wished to work with children away from home. But mother suddenly reversed the decision, sent her to work in a hairdresser's. Then worked in grocer's shop; dismissed as unsuitable after 5 weeks. Worked at shoemaker's, but mother removed her as prospects were poor. Has attempted 8 jobs in all; during this period, stole money from grandmother's purse. Eventually mother allowed her to remain at home to help grandmother, who had come to live with them and was ailing.

In intelligence test, I.Q. 97. Indolent, easily gives up after failures, embarrassed, giggles. No special abilities or disabilities.

Personality and behaviour: lies and uses bad language, is unreliable and lazy. Constantly fights with grandmother and step-brother, though professes affection for them. Fears dark, attack or murder, yet stayed out at night, sleeping on railway platforms, in open fields, or stayed out with boys. Headmistress says she was sexually underdeveloped at time of leaving school. Behaviour is childish. Shows no guilt for misdeeds; cannot tolerate frustration; steals impulsively for mild pleasure. Unless work brings her immediate satisfaction or praise, it bores her. She is selfish, impatient, a boaster; has no consideration for the property of others; in temper tantrums, shrieks and throws things about. No apparent feelings of affection or remorse. Can only be deterred from dissocial behaviour at home by deprivation of physical comforts. Main interest is boys and soldiers whom she meets when out with other girls, or at dances and films. Dislikes domestic work, unhelpful in the house; lies in bed in mornings scribbling and drawing and singing to herself. Says she wants to look after children or work with figures. When charged at court for staying out at night and wandering, seemed proud of her exploits and dramatized them.

Clinical summary: diagnosed as a case of primary antisocial conduct disorder and psychiatric treatment recommended in a hostel for maladjusted children. Sent to a remand home, where she behaved normally. Later settled down fairly well in a Church Army home where the court had sent her. Prognosis thought to be poor, since Monica's behaviour is unlikely to be changed by institutional treatment alone. The case has passed out of the hands of both psychiatrist and the probation officer.

Causative factors: grossly broken home; rejection by mother and both father and step-father; sado-masochistic relationship with mother and grandmother; inconsistency and violence in methods of handling; mother's instability and marital difficulties. Difficulties greatly increased by evacuation to two foster-homes shortly after birth of her step-brother and the break-up of mother's second marriage shortly afterwards.

Case No. 49: Daisy. *Age:* 15 years, 4 months. I.Q. 103.

A polite, well-turned-out girl, conventionally smiling in manner. Answered questions with monotonous brevity.

Referral: by probation officer as 'beyond control'; has a record of delinquent behaviour continued after 3 years in an approved school. Present reference on account of stealing, telling lies, wandering, truanting, and staying out late at night.

Family background: illegitimate, unwanted child of actress, reported to be of doubtful morals, who deserted the child when a baby. Placed with foster-parents until 2, then adopted by Mr. and Mrs. X., who were childless. Mrs. X. was then 53, her husband 52. No inquiry was made as to suitability of adoptive parents.

Adoptive mother: now a senile, helpless invalid who moves about with difficulty, never goes out, is dirty and untidy, looks repulsive; dribbles at mouth when excited. Needs medical attention, but refuses it. Treats Daisy inconsistently; indulges her excessively, paws her repulsively, then calls her a bitch. She is reported to have a violent temper, admits to rages when she does not know what she is doing. Blames girl for her bad health, though obviously she has been deteriorating while girl was away at school. Cannot control Daisy.

Adoptive father: age 65; a locksmith; respectable, hard-working, and generally liked. Distressed by Daisy's behaviour, but because of his age, unable to make any deep impression on her. Fond of her, and she returns his affection to some extent, but he is reserved and has difficulty in expressing his feelings.

Home conditions are poor, dirty, untidy, and squalid. When at home, Daisy has bed in adoptive parents' room; says that sometimes she has had to sleep on the floor.

History: little known of early years. While with foster-parents, was badly burned and neglected. She remembers nothing of her own mother. Intentions of adoptive parents probably good, but they were not mentally adapted to the bringing up of a child. Daisy remembers that she could always get what she wanted; was in some ways spoilt, in others frustrated.

School record, intelligence, and post-school work: began to do well at school, but unsatisfactory home conditions led to behaviour difficulties. At 11, brought before juvenile court as being in need of care and protection. Headmistress discovered she was staying out late at night, was wandering from house to house obtaining sympathy and material help by telling pathetic stories about herself and her home. Unknown to parents, had been truanting from school; obtained money by false pretences. Because of squalid home conditions and parents' inability to control her, N.S.P.C.C. was informed. Finally brought to court, sent to junior approved school where she remained for 3½ years. Absconded twice during first year. Lessons progressed well. Unpopular with other children as she was bossy and quarrelsome; rebellious and impertinent to teachers. Unable to make lasting relationship with adult or friend. Discipline led only to superficial adaptation to external demands. No fundamental change in attitude occurred whilst at school. Since then, unable to conform to life outside institution.

After leaving school, took job as serving maid in boys' boarding school. Work satisfactory, but made trouble. Climbed out of windows at night, wandered in parks. After quarrel with older maid, absconded. On arrival home, said she had 3 days' holiday, obtained money from father and ran away.

With help of former Headmistress, then obtained job as children's maid with understanding employer. Became lazy, defiant; jealous of babies. Spent time reading love stories; when reprimanded, pretended unconcern and bravado. Stole watch from employer. Not charged with theft, but brought before the court as being beyond parents' control. Told fantastic stories about spending days off with older girl at Brighton, meeting boy friends, going to the theatre, and of being turned away from her home on days off. Spent money from savings account.

In intelligence test, I.Q. 103; is of average standing in educational attainment. Rather moody, stubborn, easily goes to pieces. Responds to encouragement.

Personality and behaviour: was hurt and sulky after court proceedings; refused to eat, was on her guard with probation officer, who found her self-centred, difficult to please, anxious to impress. While centre of attention, can do well, but is unreliable and unstable. Moody and without application unlesss flattered and appreciated; stubborn if corrected; cannot tolerate competition. Has no friends of own age, easily disintegrated, quarrelsome with other girls. Has few interests, dislikes housework. Ruled by desire for pleasure and entertainment; avoids anything requiring effort.

Physically strong and healthy; mild degree of fibrositis in back muscles though without apparent handicap. History of nose-bleeding, tonsilitis; much histrionic behaviour. Emotional development retarded; unable to restrain her wishes; dependent upon adults' approval; wants to be admired and praised all the time; responds to minor frustrations or criticism by giving up entirely. Unable to stand tension; wishes must be granted at once. One of her greatest difficulties is that her desire to be liked is not expressed in a desire to please the person concerned, but is an attempt to see how far she can go with her provocations before being sent away.

Clinical summary: diagnosed as primary antisocial conduct disorder in unstable adolescent, with mildly hysterical tendencies. Recommended she should not return to approved school, but placed on probation and placement away from home carried out under supervision of psychiatrist. This was arranged; she maintained contact with the psychiatrist by visits and letters for over 2 years. Follow-up reports show steady progress: delinquency has not recurred, she is able to earn her own living, has boy friends, can stand more frustration. Queer moods continue, quarrels with other girls, and still has an 'uncontrollable longing for her real mother'.

Causative factors: largely environmental, in particular unhappy babyhood with failure to form genuine mother relationship; adoption by unsuitable, aged parents; grossly inconsistent handling by adoptive mother; wretched home conditions and adoptive mother's senility; failure of approved school or probation officer to achieve genuine re-education when she was first apprehended at age of 11.

Case No. 50: Joan. *Age:* 16 years, 4 months. I.Q. 104.

A plain, clumsy, worried-looking, girl, shabbily dressed. Seldom smiles, and during interviews was shy and inhibited.

Referral: by Probation Officer on account of stealing, truanting, running away and hysterical symptoms.

Family background: younger of two children whose father is dead; has had many changes of home; now lives with mother.

Mother: aged 50; an eccentric, unstable, curious-looking Irish woman, slatternly in appearance, florid complexion and thickened features. Outspoken temperance worker. Occasionally goes out to work, but poor health and instability hinder her from staying for long at job. For short periods has been shorthand-typist, cook in W.A.A.F., a V.A.D. and in the N.A.A.F.I. First joined these to get away from husband, whom she blames for all family difficulties. Inconsistent in treatment of Joan, has been frequently separated from her; unable to give children any security.

Father: unstable alcoholic who died two years ago, aged 60, from incurable disease. He was formerly in the Indian Civil Service. Intelligent, difficult and eccentric. His death left the family penniless. Widow says he had odd brain; interested in crime of all kinds, which he discussed with Joan and accused her of being kleptomaniac. Ill-treated and openly disliked her, favouring brother. Threatened her with police and with being sent away; resented any success she might have and anyone who helped her. Joan was often with him during long, painful illness; upset when he died.

Sibling: brother, aged 24. Was in Army, now serving apprenticeship. Intelligent, reliable; tries to control Joan, who is fond of him but jealous, particularly because father favoured him. Discipline in house has been divided between unstable mother, eccentric father and a number of ayahs who cared for children in India.

Mother and children now live in five-roomed house in fairly good locality. Conditions poor, house is shabby, bare and dirty. One room let to elderly lady to relieve financial strain.

History: two weeks' premature baby, mother having had malaria and heavy fall. No confinement difficulties. Refused breast. Disturbed and unhappy childhood from beginning. Father did not want child, particularly a girl; harshly treated during early years in India. Mother says she was stubborn; deliberately soiled herself day and night until 2. Forcibly tied to pot and beaten. Not clean until coming to England at 4. Teething, during hot summer in India, was late and difficult; lost weight, ran high temperature and 'nearly died'. Talked and 'ran' at 1 year. Chicken-pox at 2,

357

DELINQUENT AND NEUROTIC CHILDREN

measles at 3. Very independent; complained of father's cruelty.
At 5 and at 9, tried to run away from home. From 7–9, night
terrors; subsequently sent by N.S.P.C.C. to foster-home because
of father's ill-treatment. Against all advice, father brought her
home for holidays. At 12, began shoplifting and truanting. After
stealing bicycle, sent to approved school for 2 years. Returned
home before father's death, following which, stole books and
stationery when at private school. Sent to approved school for
further 2 years; during this time, favourite head mistress died;
began to complain of headaches, showed symptoms of rash and
ran temperatures.

School record and intelligence and post-school work: had attended five
schools before the two periods at approved schools. Always ob-
durate. Mother taught her to read; learnt quickly. Disliked school,
but is not retarded. At 10½, began stealing, truanting and running
away.

In intelligence test, I.Q. 104; appeared to have good verbal
ability, but seemed to be a depressed, deprived child.

Left school at 16; worked in nursery school where she wanted
to train for work with children. Liked this work, but was dismissed because she was, wrongfully, accused of stealing; now too
dispirited to get job, although injustice has been acknowledged.
Delivers newspapers; is a Girl Guide. Fond of reading and films,
but has no other interests.

Personality and behaviour: is now reserved, hides real feelings, is
suspicious of people's intentions; bitter towards the world; unable
to make or keep friends of own age; interested only in older
women who offer some stability. Withdrawn towards probation
officer.

Clinical summary: diagnosed as primary antisocial conduct disorder; possibly some neurotic tendencies, but these are felt to be
insufficient to explain her delinquency and the antisocial character
development is primary. Placed on probation for stealing with the
condition of attending the Child Guidance Clinic. Arrangements
made for her to undertake training in child nursing with the help
of a supportive relationship with the therapist. Follow-up shows

that so far she remains unhappy in her present situation, and has lost interest in her work. A transfer to a more suitable training is being arranged, but the prognosis is considered only fair and the outcome inconclusive.

Causative factors: general great insecurity of home background from earliest years; frequent changes of mother-substitute; open ill-treatment by father; father's abnormal personality and rejection; harsh treatment and inconsistent discipline from an ineffectual mother; death of father to whom she had a deep, if disturbed, relationship.

CHAPTER IX

Fifty neurotic children

Case No. 51: Maurice. *Age:* 4 years, 11 months. I.Q. 110.

Fair-haired, fresh-complexioned boy who had difficulty in separating from mother at clinic.

Referral: by medical officer on account of various fears and a phobia of animals.

Family background: elder of two children from stable, middle-class home.

Mother: tense, neurotic; sets high standards for children, but blames herself for Maurice's behaviour; anxious and guilty, and appears to have done the wrong things from the best motives. Rationalizes her behaviour; hostile and negative in attitude to clinic. Rigid in handling of Maurice; unable to tolerate any aggression; constantly discouraging.

Father: accountant; spends much time studying for examinations. Demobilized 15 months ago; previously at home only at odd week-ends. Rigid standards for children; impatient with Maurice about his fears, regarding them as disgraceful. Since finding that disparagement was of no avail and that phobia is now more severe, has become more protective. Mother sees little of father as he has withdrawn into his studies, has separate bedroom so that he can work late. She is aggressive towards him, and feels guilty about this.

Sibling: sister, aged 15 months. Mother says Maurice showed no jealousy until sister began to talk. Mother unable to accept his jealousy until she had talked of her own jealousy of her brother who died at 3, when she was 5. These feelings are deeply repressed; indications show her jealousy was intense.

Standards of family are middle-class, rigid, particularly about cleanliness. Some reports give impression that family are snobbish and social climbers.

History: a 'planned' baby. Born at home without difficulty. Breast-fed for 6 months; weaning difficult; always had feeding difficulties, now fussy eater. Habit-training difficult; wet until 19 months during day, until 3½ at night, despite rigid insistence on cleanliness and good behaviour. Still wets occasionally. Walked at 14 months, talked at 18 months, suddenly saying many words. At 3, sent to maternal grandmother several times to encourage independence; mother says he never minded this. Stayed with grandmother at 3½ when sister was born. Difficulties then began and increased when father was demobilized. At 4, sent to one grandparent for Christmas while mother and baby went to another. He was naughty and trying; developed dog phobia; later was panic-stricken and shrieked at sight of chickens and ducks. Ridiculed for this, deprived of sweets and sent to bed early, but without effect; reaction became more severe. Sleeps well, but has had nightmares since phobia began. Health good; no infectious illnesses; suffers from prolapsed rectum.

Intelligence: does not yet attend school. In intelligence test, was despondent and nervous. I.Q. 110. Vocabulary score low, otherwise language development good. Nervous, clinging, dependent on adults. Responses repetitive.

Personality and behaviour: mother says he clings to her at home, is easily reduced to tears, does not mix well with other children. Babyish and demanding; worries and has intense feelings of inferiority; anxious and over-polite. Marked obsessional traits in painting and drawing, but occasionally likes to mess with paints. Extremely clean in habits, takes elaborate care of books and toys, resents his sister using them.

Clinical summary: diagnosed as a case of neurotic disturbance (phobia); taken on for treatment. Defence mechanisms and phobic reactions were interpreted and underlying passive-effeminate wishes worked through. Mother also seen, and her high standards were slightly modified. Further progress prevented by mother's hostile and negative attitude to the treatment. She was unwilling to make any radical change in her attitude, expected the clinic to do all the work. Brought the boy regularly, particularly when he did not like coming. Treatment of the boy was carried on; castration fear and sibling rivalry superficially treated. Made satisfactory adjustment, symptoms disappeared. Follow-up showed that he had begun school, is progressing satisfactorily. Prognosis thought to be fairly good, but is dependent on environment.

Causative factors: mother's personality and rejecting attitude; her handling of the boy's early education; birth of sister coincident with return of stern and rigid father after long absence.

Case No. 52: Geoffrey. *Age:* 5 years, 10 months. I.Q. 143.

A slight, alert boy, very friendly to the psychiatrist; easily related his fantasies, talked in fast, excited speech.

Referral: by father on account of nervousness, fears, much crying, inability to concentrate, animal phobia.

Family background: elder of 2 boys in stable, professional middle-class home.

Mother: tall, dark, intelligent, warm-hearted woman, basically a good mother. One of a Roman Catholic family of 13 children brought up by a resident nannie in early years, then sent to boarding schools from 4½–18. Has a close, intense and loving relationship with Geoffrey; has high religious standards for him; is anxious. Spent most of war years alone with him; guilty about having given him too much attention and affection, and is now out of touch with husband.

Father: professional man; 4 years in Services; served overseas. C slight build; since demobilization suffers from severe arthritic condition for which he receives 40 per cent disability pension. Difficult and moody on return, periods of heavy drinking. Found to be suffering from well-developed, long-standing obsessional neurosis. Always felt himself to be a failure; nervous symptoms have existed since childhood. Parents died when he was young; brought up by a relative in whose family he felt an outsider. Went overseas when Geoffrey was 10 months. Son resented and ignored him on his return, recognizing only mother's authority. Argued with father, regarded him as interloper. Jealous of parents being together; developed phobia when brother was born 15 months after father's return. Father cannot tolerate Geoffrey's noisiness or his aggressive but skilful and highly intelligent remarks. Expects high standards of orderliness and quiet from him. Argumentative and quarrelling relationship of father and boy amuses and distresses mother. Father has obsessional fears, which are unsubstantiated, that boy may have T.B. Period of marital difficulty after father's return; he had tried to combat loneliness and boredom of tropics by heavy drinking. He is Protestant; Geoffrey is a Roman Catholic.

Sibling: brother, aged 9 months. Healthy, well-developed. Geoffrey acutely jealous. During her pregnancy, mother says she and father were slowly reunited; this has been consolidated during Geoffrey's treatment. She has insisted, supported by the clinic, upon more lenient ways with younger child, despite criticism from her mother, a strict Roman Catholic who periodically stays with the family, and who criticized her handling of Geoffrey when baby was born. Father and Geoffrey take great interest in baby's training, particularly in toilet habits; want mother to be stricter.

Family lives in suburban professional home. No poverty or over-crowding; no changes of home.

History: much wanted baby; pregnancy good, but mother had fears that child might be abnormal or blind. Three weeks premature; weighed 5½ lb.; breast-fed until 9 months; disliked weaning, although this was gradual. Short period of spitting out food; appetite poor, no interest or enjoyment of food; still has food fads. Sat up alone at 9 months; walked at 16 months; talked at nearly 2. Mother says temper tantrums were so severe that he was sick with temper at 18 months. Habit-training over-strict; punished when dirty or wet. No breakdown since he became clean at 13 months and dry at night at 17 months. Sleep good; several short periods of fear of dark. Now shares room with brother; likes to get into parents' bed, especially to sleep with father. Severe nightmares recently. At present is resentful and hostile towards father. Terrified of dogs and fire. Nervy; has bad dreams; occasionally temper outbursts or panics, which appear to be feverish attacks for almost no known reason. Recently made scene on railway platform with screaming and phobic reactions to father's disappearance to attend to luggage. Became hysterical when teeth were to be extracted; has phases of being indecisive. Stammered for brief period during treatment; suffered from temporary inhibition in drawing and design in which he is talented. At 5, very upset when mother breast-fed baby; only consoled when allowed to 'feed' and dress his teddy. At 5, 4 days in hospital for tonsillectomy; at 6, underwent emergency appendicectomy during treatment. Reacted badly to both periods of hospitalization.

School record and intelligence: began school at $4\frac{1}{2}$, shortly after father's return. Soon afterwards, broke arm, had measles and tonsilitis. Did not get on well with other boys, returning home with bruises and scratches and stories of being beaten. At time of referral, had been at school for a year, but had made little progress, concentration poor.

In intelligence test, I.Q. 143; superior intelligence, very sensitive and excitable, observant, alert and well able to use his high abilities. Less control in emotional responses.

Personality and behaviour: Mother describes Geoffrey as over-excitable, imaginative, very talkative and boastful. Daydreams, is highly strung, emotional and cries easily. She says he can be alert and active, but is slow, and at times irritating. Likes drawing and reading, active games and sports; enjoys helping father in carpentry. Is serious and religious, likes his mother. Phobias focused upon dogs and fire, but recently has become afraid of lightning, thunder, noises, railways and Underground trains.

Clinical summary: diagnosed as primary behaviour disorder with pronounced neurotic trends (phobic type). He and mother taken on for treatment over period of 15 months. Geoffrey made good progress, symptoms disappeared. Mother's insight into reasons for Geoffrey's behaviour greatly increased; able to modify her handling both of him and of the baby. Both parents cooperated fully in treatment, kept in touch with clinic for some time afterwards. Follow-up shows Geoffrey's improvement has been maintained; relationship with father has improved, and has made enormous progress at school. New sublimations, particularly a biological interest in life history of animals, have opened up. Mother says that now a dog is just a dog, phobia having disappeared, and boy has puppy. During treatment, he became 'engaged' to a girl friend of his own age, was able to give up intensely jealous feelings for mother and adjusted happily to school life.

Causative factors: thought to lie in intensely exclusive relationship which boy developed with over-anxious mother during fathers' absence; return of father and birth of brother at height of this relationship; father's obsessional neurotic character structure and physical ill-health; mother's over-strict and rigid cleanliness training, her intolerance of jealousy towards father and baby. Prognosis thought to be good. Follow-up shows that Geoffrey is popular and holds his own at school with other boys; has begun to read widely in elementary science and biology. Takes part in active outdoor sports; has boy and girl friends of own age.

Mother states that all family relationships, including marital one, have improved during course of Geoffrey's treatment, and she has increased confidence in methods of handling baby.

Case No. 53: Colin. *Age:* 6 years, 2 months. I.Q. 100.

An odd-looking though attractive boy with thin legs and large head. Conversation engaging, but childish; he confuses fact and fancy.

Referral: by headmistress on account of wandering and backward, dreamy behaviour at school.

Family background: at time of referral, was believed to be elder of 2 children whose father is in India for long periods.

Mother: tall, dark and intense; intelligent, musical, fond of reading. Youngest of 7 children, says she was unwanted. At boarding school from 5-18, then trained as nurse and masseuse. After marriage, lived in India; lost her first child. When Colin was baby, she suffered from malarial attacks, so returned to England with him. Constantly ill; has regular injections; phases occur when she fails to recognize acquaintances, neglects Colin, and remains in bed. Suspected drug-taking (unconfirmed). Relationship with Colin is difficult to assess; several separations, several long periods of being alone with her. He is frequently sent to relations and neighbours for care or meals. Mother seems guilty about the child, is untruthful in dealings with clinic, deliberately evaded P.S.W.'s visits, though professes to be worried about him.

Father: industrial engineer. Quiet, sympathetic; obstinate, slow and methodical rather than clever. Mother describes him as dumb but deep. He expects to be abroad for further $2\frac{1}{2}$ years; urges mother to send Colin to boarding school if she is so ill. He visited family in England when Colin was nearly 3, and again at 5 and 3 months.

Sibling: 2-month-old baby. Colin has never shown overt jealousy, according to mother. Later, hidden aggressive fantasies and sadistic ideas towards the baby were discovered.

The two children live with the mother in small, comfortable coastal cottage, having had many changes of home. No poverty or over-crowding. Standard of home is professional, upper middle-class.

History: pregnancy and birth normal, weighed $8\frac{1}{2}$ lb. Progress good. Bottle-fed, good appetite, but suffered from acidosis. Teething normal. Never crawled. Heavy baby with (apparently) flat feet. Walked and talked at 2. Habit-training lenient: clean and dry at 2. At 2, when mother went to India, sent to small, residential nursery; settled well, but developed gastric symptoms and acidosis. On her return, she removed him; he failed to recognize her; very attached to nursery staff. Mother pregnant and suffering from malaria in benign tertiary form, lost baby. She still has many temperatures and attacks of delirium, necessitating large doses of

quinine. Colin's health good except for tonsils. No sleeping
difficulties; shares room with baby. Has had much orthopaedic
treatment for feet, which mother constantly massages and bathed
in salt water. Measles 2 years ago.

School record and intelligence: went to school at 5. Mother declares
he knows less than when he was 3. Soon had periods of returning
late and wandering. Now attends local infants' school, is backward, fidgety, restless and talkative; dreamy and inattentive.
Attendance irregular. Left-handed, tends to mirror-write, poor
wrist coordination. Solitary and friendless, tells tales. Work below
average. In P.T., physical control poor. Art work merely large
messes.

In intelligence test, I.Q. 100. Dreamy, anxious child. Evasive,
placatory attitude. Thoughts wander.

Personality and behaviour: at home, described as active and independent, but slow and dreamy. Sometimes plays with younger
children, but prefers to play alone. No temper tantrums, not
difficult to manage; vague. Not demonstrative, though pleasant
and affectionate; likes to help mother in house. Reports that other
children hit him. Lives largely in world of fantasy; pretends to be
giant, rides imaginary bicycle into school shed. Had been neglected; wanders about the beach as he pleases. Childish in his play,
with little relationship to any other child, and has few interests.
Fond of Sunday school teacher. When a toddler during war,
house was bombed; no fears, denies having any worries.

Clinical summary: diagnosed as case of primary behaviour disturbance with pronounced neurotic trends. Passive child who re-
treated into fantasy. Taken on for observation; attempt made to
find stable home environment which would make treatment
possible. Mother refused to cooperate; uncle agreed to bring
Colin to clinic; or boy came by himself, making long bus journey
alone. Mother completely irresponsible, pleading illness which
prevented her from attending clinic even at first interview. Colin
was found to be very disturbed with severe castration anxiety.
Made strong relationship with therapist and was hungry for
affection; began to bring material about conflicts on an anal level

when treatment was interrupted, as mother, without informing clinic, had made plans to take child to another county. Case closed as incomplete and unsatisfactory with poor prognosis. About a year after Colin's last attendance at clinic, a health visitor came in touch with the boy as a foster-child in a neighbouring county. He was then said not to be mother's child, but a foster-child. A report followed that mother was recently divorced by her husband, a local professional man being cited as co-respondent. The couple lived in a remote town for some time while Colin was fostered out; 'father' given custody of children. Mother then prepared to leave the man whom she does not intend to marry, wanting to reopen proceedings in order to get custody of children. The case is not settled. Meanwhile Colin remains in a foster-home; the case will be followed further.

Causative factors: mother's personality; early separation from mother; her continual illnesses and her 'odd' phases; great insecurity in upbringing; strong and intense relationship with mother followed by detached, odd moods; repressed sibling rivalry; frequent changes of home and possible neglect.

Case No. 54: Jackie. Age: 6 years, 7 months. I.Q. 108.

A friendly though subdued boy, thin and heavy-eyed, with a low, moaning voice.

Referral: by school medical officer on account of pilfering, lack of concentration, temper tantrums, irritability, imaginative lying, whining, babyishness and subdued, inhibited behaviour.

Family background: older of 2 boys in unhappy, estranged family.

Mother: aged 30; active, intelligent, thoughtful, well-read, with many social interests. Describes herself as highly strung. At 20, nervous breakdown; has hypochondriacal fears; appears to be hysterical. Recent hysterectomy. Early life spent in unhappy home with step-father, who had impossibly high standards and a disturbed relationship with her. Worked as a cook. Basis of marriage was to convince her father and spendthrift mother that she was a person in her own right. Now conscious of husband's failure; dominates and resents him, and from beginning, marital relationship disturbed. Unfaithful to husband during his absence. Now says she could not manage without support and friendship of her lodger, who is estranged from his wife and whose son is with him. Mother is a severe disciplinarian, over-restrictive, anxious, and emotional. Physical care of children is excellent.

Father: aged 33; tall, of pleasant, boyish appearance, looks unhappy, has many irritating habits and mannerisms. Dreamy, lazy, slow-witted; speaks in slow, long-winded, aggressive way. Has number of suicidal ideas. Suffers from leg injury. Works as unskilled labourer; calls himself fitter by trade. Wife says he is almost illiterate. In Army for 5 years as private; home about once in 3 weeks. He denies his wife's allegation that he regards her as his mother. He has unhappy personal history; number of sexual difficulties; partially impotent since return from Army. Constantly quarrels with wife who refuses to let him near her. Apologetic and hopeless about solving difficulties; adopts passive, masochistic attitude towards wife. Frequently loses jobs, fails to support family. Admires lodger; during treatment, revealed latent homosexual relationship between the two men. Jackie recently surprised father by asking him to put him to bed. Loves the children, especially Jackie, but doesn't know how to treat them. Great tolerance is unexpectedly followed by loss of temper, shouting, and histrionic bombast. The lodger suffers from neurasthenia and heart pains. Mother makes no secret of her being unfaithful to husband with him. Father accepts her behaviour and refuses divorce. Lodger is scoutmaster; mother has become scoutmistress. Father excluded from these activities, as he also is when mother and lodger have pseudo-philosophic conversations. Romping and horse-play between mother and lodger in presence of children.

Sibling: brother, aged 4. He and Jackie get on fairly well. Mother describes him as lovely and tractable. Much hostility between Jackie and lodger's son of same age, who is blustering, unheedful, cruel. The children are supposed to call him their brother.

Family lives in crowded conditions. Mother shares bed with 2 boys, father sleeps in same room in single bed. Lodger and child share second bedroom. Mother admits harmfulness for the children of the triangular situation, but maintains that she would be a worse mother without it.

History: mother had difficult and unhappy pregnancy; baby bruised and scratched at birth; very long. Bottle-fed because mother's milk caused rash. Progress slow; feeding difficulties leniently dealt with; appetite now good. Walked at 14 months; speech not understandable until 3. Systematically trained, no napkins day or night after 14 months. As toddler, had temper tantrums; later was frequently constipated. Health poor. At 3 months, eczema, which continues. At 4 months, bad whooping cough. Between 3 and 4 years, bronchitis. At 4, chickenpox (mother says she gave it to him); at 5, German measles, followed by tonsillectomy (because he snored); in hospital 2 days. Since then, anxious about being away from mother. Is irritable and babyish, whines and cries. Likes to play with fire, to burn paper and string; always 'finding' things at school.

School record and intelligence: started school at 5; disliked it. Cannot concentrate, says teachers bully him. Is destructive, cries for attention, is easily distracted, and a nuisance in class. Teacher says he is unsociable, does not play normally with other children. Year older than average age of class; mirror-writer, below average in every subject, including all practical work. Described as resisting all formal education.

In intelligence test, I.Q. 108; unwilling to separate from mother, but quick and cooperative. Good verbal facility; easily fatigued. Some constructive ability.

Personality and behaviour: mother says he is irritable, grizzling, moody; has vivid imagination; constantly fears things; demands whether she loves him. Insecure, likes to be boosted; responds to praise, does not stand up for himself. Protective towards babies; lovable and helpful if mother is ill. Does not mix with other children. Clever with hands, wants to be plumber, likes mending pipes, which father dislikes, and can do this better than father. Until recently, avoided playing group games; can be unpleasant to other children, who bully and attack him, then he cringes and fears their touching him.

Clinical summary: diagnosed as primary behaviour disturbance with neurotic trends; taken on for treatment. Found difficulty in making relationship with psychiatrist; treatment was difficult because of irregular home situation. Is in extreme rivalry with lodger's son, aggressive and disparaging towards father. Frequently miserable and unhappy—would sit painting and crying at same time, or would talk about wanting to jump out of window. Strongly identified with mother; wants to do the cleaning and cooking, imitates mother's disparagement of father. In speaking of father said, 'If he was my wife, I wouldn't drink the tea if he made it.' Played games of war in which everyone was killed, or Indians were attacked from behind. Referred to himself always as useless and no good. Treatment is now progressing; he has made some response, has become more manly; behaviour at school has improved in all ways. Prognosis thought to be fair, dependent upon home situation and continued treatment.

Causative factors: personality of mother and of father, their disturbed relationship to each other; their unwise handling of Jackie and the unstable, irregular home circumstances.

Case No. 55: Billie. *Age:* 6 years, 11 months. I.Q. 123.

A tall, clumsy boy, reluctant to run because of foot supports worn for flat feet and weak ankles.

Referral: by school medical officer on account of day-dreaming, romancing, forgetfulness, crying, lack of concentration and inability to mix with other children or to stand up for himself.

Family background: father killed in war; boy now lives with mother, step-father and 3-year-old step-sister.

Mother: Canadian; pleasant young woman of average intelligence, pale, thin, but attractive. At first, seemed casual, showing little warmth towards Billie; later showed understanding, intellectually rather than emotionally. Made hazardous journey across Atlantic in convoy when Billie was 4½. Neither she nor the boy is well-adjusted to life in England. Lived with second husband's parents. Now concerned about reports received from school about Billie. She is impatient with his fantasies, says he is a tell-tale and will go 'mental'. The boy has obviously become passive to satisfy mother's needs.

Father: in American Army; killed when Billie was 2. Marriage unhappy and unsatisfactory due to domination of his mother and untruthful sisters. Divorce proceedings pending at time of his death. Mother describes him as big, quiet-natured man, easy to get on with; unfaithful to her. Billie resembles him in appearance and temperament; good relationship between them. Billie does not remember him, has photograph, knows he was killed, speaks of him occasionally as Daddy Tommy. Says good night to a star which he says is his father, and is comforted by this.

Step-father: English, married mother when abroad during war. Skilled artisan. Good-natured, easy-going, fond of Billie with whom he has teasing relationship. Billie likes to rough and tumble with him until it becomes too tough, then Billie cries. At clinic, Billie tells, in a confused way, of parental squabbles.

Paternal grandparents: Billie their first grandchild, so made great fuss of him, and mother feels they spoilt him. A very united family.

Maternal grandparents: met in Canada where Billie's mother was born. Grandfather came to England as a horse-trainer; emigrated to America and started building business.

Mother, husband, and children now live in rooms. In the house there is a delinquent boy on probation who mother thinks has bad influence on Billie. Family have had many moves, usually live under unsatisfactory and crowded conditions. No great financial stress.

History: pregnancy poor because child so big; 60 hours in labour, instrumental delivery. Baby weighed 11 lb., cut and bruised on face. Breast-fed; no feeding or weaning difficulties. Greedy as young child; appetite now poor, still greedy though not faddy.

Sat up at 7 months, walked and talked at 18 months. Habit-training standards high; clean by day at 10 months, day and night at 14 or 15 months. Hated wet bed; now particular about cleanliness, especially of genitals. No sleep disturbances, has own room. At 18 months, in hospital with scarlet fever; upset by mother's visits. As toddler, period of being religious when he visited woman whom mother regarded as religious maniac. In early childhood had temper tantrums; wandered from home; told lies. Slight nose and lip twitches; enuretic when he had a cold. Had bronchitis when teething; many chest colds and coughs. Reacted badly to diphtheria immunization. Scarlet fever at 5, followed by measles. Some nasal obstruction. Has orthopaedic treatment for weak ankles and flat feet.

School record and intelligence: began school at 5 in England; after 2 days, developed scarlet fever. Likes school, especially reading, but does not concentrate, and makes only average progress. Truanted once; does not get on with other children. Because of frequent moves, has had about 1 year's schooling in all.

In intelligence test, I.Q. 123; superior all-round ability, but poor memory. Preoccupied with aggressive stories and fantasies during test.

Personality and behaviour: according to mother, is a day-dreamer. No friends; complains that other children set on him, unable to fight back, liable to cry if touched. Timid; clumsy, possibly because of size. Loving and affectionate; thinks others do not like him. Easy to manage, not shy with strangers; willing to go on errands. Tells lies to get out of minor troubles; vivid imagination. Slow; maintains he cannot do things, such as tying shoe-laces. Possibly over-restricted at home, with no outlets, since many of his wants seem to be unsatisfied. Goes to films every week-end; buys books with irregularly given pocket money. Memorizes stories easily; writes good stories and spells well. Likes to play with step-sister's dolls; gets on well with her and helps mother. Jealous of her at first, had aggressive fantasies, but this now hidden. The sister is noisy and demanding, and mother sets high standards of unselfishness for the children but thinks both are greedy.

Clinical summary: diagnosed as primary behaviour disorder with neurotic trends; taken on for treatment. In observation period, general lack of gratification was revealed. Attendance at clinic partly compensated for this deprivation at first, and his loquacity and romancing were given full rein. His attitude to 'cissies' was discussed and his knowledge of adults' opinion of them. Had begun to respond to treatment when his attendance was interrupted through illness of both Billie and his sister, and later on account of family's sudden decision to return to America. The treatment was incomplete; prognosis thought to be fair, but with further treatment it should have been good.

Causative factors: general insecurity and frequent moves; mother's personality; her fear that he takes after father's family; absence of father or father-figure for him to identify with in infancy; mother's handling of his 'sensitiveness'; possibly a very sensitive nature on constitutional grounds.

Case No. 56: Roger. *Age:* 7 years, 6 months. I.Q. 105.

A worried, pale-faced boy who looks as if he had been crying. Unable to play with or touch the toys; tried to hide anxiety and worries by talking about trivial things and with long-winded, irrelevant descriptions. Totally defeatist in discussing problems.

Referral: by mother on account of inordinate crying, reluctance to go to school, fears and babyish behaviour.

Family background: fourth of five children from stable home of skilled working-class level.

Mother: friendly, talkative, not very intelligent woman with little insight. Describes herself as worrying, with faith in doctors and clinics. Warm, suggestible, fond of children; managed other four without difficulty. Was run down in health at time of clinic visit. Finds Roger different from others and baffling, saying that without him they would all be happy. Concerned about his behaviour, says worry of this threatened her health. Fond of boy, and the relationship between them is fundamentally good.

Father: still in Services. Wounded, now has stiff leg. Roger is attached to him, pleased to see him come home. Father impatient with Roger, becomes angry when he cries; stricter than mother. Absent for long periods; soon to be demobilized.

Siblings: eldest brother, 16, and sister, 12, have shown no problems. Roger jealous of next brothers, aged 10 and 2. No open expression of hostility or aggression. Behaviour regressed two years ago on birth of baby.

Family lives in comfortable working-class circumstances; no financial difficulties.

History: pregnancy and confinement normal. Breast-fed without difficulty. Walked and talked at about 1 year. Habit-training fairly lenient; reliably clean and dry by 18 months without undue difficulty. Between 18 and 24 months, period of having to be coaxed to eat. Mother then gave up coaxing, eventually child overcame difficulties; now eats well. Between 2 and 4, like other children except that he did not get into tempers and put everything into his mouth, was more independent of his mother, would go to strangers. No sleep problems; shares bed with brother. Sucks thumb in bed; no fears of dark. Babyish behaviour began at birth of baby, though no overt jealousy. Became tearful, whereas family is cheerful. Now cries inordinately, sucks thumb and grizzles in public. Health good. No separation from home.

School record and intelligence: began school at 4, shortly before baby's birth and father's return, going to local school. Made excellent start; now reluctant to go, cannot do his best for fear of failure. Crying attacks started soon after birth of baby; returns from school red-eyed. Recently complains less about going. Teachers say he works well and is not backward.

In intelligence test, I.Q. 105; needed praise and encouragement to continue working in test; suddenly started to weep miserably when confronted with task he could not do. Docile in manner, worked quickly and expressed himself clearly.

Personality and behaviour: mother says it is impossible to know what he is thinking about. He has never been seen in a temper. Likes to help mother when other children are absent; has no friends. Blames others when things go wrong. Never fights or sticks up for himself; cries as soon as others touch him; children call 'cry-baby' as he passes. Spends time making things out of wood, doing puzzles. Afraid of adults, cannot stand up for himself with them. Seems afraid of his feelings or of any form of violence, of caning or of being punished, so blames others. Gets dirtier than other children.

Clinical summary: diagnosed as primary behaviour disturbance with neurotic trends; taken on for treatment. Made good relationship and showed insight into most immediate conflicts and strong wish to be helped. Main problem sibling rivalry and difficulties round position in family. On one hand, wish to be protected and treated like baby (regressive behaviour) on other, wish to be respected and have freedom of older ones. Not deeply disturbed; treatment carried out on conscious level and in working through present situation with him. No attempt made to change passive personality structure. Adjusted well, good insight, told friends he went to see lady doctor who 'helped him with his miseries'. Mother pleased with improvement, says he now leads normal life, gets on well at school. Follow-up showed progress had been maintained, prognosis thought to be good.

Causative factors: mother's anxious handling; boy's position in family and intense sibling rivalry which was intensified by birth of baby after his having been baby for 5 years. Before birth of baby, during absence of father, probably mother made more intense relationship with Roger and at same time kept him more babyish and dependent upon her than the other children.

Case No. 57: Bertie. Age: 7 years, 11 months. I.Q. 89.

A friendly, talkative boy with an engaging sense of humour.

Referral: by head teacher on account of general nervousness, many fears, truanting, refusal to attend school and long-standing enuresis.

Family background: illegitimate; lives in lodgings with unmarried mother.

Mother: over-anxious, insecure and very disturbed; probably main cause of child's difficulties, and in need of treatment herself. Says she had breakdown at 26 when she wept for 4 months. Works all day, often tired, ill or irritable at night. At present, is depressed, on the defensive and resentful at having to bear sole responsibility of boy. Wants to send him to special school. Anxious to hide his illegitimacy, yet kept him with her when she could have sent him to institution. Talked much about their early deprivations and misery at having to put him in a home temporarily at 5 weeks. She and boy now live with noisy family where there is much friction, and 4 spoilt children who resent him. Mother over-coddles him. During the war, she worked in a factory; now works as daily help in 4 different places, but is out all day.

Father: aged 55, married man who works in London. Wife in an asylum; grown-up family unknown to Bertie. Mother secretive about father and his occupation. He visits boy regularly. Did not marry mother as he did not wish to upset his family. May retire soon and live with mother and boy, but makes it clear that even if free, will not marry. He is morose, rarely takes mother out, visits them at alternate week-ends, allows them £1 a week without legal pressure. Takes great interest in Bertie, who 'worships' him, calls him father, but now says he has not got a daddy.

Mother and boy have had many changes of home; now live in 2 furnished rooms, but have had notice to leave and have applied for council house. Father, mother and boy share room on father's visits. They have never had stable home; living conditions are unsatisfactory.

History: unwanted baby. Pregnancy normal, instrumental delivery, residual scars. Breast-fed for 5 weeks, then had to be put in residential nursery. Upset when taken from there. Mother visited him every 2 weeks, suspects he was harshly treated and strictly trained. Removed him to foster-mother, who was disturbed by death of her own son and took it out on foster-children. Mother knows little of Bertie's early history; found he cringed when she visited him. Later, he had to go to other institutions. From 18 months to 5½ years, lived in Waifs and Strays nursery where he was one of 13 children in charge of one nannie. At 5½, mother fetched him to send him to school. Since then he has been living in rooms with her. She has frequently threatened to send him away. On his return to her he was enuretic; apparently has not been completely dry since infancy. Behaviour was aggressive; temper tantrums. Mother tried to keep him away from other children to 'keep him nice'. Had severe mumps, then whooping cough and measles. Mother, but not child, experienced air-raids; later he was unduly afraid of hit-and-run raids though did not experience them directly.

School record and intelligence: at 5½, went to village school; since then, several changes. Scared and backward; virtually a non-reader, likes arithmetic and nature-study, although backward in these as in all subjects. Behaviour variable; upsets class, has tempers, refuses to work alone, obey teachers, or observe school rules. In difficult periods, lies on floor, kicks and screams to attract attention. Head teacher declares Bertie is worst boy he has had in 40 years' of teaching, and now refuses to have him in school.

In intelligence test, I.Q. 89; basal age 4 years. Poor concentration, unperturbed by failure, 'shrugs it off'.

Personality and behaviour: mother says he used to be girlish, but is now less so. Worries about dirt, hands must be clean. Affectionate and demonstrative, helpful towards her, willing and unselfish, but clings to her and does not stand up for himself among equals. Honest and truthful, uses fists against smaller children, is a bully, and other children exclude him from their games. Says he wants a gun, a knife and a bicycle; writes to father asking for these. Definite obsessional tendencies. Mother repressive in standards for the child, partly exaggerated by fear of being turned out of lodgings.

Clinical summary: diagnosed as primary behaviour disturbance with neurotic trends; both he and mother taken on for treatment. Mother, a withdrawn woman of depressive type, now approaching middle-age, failed to cooperate with treatment and repeated a pattern she apparently made with her numerous employers. Good progress at beginning, then felt people expected too much of her, so threw up job. Repeated this in treatment, made no real attempt to change her handling. Bertie had responded well to the psychiatrist, made some progress, but it was found impossible to carry through his treatment under existing conditions; attempts to change these were not satisfactory. Outcome inconclusive. Prognosis under present conditions thought to be poor.

Causative factors: irregular and disturbed early years; interrupted relationship with mother; repeated change of mother-substitute and abnormal family conditions, particularly absence of father.

Case No. 58: Anthony. *Age:* 8 years, 1 month. I.Q. 89.

Anthony is a pale, anxious boy.

Referral: by School Medical Officer for behaviour difficulties which have existed for a long time. Chief amongst these are irritating behaviour at home and at school, playing the fool, making noises and faces, backwardness at school, a speech difficulty, fears and temper tantrums.

Family background: second of three children from stable, lower middle-class home.

Mother: warm, maternal woman with close emotional relationship with Anthony; at a loss to know how to deal with him; feels she should give him more attention, yet be more strict; threatens to send him away if he does not improve since that alone frightens him. Not over-harsh in handling of him. A capable, managing woman, goes out three days a week doing home nursing. Until recently had a mother and two children staying with her. From 1939, cared for twin evacuees (for 2½ years), which she enjoyed.

Father: nervy; has chronic illness. Work as salesman requires much travelling, but spends spare time at home. Fond of children, but strict; cannot stand noise or riotousness. Concerned about Anthony.

Maternal grandmother: has always lived with family; Anthony and she are at loggerheads.

Siblings: two brothers, aged 13 years, and 1 year and 5 months. Older one is expected to win scholarship at school, sings solo in church, plays violin. Mother very proud of him. Anthony is fond of younger brother, but will not let him touch his toys. Mother denies jealousy, adding that younger one is already brainier than Anthony. Anthony provokes his older brother, and likes to irritate his mother.

History: mother dreaded Anthony's birth because of previous difficult confinement. Anthony's birth also difficult. Healthy baby, weighed 8 lb. Breast-fed for 9 months; vomited a great deal, especially during first week. Always backward; crawled at 18 months, walked about 2 months later. Over 2 when he began to talk, and then indistinctly; still has slight speech defect. Habit-training achieved by 2. No outstanding illnesses, but frequent sick turns. Afraid of dark, refuses to go to bed alone. No feeding difficulties. Has habit of making stupid faces and dancing around, irritating everybody; likes pulling faces in front of mirror and laughing. Unable to dress himself or tie shoelaces. Loves to be dirty. Started to be naughty when mother had evacuees when he was 2.

School record and intelligence: likes school, has special friends. Stands up for himself, is not teased; anxious to be liked, so gives away his sweets. Does not worry about work or make any effort; year older than those in his class, far below average in reading and arithmetic, but average in practical subjects. Teacher says speech defect does not interfere with work.

In intelligence test, I.Q. 89; failed to concentrate, remained as passive as possible; gave impression of being a much younger child. His silly behaviour seemed to be an attempt to get attention by being a booby, since he was unable to get it by being clever.

Personality and behaviour: when alone with her, mother says he is good-natured and generous, and no trouble. She is convinced he is unhappy despite clownish behaviour, and wants to behave well. Cries easily when reprimanded, complains that she is always 'on at him'. Likes to pretend he is driving a car about at home. Seldom draws or does anything constructive; spends time day-dreaming.

Clinical summary: diagnosed as primary behaviour disturbance with neurotic trends; he and mother taken on for treatment. Mother, although stable and good-natured, found to be facile and thoughtless, tending to deal with every emergency by threatening to send Anthony away. Was shown step by step why Anthony behaved in a silly way and the educational means by which she could deal with it. Responded well when she saw positive results of this, became more patient. In interviews, Anthony became rapidly more aggressive, more aware of his hostility to brother and reasons for temper tantrums, and of the unsatisfactory nature of the defence mechanisms used against them. Jealous of brother's superior achievements, intensely guilty about aggressive tenden-cies. Adjustment greatly improved, and prognosis, within limits of his dull intelligence, thought to be good. Follow-up reports show considerable improvement at school, almost normal be-haviour at home and at school; is happier, has only occasional outbursts of temper when mother does not give him as much of her time as he wishes.

Causative factors: position in family in relation to his intellectual dullness, which forbade his excelling in a positive way; mother's carelessness, lack of understanding; her rather masochistic rela-tionship with boy and father's anxious attitudes prevented him from obtaining adequate outlet for aggression. After treatment, boy's behaviour seemed to be adequate in a difficult reality situation.

Case No. 59: Clifford. *Age:* 7 years, 1 month. I.Q. 85.

A small, fair-haired boy with a pronounced stammer which is mainly a complete halt in speech; unable to say anything, the boy holds his breath and grimaces.

Referral: by speech therapist on account of his speech disturbance, disobedience, temper tantrums and enuresis.

Family background: elder of two children, the other a girl, from stable, working-class home.

Mother: intelligent, soft-voiced Welshwoman, anxious about the boy, willing to be cooperative in treatment. Standards and ideals high, wants Clifford to be polite. She is easily excited and worried. Parents died in her early childhood; still dependent upon older sister who brought her up and with whom she quarrelled. Both are neurotic; mother has had suicidal ideas. Identifies herself with Clifford, feels his difficulties are hers, shares his emotions but becomes overwrought when father and he have rows, telling the boy he is not worth the trouble he causes. Clifford is more obedient to mother than father, says he knows how disappointed she is in him. She has a morning job to supplement family income.

Father: builder; comes from more stolid working-class background; throws cold water on wife's idealism. Chronic sufferer from gastric complaints which caused his being off work for 16 months; does only light work now, such as being night-watchman. He is moody, difficult and hard; frequent rows with wife with physical fights, sometimes not speaking for days. Separation has been threatened; sexual relations disturbed for some time; frequent periods of sleeping apart. He is irritated by Clifford, 'explodes' at him, enjoys punishing him. Preoccupied with frequency and regularity of his own and boy's bowel movements; gives boy many laxatives.

Sibling: sister, aged 3, favourite of parents. She and Clifford fight. Parents say she is more stable and appealing than Clifford. He was sent away when she was born; on return tried to conceal his jealousy. Mother says he now adores her.

Family lives in small house, invariably muddled, as mother is poor manager. Father's illnesses and inability to work have meant recurrent financial difficulties.

History: mother had bad fall during 6th month of pregnancy on which she blames boy's stammer. Had isolated and overwhelmingly intense wishes during pregnancy, e.g. for a pomegranate, but through lack of money, longing was not satisfied. Birth normal; breast-fed, no feeding difficulties. Superstitious beliefs

382

played large part in mother's handling. During early months, boy hung his tongue out; mother worried, believing this denoted an unsatisfied longing similar to that of hers for special foods. Old woman told her to give him something sweet, something bitter, and the juice of cherries mixed with rabbit brain. This she did, and he no longer hung out his tongue. Added to superstitious ideas were modern ones, which meant doing exactly what the nurse had told her, e.g. never picking him up when he cried, nor playing with him. He was left alone for hours. Late in sitting up; walked at 18 months; little talking until 2½, always stammered, mostly when excited or angry, or with sister. Speech therapist has seen him over long period, is unable to do anything with him. Toilet-training one long struggle over bowels; purge every week; frequent soiling and wetting incidents which were dealt with harshly. In napkins until 3½; bed wet until 4. Sleeping difficulties until 2½; has own bed in bedroom with parents and sister. Appetite always poor. Usual childish illnesses in mild form; catches cold easily; since 18 months, frequent worms; often given tonics. Enuretic until 6 months ago; fears the dark, picks nose, has jerky head movements. Masturbated openly for years despite punishments and threats.

School record and intelligence: began at 5; cried a lot at first, frequently ran home. Now likes school; backward, unable to read or write. Attendance irregular because of colds, etc. Below class average in all subjects. Bullied by other children, easily led, often in trouble. Has exposed himself at school.

In intelligence test, I.Q. 85. Assertive and aggressive, but insecure, constantly demanding reassurance. Difficulty in making adequate verbal responses; flow of speech seems to be dammed up, and at same time holds breath. Vocabulary excellent for mental level. Expressed fantasies about his powers, betrayed marked fear of authority. Mental age on assessment is 6 years.

Personality and behaviour: at home, affectionate, lively and restless, easily upset; temper tantrums. Dislikes playing on his own, follows other children around, but is sulky, quarrelsome and aggressive and usually left to play alone. Upset if dirty; cries easily, will not let parents smack him. Quarrelsome and aggressive in all relationships with adults and children.

Clinical summary: diagnosed as primary behaviour disturbance with neurotic trends. Thought to be extremely disturbed and badly handled in a disturbed home. Mother and child taken on for treatment with object of helping her to understand his behaviour and to attempt to alter her handling, and to help him to deal with his aggression in a more satisfactory way. Mother attended irregularly, tried to make a disturbed relationship with therapist. Made some progress, genuinely tried to change her handling. Attitude to boy became less harsh and unsympathetic; at end of treatment, preferred him to the girl. Clifford became aggressive immediately in first interviews which were full of fantasies of death and killing people. Individual treatment was continued for 1 year; satisfactory progress was made, behaviour improved on all levels. Follow-up reports show that he is progressing well at school, is easier to handle at home. More grown-up and protective rôle towards mother has developed, anxious to help her in many ways. Jealousy of sister less intense; no further stammering. Prognosis thought to be good within limits of boy's ability.

Causative factors: unsatisfactory home conditions; disturbed personalities of parents and their disturbed relationship; extreme strictness and rigidity of handling by mother in infancy; father's poor health and failure to play dominant rôle in family; mother's wish that Clifford should be a girl.

Case No. 60: Irving. *Age:* 8 years, 9 months. I.Q. 105.

A red-haired, freckled boy, big for his age; heavy-eyed, anxious, inhibited but friendly.

Referral: by grandmother for variety of symptoms, including violent tempers, nightmares, headaches, unhappiness at school, persistent cough and head movements, asthma, bad language and disobedience.

Family background: lives with maternal grandparents with whom mother left him when he was 3. Mother, who is separated from her husband, rejected Irving; lives nearby with an American and their 2 children. Father also lives nearby with Irving's sister.

Mother: aged 28; very unstable; described as 'nearly mental' after last confinement. As a girl, reported to have been uncontrollable, used bad language, stole and went out with boys. Afraid of husband, though not ill-treated by him. Disappointed that Irving was not a girl, soon turned against him. Irving has been told of her rejection, of her living with another man. She visits him regularly.

Father: aged 29; artisan. In Army for 5 years, abroad until recently. Marriage a failure from beginning; wife unfaithful. Grandparents disapproved of marriage; grandmother describes father as sleepy, unexciting man who bored his wife and was mean with money. He was prepared to adopt illegitimate children, but she hated him, refused to return. Irving sees father, who has no insight into boy's difficulties; blames grandparents for these.

Grandmother: elderly, ineffectual, poor intelligence, limited insight. Was formerly a nurse. Deals with Irving with half-hearted threats, is easily excited and exhausted, feels situation is beyond her control. Guilty and anxious about her handling of him, provokes scenes and fights him on his level; has curious sado-masochistic relationship with him (similar to her disturbed relationship with his mother). She and the boy have physical fights; he threatens to kill her. His attacks of rage cease when she is away. She has sado-masochistic fantasies of his becoming insane and attacking her. Her childhood was unhappy with brutal father, reserved, distant mother. Suffers from rheumatoid arthritis. Excessively anxious about Irving, likes to keep him ill or babyish.

Grandfather: fond of Irving; is steady, good-humoured and patient, with more insight than grandmother, but takes passive rôle, and occasionally finds boy a nuisance. Grandparents quarrel with people, have few friends.

Also in household is maternal great-grandmother, aged 82, whom Irving treats rudely; and mother's brother, aged 20, a borderline epileptic. Maternal great-uncle was certifiably insane, refused to go to mental hospital, died several years ago. There have been frequent changes of home and some financial strain.

History: pregnancy and confinement normal, but he soon pushed mother away. Feeding difficulties from outset; became difficult to manage as he was neglected by mother. Little known of early life. Rejected by parents, left on own for days on end, would be found waiting feverishly when grandfather visited him. Witnessed many violent scenes between parents, then cried and was frightened. At 3, supposedly went for holiday with grandmother, has remained with her since. Not been adopted, lived insecurely, not knowing when he would return to mother. Appetite and sleep good, occasional night terrors. Fights with other children. During last 9 months, daily headaches. Wet bed until 6. Since 2, head movements and grimaces; shoulder-shrugging tic now evident. Left-handed. Temper tantrums since birth; romances and lies. After emotional upsets, he and grandmother have psychosomatic symptoms. Has had whooping cough and tonsilitis; visited numerous doctors and clinics about pains and asthmatical cough, feet, possible worms. Takes pride in numbers of medicines and treatments and in level of nutrition. Worries about his health.

School record and intelligence: reluctant to go to school, dislikes it; teacher has no contact with him. Destructive and difficult with other children. Many absences because of asthma, numerous hospital consultations and grandmother's fussiness. Head teacher describes him as a nervy child who does wilful damage during his 'brain storms'. Backward in arithmetic, fairly good at handwork, reading much below average. Average age of class 7–8.

In intelligence test, I.Q. 105. Ambidextrous, but prefers to use left hand. Slow and clumsy in drawing. Apprehensive and lacking in confidence. Responds to encouragement.

Personality and behaviour: quietly and calmly disobedient at home. In tempers, kicks, spits, scratches, threatens and screams; rages end quickly. Quarrels with other children because he is so demanding, but has one friend with whom he goes tree-climbing. Affectionate as well as aggressive; honest and straight; cruel, then asks to be kissed and helped to be good. Slow and clumsy in movement. Likes aeroplanes, soldiers and farm things; wants to be farmer or market gardener. Deeply interested in flowers and animals. Likes Cub meetings. Careful with toys. Vivid imagination; every horror he sees concerns himself. Number of passive fantasies, e.g. damaged car is mad and surrounded by other cars.

Clinical summary: diagnosed as suffering from a neurotic disturbance; grandmother and he taken on for treatment. Boy very inhibited at first, unable to play or talk; after 2 months became slightly aggressive. Play revealed severe castration anxiety, sexual fears and pleasure in passive fantasies. Later, he became provocative towards the therapist, tried to make her respond to provocations as grandmother did. Prognosis for child thought to be good if grandparents did not give satisfaction to his provocation and wishes for passive attack. After prolonged period of work with grandmother who superficially tried to cooperate at the clinic, it was decided that no further improvement could be expected in her erratic handling, and that while he remained with her he would be constantly stimulated to continue his present behaviour. Her personality is such that further response cannot be expected. Boy attended clinic for some time with group of boys; he was disrupting element, playing wild games, pushing boys about in cart, throwing plasticine, chasing and fighting. When others wanted constructive activities, he played the fool and disturbed their games. Presence of other children appeared to put him into state of intense excitement which he could not control; he dared and provoked them until they participated in equal excitement. In such states, his face turned purple, eyes grew big with irises turned upwards so that only the whites showed, held up his hands as if they were claws, made animal noises. On such occasions, he was almost inaccessible, beyond his own control. Gave impression that he was acting out some animal fantasy.

Irving was thought to be an extremely neurotic boy; disturbance closely related to his relationship with grandmother, since he appears to be relatively undisturbed in his ordinary life apart from her. Yet relationship with grandmother is the only secure one he has. It was considered important to try to preserve this strong relationship; grandmother was urged to complete his adoption instead of tantalizing him about possibility of his return to his mother. She finally completed the adoption, was able to modify her handling slightly and now permits him to attend clubs. Her age precludes her being able to change her basic attitude to him. Recommended that Irving should be sent to a hostel for maladjusted children. So far this has not been practicable. Present aim of treatment is slowly to get grandmother to help accept and support this project. Meanwhile, father has divorced mother. Outcome inconclusive.

Causative factors: disturbed early life; grossly disturbed inter-family relationships; rejection by both parents; violent scenes he witnessed between them; mother's and grandmother's personalities; eccentric and irregular handling from grandmother since age of 3 which has led to intense sado-masochistic type of relationship between them.

Case No. 61: Richard. *Age:* 8 years, 1 month. I.Q. 110.
A boy of average height and weight, with hesitant manner.

Referral: by School Medical Officer on account of exaggerated fears and shyness. Reported to be very nervous at school, shy with strangers, afraid of being alone, refuses to go upstairs in dark. Very dependent on his younger brother, does not mix with other children.

Family background: older of two brothers from stable, lower middle-class home.

Mother: stable, sensible woman, motherly and kind, anxious to do her best for Richard; being shy herself, has sympathy for him though occasionally considers his behaviour silly. Finds him like her 8 years younger brother whom she mothered. Rarely smacks or punishes him, or forces him to do things; clearly has close emotional tie with him.

Father: a professional man; engaged on essential work in war-time so never in Forces. Not shy; some of family rather odd, especially a sister, who is extremely shy and sensitive and very attached to Richard, seeing herself in him. An uncle is also very shy. Father is interested in and fond of children, plays a lot with them. Worried about Richard, encouraged mother to take him to clinic. For two years during war, family stayed with father's family who made great fuss of Richard. Returned to their own home a year ago.

Sibling: unlike Richard; happy, forthcoming. The boys get on well; when together, Richard is sometimes naughty, but never without brother's support.

History: pregnancy and birth normal; easy baby. Breast-fed, developed normally. Walked at 16 months, started to talk a year later. Speech not clear until 3. Habit-training not unduly difficult; early developed constipation, which was a problem until a year ago. Eats and sleeps well, no food fads. No mischievous behaviour as a toddler; always excessively shy and passive, now relies completely on brother. Day or night, dislikes being in room alone; must have door shut, except in lavatory when door must be open and window shut. Has night-light, calls out before going to sleep. This has been more marked lately when, as result of illness, brother did not sleep in his room. These long-standing fears have become more severe during last year. No outstanding illnesses; year ago, tonsils taken out, but he was not greatly upset.

School record and intelligence: gives no trouble; work is good average in all subjects. Blushes easily; shyness and nervousness prevent him from mixing with other children, though he likes school, and never complains. Never bullied, as he remains apart; physically timid, never fights or sneaks.

In intelligence test, I.Q. 110; dreamy; rocked, and sucked fingers. Failed on tests requiring prolonged attention or formulation of longish replies. Performance uneven; very preoccupied with own ideas.

In psychiatric interviews, shy and reserved, unable to discuss fears, generally uncommunicative. Disturbed, cannot make full use of intellectual capacities.

Personality and behaviour; affectionate, slow and dreamy; will do anything to keep mother in house; plays for hours with brother; no signs of overt jealousy or resentment. Until recently, would play by himself with dolls and girl's toys. Passion for babies. Easily managed, quietly obedient unless brother is with him. If asked to recite or anything similar, becomes self-conscious, gets under table. Slow to speak to anyone new, excessively shy with strangers or in new social situations.

Clinical summary: diagnosed as primary behaviour disturbance with pronounced neurotic tendencies; mother and boy seen regularly. Mother attained good insight into his problems, able to modify handling. Richard seen in group of boys; at first completely withdrawn, played alone, rocking at same time. When other children commented on his behaviour, became self-conscious and stopped. With help of therapist, became more interested in others' activities; after time, took active part in fighting when it was acted; became defiant towards therapist with whom he had established good relationship. Conflicts about other boys were interpreted; behaviour at home and at school changed. Fears disappeared, reported to be better in every way at school; sings, mixes better, plays with other children. Individual treatment not indicated; follow-up showed that improvement had been maintained.

Causative factors: partly constitutional, following the temperament of many shy and 'queer' members of father's family; pronounced sibling jealousy; over-dependence upon mother and an early passive identification with her; attitude of parents which from early years has not allowed the boy normal outlets for the expression of aggression.

Case No. 62: Phineas. *Age:* 8 years, 3 months. I.Q. 105.

A thin, round-faced boy, anxious and diffident. Slight limp, as left leg is permanently affected by poliomyelitis. Wears splints at night, still has massage. Easily tired. Tip-toes round room; talks very little.

Referral: by parents on account of babyish behaviour, backwardness at school and crying easily.

Family background: third of four boys from a cultured, middle-class home.

Mother: hard, disagreeable expression, fidgety and intense, on the defensive, but not unattractive. Good intellectual appreciation of Phineas's difficulties, but unable to show him warmth of feeling. Talked about her unhappy childhood; only child of parents who lived in Malaya; spent most of life in boarding-schools or with relatives; up-bringing was old-fashioned; felt unwanted. Never shows affection for Phineas, finds his babyish ways irritating, yet feels guilty about him. Each child has been a problem to her; conflict over leniency and severity. Says she takes after her father in being undemonstrative. Attitude is rejecting towards all boys, but most markedly so towards Phineas.

Father: officer in regular Indian Army; absent for most of children's lives, now at home on 2 months' leave. Tall, good-looking, shy, aloof and sensitive, appears stable and reasonable. Uneventful childhood. Tendency to wear effeminate clothes, lets mother handle most of interview. Fond of the children, but fails to understand them; shares interest in nature and horticulture with Phineas. Wanted to have a profession; not actively unhappy in army. Many differences of opinion with mother about handling of Phineas.

Siblings: two older brothers, at boarding-school; younger brother, aged 6. Eldest boy is solitary, reticent and nervous, backward at school; jealous of more popular brother. Mother describes second boy as live wire of family; nervous, restless, and talkative. Eldest considers himself too old for Phineas, who is devoted to second boy. Youngest is lively, more stable, stronger and more mature than Phineas, and more advanced at school; mother's favourite. Phineas is jealous of him. They are rivals for popular second brother's affections.

Family has never had settled home. Lived in India until Phineas was 6, now live with paternal grandmother, who is strict. Phineas dislikes and is rude to her. Each child cared for by nannie until 3.

History: unwanted baby. Pregnancy and birth normal; mother disappointed he was not a girl. Weighed 10 lb.; breast-fed for

3 months. Tongue-tied at birth; this was snicked at one month. Easily weaned, good appetite. Feeding difficulties developed later. Until 3, series of unsatisfactory nannies; never had close relationship with mother. Walked at 17 months, babbled at usual age, not speaking clearly until 4. Toilet-training easy; clean and dry at 3 when family moved to India, then cared for by ayah until 7. Has room to himself, sleeps well, sometimes 'wails out' in sleep. Mother says babyishness more pronounced since 3; speech is still babyish; nails badly bitten. Feeding difficulties have now returned and failure in school more evident. Mother thinks he masturbates considerably. Health good at present. At 5, broke arm; at 6, anterior poliomyelitis; one month in hospital. Missed school for 6 months while leg was treated. During past year, many accidents and illnesses. At 7, ringworm and greenstick fracture of arm. More accident-prone than brothers.

School record and intelligence: began school at 4 years in India, mornings only. Attainment poor, especially reading and spelling. Writing is mixture of script and capitals. Below average in all subjects; inattentive and fidgety; no desire to do well, concentration poor.

In intelligence test, I.Q. 105. In some tests, responded in stupid, bewildered and uncertain manner. Cried, was miserable and rejected. Unable to use full intelligence at present.

Personality and behaviour: at home, is said to act and speak as though he were simple, which parents find difficult to describe. Slow in uptake, cries easily, little control over emotions. Stands up for himself in scrapes with brothers, though generally avoids these. Less responsible when brothers are at home, adopting miserable, dejected and whining attitude. Dreamy; dribbles; 'don't care' attitude about school work. Likes being read to; interested in animals, insects, gardening. Has friends; dislikes being alone. Preoccupied with sado-masochistic fantasies.

Clinical summary: diagnosed as a case of chronic neurosis. Taken on for treatment. Found to be very anxious, insecure, worried, passive and effeminate, absorbed in fantasy life. Made good progress. Mother gained some insight from treatment, was able to change attitude to boy. It became clear that Phineas was always father's favourite and has identified with his passive-effeminate attitudes. Treatment satisfactory but incomplete when terminated through family leaving the district. Prognosis for adult life thought to be only fair and boy's personality remains passive. Follow-up shows he has settled well in new preparatory school as a day boy. Attends different school from younger brother, is making slow but satisfactory progress. Is more self-confident, has many friends, enjoys games.

Causative factors: impaired early relationship with mother; lack of enduring mother-substitute in her place together with mother's personality; her handling of all family and special emotional rejection of Phineas; absence of father for long periods.

Case No. 63: Charles. *Age:* 8 years, 5 months. I.Q. 130.

A slightly effeminate, neat, tidy boy, with sharp features, small for his age, over-polite in manner. Not spontaneous, but glib and anxious to please. Emotional reaction probably masked.

Referral: by step-mother on account of behaviour difficulties, lack of bladder and bowel control, lying, sexual offences, nail-biting and queer, 'awkward' behaviour with other children.

Family background: only child whose mother is dead, and whose father is abroad. Lives with step-mother.

Mother: step-mother describes her as excitable, mischief-making, promiscuous, unstable, neglectful and cruel to Charles, leaving him alone when she went out with men during husband's absence, or carried on with them in his presence. She died 2 years ago.

Step-mother: pleasant woman who knew mother's family. Thin, nervous, harassed, anxious and guilty towards Charles although she has given him sensible and sympathetic treatment. Has affection and limited understanding for him. He clings to her, is frightened she will leave him. Her treatment of him is alternately aggressive and harsh, tender and spoiling. She is unable to have children. Works daily as waitress.

Father: hospital caretaker in civilian life; been in Army for 4 years, some time abroad, expects to be demobilized soon. Described as weak personality. Beats Charles when he wets or messes; probable that Charles provokes these beatings. Boy never cries, but is cheeky and deliberately provocative towards father, who has been completely absent from the family for 3 years. Uncooperative towards clinic.

Family lives under ordinary working-class conditions.

History: little known of early history; led irregular life with mother, with little security and much illness. On death of mother, cared for by woman who was living in same house. She left suddenly, so father took boy to his sister's home. At 6, returned to father when he remarried. Then lacked bladder and bowel control; slow to fall asleep; enormous appetite. Health has improved since living with step-mother. Two years ago, tonsillectomy. Incontinence lessened after step-mother took him to private doctor. Now has night fears, periods of sleeping badly, bouts of lying and fantasying. Follows punishment (i.e. for wetting) by staying out all night. Bites nails; when reprimanded said mother had done the same. Complaints made about his kissing girls. Step-mother says he is not like other boys, fears he will show sexual precocity. Has undoubtedly witnessed sexual, possibly violent, scenes during period when he lived with mother.

School record and intelligence: is in class of average age a year older than his own; 2nd in form of 42. Reports good, progress satisfactory; begs head teacher to give him homework. Before living with step-mother, unable to read despite high intelligence. Rather solitary; sometimes returns home with bruises on face. Teacher has noticed that he is accident-prone.

In intelligence test, I.Q. 130. Quick in response, enjoyed the test. Score upon Koh's Block Design Test indicated mental age of 14 years. Over-confident, thrown into confusion by failure, accustomed to praise for being 'small and bright'. Rather glib, not spontaneous; emotional reactions masked.

Personality and behaviour: at home, step-mother says Charles is always bumping into things and hurting himself; never cries. When threatened with punishment says it will do no good, that

there is no feeling left in his bottom or his head. When reprimanded for kissing girls, said his mother used to do it. Step-
mother is disturbed because his kisses to her are sensual. No
friends of own age; reluctant to play outside, prefers to read
comics or do cross-word puzzles so as to be with his step-mother.
Sometimes gets very dirty. Step-mother says he expresses peculiar
ideas, especially about death. He is sulky, abnormally quiet, over-
anxious, unable to show real feelings; has no field of self-expres-
sion; tendency to self-punishment, frequently gets hurt, otherwise over-good child. Loves brushing step-mother's hair; likes
reading, collecting stamps. Preoccupied with masochistic fantasies; tells lies about other boys to get them into trouble. Unable
to play, prefers girlish activities. Often says people are working
against him or ill-treating him.

Clinical summary: diagnosed as a case of neurotic disturbance.
Charles might, in later years, develop grave psychopathology.
Passive, effeminate boy, showing masochistic behaviour and
abnormal sexual development. Taken on for treatment with the
object of making him more aware of his wish for self-punishment.
Step-mother also seen in order to help her alter her handling and
refrain from being provoked by his wish for punishment. In the
treatment situation, Charles displayed many sado-masochistic
fantasies, was preoccupied with fantasies of bodily injury. Following an accident in which he broke his arm, his behaviour improved greatly. Became more active, played normally. Resistant
to any interpretation of his need for punishment, or his obvious
wish to injure his arm again. His symptoms of wetting and soiling
cleared up in response to interpretations of their unconscious
motivation, but he was thought to be still disturbed and in need
of treatment. When he became reluctant to continue deeper
treatment, step-mother was satisfied with the symptomatic improvement, and did not wish to continue clinic attendance. He
made excellent progress in school during this time, and his behaviour there improved. The prognosis, without further treatment,
was thought to be poor. It is likely that Charles will have a severe
character disturbance and probably an abnormal sexual life.
Treatment incomplete and outcome inconclusive.

Causative factors: abnormal early background; mother's open promiscuity and ill-treatment of him; desertion by two mother-substitutes. Follow-up showed that on father's return he at first appeared to make good relationship, but is now obviously provoking father to hit him as punishment for soiling and cheeky behaviour, and he has injured his arm again. Outcome of this case is considered unsatisfactory, but father has refused to allow the treatment to continue.

Case No. 64: Fred. *Age:* 8 years, 9 months. I.Q. 89.

A rather small, healthy boy.

Referral: by school medical officer on account of 'odd' fears, headaches, nervous behaviour at school and not mixing with other children. He is said to refuse his school dinner if anyone else is in the room and will never play with the other children.

Family background: illegitimate; reared by grandmother who is known to him as his mother.

Mother: aged 27, known to Fred as his sister. Had wanted to marry boy's father, but grandmother intervened because of father's instability and unsuitability. Mother, now married, has child of 2. Fred sees her occasionally, but she has little interest in him. Grandmother is certain he does not realize their relationship. Father unknown to Fred.

Grandmother: aged 50, young enough in appearance to pass as boy's mother. Warm, maternal, loves Fred. Likes country, hates city and noise; dislikes eating away from home; her irrational fears dovetail with Fred's. Heart attacks and asthma coinciding with 3 years she has been most worried about Fred. Severity of attacks prevents her moving in morning, so Fred is often late or absent from school. Her own family, now grown up, say that she spoils Fred by giving in to his odd fears, that her handling should be different, and that she gives him preferences denied them. She excuses her behaviour by saying she wants to make up for all he has lost.

Grandfather: works at fairly distant factory; much away from home. Said to idolize and spoil Fred, but impatient over his food fads and odd ideas. Negative towards psychological treatment.

Grandparents' 27-year-old son lives at home and is supposed to be Fred's brother.

History: at 2 weeks came from hospital to grandmother; gave minimum of trouble; led regular life until 2½ when air-raids began; 2-3 months of shelter life; upset, cried a great deal. Habit-training normal, achieved at 1 year. Sleep restless; often afraid to sleep alone; shares room with grandmother's son, cries out in sleep, and grandmother goes to reassure him. Lies awake listening for noises, imagines things. Appetite always excessively faddy; between 2 and 5, constant battles over meals, now given only what he will eat. Dislikes having school dinners, vividly describes them as horrible in colour and smell. Health good; periodically complains of headaches and looks pale and exhausted.

School record and intelligence: always disliked school, but no longer complains. Progress average; has no friends, never talks about school. Teacher says he seldom spoke during first year; for 2 years spoke only to teachers, who find him nervous and difficult to understand. Attendance irregular because of grandmother's asthma. Idle and inattentive during lessons, self-conscious when spoken to, often unable to speak. Reading quite good, arithmetic and spelling poor, unable to grasp idea of tables. Learning hampered by preoccupation with fantasies. Never fights, prefers to play with girls. Usually quiet in playground though occasionally bursts forth into wild, rough behaviour and war games.

First intelligence test unsuccessful owing to Fred's not talking. Average scores on several performance tests. After 3 months at clinic, re-examined. I.Q. 89; speech jerky, stilted in phraseology; poor results in all verbal tests. School work competent within limit of abilities; reading age 7-8 year level. No spontaneous reactions.

Personality and behaviour: likes to stay indoors and play with Meccano set; always good. Dislikes separation from grandmother, needs much persuasion to go on visits; often behaves as though afraid grandmother will not return. She can now get away to cinema; when she goes visiting, he sits on step outside. Afraid to stay away for a night. Interested in smell of things; refused school milk because of smell of beakers. Never cries; no talking difficulties at home. Grandmother finds it strange that she is never angry with him as she was with her own children.

Clinical summary: diagnosed as suffering from severe obsessional neurosis. Various factors in his history led at first to a suspicion that the boy's difficulty in talking may be caused by a pre-psychotic condition. Detailed psychiatric observation over more than a year, however, made this appear unlikely. In psychiatric interviews there was at first a complete inhibition of play activities and speech; some contact was established. Gave impression of wishing to talk but could not succeed. His fears, especially fear of grandmother leaving him, were played out through medium of plasticine models. After this, he began to talk spontaneously at the clinic and began to go out at home. When deeper anxieties were discussed, the necessity became clear for Fred to be told whose child he really is. This was finally done by the grandmother under the psychiatrist's supervision, and Fred's behaviour, especially his talking, showed immediate improvement. Grandmother and boy were seen regularly; certain of his fantasies were understood by both of them. After improvement in his symptoms, however, boy did not come regularly; treatment ceased owing to combination of external circumstances and grandmother's unconscious lack of cooperation. Follow-up shows that he has improved in behaviour, is more boyish and more mature at home. Social relationships have improved, night fears have cleared up and school improvements maintained.

Causative factors: grandmother's deeply disturbed personality; her unusual handling; his suspicions about illegitimate birth and family attitude to the secret about his birth; possible constitutional factors.

Case No. 65: Julian. *Age:* 8 years, 4 months. I.Q. 109.

A shy, quiet, retiring boy, above average in height and weight.

Seldom smiles, has sad voice, slow and hesitant in speech. Walks stiffly with arms pressed to sides.

Referral: by teacher on account of extreme shyness and inability to talk at school. Teacher had difficulty in obtaining Julian's cooperation in oral work and dramatics.

Family background: 3rd child in family of 4 from stable, upper-middle-class home.

Mother: aged over 40; pleasant, sensible, apparently stable; warm-hearted, enjoys her family and handles them well. Julian shares her high moral standards. A year older than her husband, she is a powerful personality in relation to him. Dominates her family.

Father: professional man; shy, expects much of his children, especially that they should be intelligent. So far, they have come up to his expectations. Julian's relationship with father is strained; boy is frightened to express aggression towards him.

Siblings: brother, aged 12, also shy; does well at private school. Sister, aged 10, artistic and musical; shy and timid. Sister, aged 5, very intelligent and musical; much fuss made of her. Children are all good friends and family is a happy one; Julian not regarded as problem at home; whole family are of shy and timid disposition. Father has several aunts, all teachers. A number of members of mother's family also teach, so Julian is expected to be bright and do well at school.

History: mother says he was nice baby; breast-fed, but weaning sudden and difficult because of mother's having to attend two confinements among relatives. During 1st year, mother over-wrought by war work and family responsibilities; Julian had difficult time; had to be rocked in cradle day and night from 9–12 months. No feeding difficulties; talked and walked at normal age, but crawled for longer than other children. Speech development slow, hesitant from outset, almost as if defective. Unco-operative as small child, still inclined to drop out of activities. Before 6, period of being difficult in playing with brothers and sisters, preferring to be on his own; this attitude has now improved. No sleep problems; shares room with brother. As a baby,

399

talked and played with himself when he woke; now often talks and giggles to himself before going to sleep. Worries about illness and accidents to family; frequently has accidents with play material. During last 2 years, occasional phases of face-twitching and grimacing; nervous cough; picks nose. In infancy, short attacks of bronchitis, though not serious. Health now good.

School record and intelligence: went to local school, works well. Reading above average, arithmetic and practical work of average standard; backward in spelling, and father coaches him. In response to direct questions in class, bites lip and is unable to reply. Shy and retiring in playground, quiet and well-behaved in class. Family are Methodists, and head teacher considers they are extremely intelligent but over-strict in religion.

In intelligence test, I.Q. 109. Unable to talk freely; apprehensive and withdrawn, spoke in monosyllables, giving little information. Pencil work careless, results very scattered as he had failures very early upon tests of immediate recall.

Personality and behaviour: mother says Julian differs from other children in that he likes mechanical things while their interests are artistic. Julian is lively at home, no shyness with brother and sisters; talks to strangers who visit them. Plays with friends of own age at their house. Family are all quiet-tempered, undemonstrative, but Julian can show anger when frustrated. Goes to Cub meetings; is frightened of other boys and would not fight. Blushes if afraid of being forced to do something. Poise and posture clumsy; many accidents. Had interest in making doll's clothes in fine needlework. Plays piano, shares family love of classical music.

Clinical summary: diagnosed as suffering from a neurosis. Difficulties very deep-seated, and he has identified with mother's strong moral code. Silence results from fear of his own aggression; he appears to have turned his fierce super-ego against himself. He is responding well to treatment, behaviour has improved; he shows new interest in flowers and animal life. Prognosis as far as his symptoms are concerned is thought to be good, but underlying neurotic personality cannot be changed without more intensive psycho-analytic treatment than is possible in a child guidance clinic.

Causative factors: mother's personality, unequal relationship between parents, together with a strong neurotic family pattern which Julian has followed.

Case No. 66: Mark. *Age:* 9 years, 2 months. I.Q. 96.

A large, well-built but clumsy boy; wears glasses. He is easily distracted, disparages what he does.

Referral: by School Medical Officer on account of failure at school, enuresis, violent behaviour towards other children, quarrelling and truancy.

Family background: illegitimate; lives with mother and step-father whom she married when Mark was 6 and who intends to adopt him legally.

Mother: aged 30, attractive, open-natured and intelligent. Has month-old baby; during pregnancy was worried and nervous, had fainting fits and night terrors in which she 'saw things'; looks anaemic. Depends on husband for support and advice. As child, was ill-treated by mother, punished, then withdrew into daydreams, just as Mark now does. Has ambivalent relationship with Mark; unable to make him obey her; appeared to be indifferent to him in accounts of his behaviour, but he is very loving towards her, appeals to her for help against father. Mark knew his maternal grandmother as mummy until he was 2, while his mother went to work.

Father: married man whom mother hopes never to see again.

Step-father: aged 38; intelligent, humorous, sensible; has initiative and drive. Runs small business. Standards are high; is cooperative but likely to hit out in temper. In Army for 5 years during war; no overseas service. It was he who gave full case history at clinic. Relationship with Mark unsatisfactory, on which mother blames present trouble. She says step-father started off badly by hitting Mark with a slipper when the boy was rude; the boy has never forgiven this, and has always resented him. Father tries to be patient, but boy provokes him so much that he shouts; loses his temper then takes strict measures. Has little insight. He refuses to tell the boy he is not his real father, although the boy has questioned the reason for his old name being on his ration book.

Sibling: step-sister; Mark said to love her, but has thrown pepper over her so that he could laugh when she sneezed. Once put stocking over her head and left her.

Family lives in overcrowded conditions in two rooms.

History: confinement long and difficult; birth normal. On grandfather's insistence, child passed off as grandmother's for 2 years. Grandmother spoilt him. Early years disturbed; life insecure until 6. Mother unable to breast-feed him as she was nervous and depressed. At 2, refused to call grandmother 'mummy', became difficult, developed temper tantrums. Early toilet and habit training difficult, never gaining complete control. Grandparents dealt strictly with this. Eats well; usually sleeps well; shares parents' bedroom; restless in sleep. Sometimes jealous of mother towards father. Developed strong hatred for 4-year-old cousin who replaced him as grandmother's favourite. Rude to step-father prior to marriage; this continues. At 3 or 4, developed asthma; continues to have temper tantrums; wets bed about once a fortnight, occasionally soils knickers and hides them. Often hurts himself; kicks and hits other children. Apart from asthma, health good.

School record and intelligence: started school at $4\frac{1}{2}$; owing to moves during war, many changes, and has attended five schools in all. Poor progress, bad reports; is now in class with twenty-five backward children. All teachers query his mental ability, say he has strange temper, waves arms in class, distracts other children. Fights with boys, chases girls about. Unable to read, educationally one year retarded; good at handwork and drawing.

In intelligence test, I.Q. 96; very distractable, failed to use full abilities; uninhibited, emotionally disturbed. Confused in mental processes. Chatted brightly during test.

Personality and behaviour: mother says he can be model child, but is usually disobedient and difficult. Day-dreams, is shy and retiring, slow to show affection except towards mother. Sensitive, cries easily, never answers back; often hurts himself without complaining. Friends are younger than himself; over-generous to other children. Prefers to be with parents than with children. Likes all forms of nature study. Truancy occurred at time of baby's birth.

Clinical summary: diagnosed as primary behaviour disorder with neurotic tendencies; taken on for group treatment. Attendance irregular, came late, usually had to be supported by some object such as a mouse or knife in his pocket, or accompanied by a friend. Anxious, never really formed group relationship. When individual treatment was offered, too afraid to come alone; eventually failed to come with group. Parents indifferent and refused to send him for individual treatment; case closed as unsatisfactory.

Causative factors: illegitimacy and parents' concealment of this; inconsistent handling in early years between mother and grandmother; quarrel relationship to step-father; mother's personality and parents' basic rejection and ambivalence. The indifferent attitude of the mother, and high standards of step-father, make prognosis poor unless individual treatment can be carried on for a long time. This seems to be impossible at the present time since family lives far away from the clinic, and the parents refused to allow the boy to attend.

Case No. 67: Portland. *Age:* 10 years, 1 month. I.Q. 110.

A small, healthy boy with an obvious scar on nose and forehead.

Referral: by Speech Therapist, with whom he had failed to make any progress, on account of stammering, inhibited behaviour, jealousy, enuresis, school retardation and speech and sleep disturbances.

Family background: second of three children from stable home.

Mother: middle-aged, twice married. First husband, father of Portland's 24-year-old step-sister, is dead. Mother is well-dressed, efficient and managing; has ideals and ambitions, but is reserved, self-satisfied and deeply neurotic, with great emotional problems.

Is intelligent and hardworking; defences of respectability and rigidity limit the extent to which her outlook and attitudes can be modified. Childhood very hard; bore all household responsibilities at 13. Since girlhood, has had many fears; severe mouse phobia. On death of husband, started her own small shop, which she enjoyed. Intended to continue this, but pregnancy with Portland hindered the plan, which displeased her and made her resent her husband's making her pregnant. Relationship with Portland is disturbed; he has excessive anxiety about her. She is genuinely anxious to help him, but unable to be consistently firm. She now takes seasonal work or boarders in summer.

Father: shop assistant. Easy-going; had deprived childhood, no family life. Liked to spoil the children but now has little time in which to play with them. Mother describes him as thin, wispy, timid and diffident. Marital relationship obviously unequal; mother secretly despises him. He does much domestic work while she gardens. Though fond of Portland, he is easily irritated by him and his unreasonable demands; tries to offset what he considers is mother's over-indulgence by thrashing. Portland is a frequent cause of quarrels, and plays one parent off against the other.

Step-sister: married; lives at home with 2-year-old child.

Sibling: brother, aged 6; different from Portland; independent, said to be father's favourite now, and father rejects Portland whom he spoiled during early years. Portland jealous of brother.

Family lives in good, lower-middle-class conditions.

History: birth precipitate, 2 weeks premature. Unwanted baby, mother still feels guilty. Bottle-fed; no weaning or feeding difficulties. Walked and talked at normal time. Severe temper tantrums as toddler. Clean and dry at 2; harshly treated in this. Occasional bed-wetting continued until 18 months ago. Sleepless until late at night, wakes early; sleep-walks. Sedatives given by private doctor. Has nightmares, dreams of murders or women in men's clothes, or of falling from high up over a cave on to rocks. At 5, severe stammering began, also sucking and chewing of sleeves and lapels. Between 7 and 8, nervous sucking and biting habits became severe; at same time, afraid of being bullied. Twice beaten up by neighbouring evacuee. Has fears of being assaulted or attacked and of any form of violence, particularly in films. Dislikes meeting people, becomes embarrassed and flushes, refusing to speak to visitors. Several traumatic experiences: at 2½ attacked and frightened by dog which clawed him, marking his face; now terrified of wild animals. At 4, at time of precipitate birth of brother, about which he had been told, he was terrified, refusing to go near mother for several days and believing she had lost her legs. After 6, acute earache, developed fears, witnessed machine-gunning, which frightened him. Health good; no separation from home.

School record and intelligence: likes school and is popular. Works and plays well, progress is good average; hopes to gain scholarship. Regarded as highly strung. He is well-mannered and helpful, over-anxious and conscientious. Weak in spelling, good at manual work; hopes to go to technical school.

In intelligence test, I.Q. 110. P.C.I. score indicated mental age of 12 plus. Inhibited in emotional response.

Personality and behaviour: at home, is willing and pleasant, popular with neighbours, but shy, diffident and anxious, lacking self-confidence. Restless and demanding, cries easily, readily becomes sullen, often moody and bad-tempered. Plays family up if particularly anxious to have his way. Likes to ride bicycle, go fishing or to Cub meetings. Occasionally makes intense friendships. Secretive about sex matters, is exaggeratedly modest, like his mother. Weepy, fearful and anxious when at films.

Clinical summary: diagnosed as suffering from a neurosis; taken on for observation and advice on handling of his behaviour difficulties. Thought to be doubtful if anything could be done for his stammer without full psycho-analytic treatment. Sibling rivalry worked through and became better able to deal with it. His ambitions and achievements and his parents' attitude to these were discussed. Helped in a number of school difficulties, given coaching in spelling. Interviews with mother helped her to become

o

more tolerant and more able to adopt consistent methods. At end of treatment, said she had benefited as much as boy. It is doubtful, however, whether or not she is able to alter her deep-seated attitudes as, basically, she is smug and well-satisfied with herself. Portland's behaviour improved; follow-up shows that progress has been maintained, behaviour difficulties have satisfactorily cleared up. Stammer, as was expected, remains unchanged. Prognosis thought to be fair.

Causative factors: mother's neurotic and dominating personality; her consistent rejection of boy; his sibling rivalry, aggravated by mother's preference for brother; disturbed parental relationship; rather ineffectual father; several gross traumatic experiences in early years.

Case No. 68: Roy. *Age:* 9 years, 7 months. I.Q. 99.
   An attractive, self-possessed boy.

Referral: by teacher and mother on account of learning difficulties. He is judged by everyone who has to deal with him as very intelligent, but he cannot get on at school, does not concentrate and is backward.

Family background: only child from stable, professional home.

Mother: in late 40s. Quiet, depressed, competent and intelligent. Has had many serious illnesses; now speaks in odd, hoarse, low voice. Ambitious, but lacks insight and understanding of Roy; anxious to give impression that Roy is intelligent and has no difficulties beyond inability to learn.

Father: highly trained professional man, much away from home leaving management of the boy to mother. Gets on well with him, thinks he has outstanding abilities; allows him to help in work that involves drawings and drafts. Both parents regret having only one child. First child was still-born; second, a girl, died 10 years ago, was weakly child who died of an infection at 7. Third pregnancy was terminated because of mother's health. Roy was fourth pregnancy.

The family has had many changes of home; for period lived in an hotel.

History: birth normal and full term; bottle-fed. Walked at 16 months, talked at 2. No specific difficulties. During first 5 years, mother was in hospital several times for periods of 2 or more months; Roy undisturbed by her absence, and visited her. At 5, mother again ill; resident nurse cared for him. When 6½, mother had major operation in hospital; Roy spent 9 months with aunt in country. He loiters over food, though has good appetite. Sleeps alone, shows no fears. Had pneumonia badly, otherwise health good. Day-dreams a great deal.

School record and intelligence: started school soon after 5; has had many changes and liked none of them. At 6½, started at present one, likes it. Head Teacher says he is incapable of learning and can scarcely read. Former teachers said he could not concentrate. He is one year retarded; difficult to make him work because of talking to other boys. Head and class teachers consider mother is odd; she frequently visits school; expects too much of Roy.

In intelligence test, I.Q. 99 with poor verbal ability. Perform-ance scattered and uneven; rushed into tests without waiting for instructions. Scores were best in group performance tests. Prac-tical bent borne out in enjoyment of drawing and painting, which he likes. Dislikes reading, weak in arithmetic. He said he liked school, but preferred to play by himself at home with soldiers and ships, or making up stories to himself in bed, which is probably what he does in class time.

Personality and behaviour: mother finds him no trouble; he is inde-pendent. Has learnt violin for a year, practises spontaneously, arranging lessons for himself. Mother implied he was a musical genius, but teacher reports that he shows average ability with more than average interest in music. Mother insists on attending violin lessons, is harsh and exacting, hits him when he is inatten-tive. Teacher thinks his day-dreaming is an expression of relief at being away from mother; she has observed many examples of mother's over-protective, coddling behaviour. Roy is ambitious, wants to be good at things, worries about his reading. He likes to make things to help father. Has one particular friend of own age.

Clinical summary: diagnosed as a case of primary behaviour disturbance with neurotic trends. In psychiatric interviews, Roy appeared to be socially mature beyond his years and talked with pleasure about some of his day-dreams. Analysis of these indicated presence of neurotic learning inhibitions. He was taken on for individual treatment. In subsequent interviews, he showed that he cannot stand not being able to do a thing; gives up immediately without admitting that he cannot do it. Disturbed in all activities; play entirely a defence against admitting his true thoughts and feelings. Kept himself aloof from therapist, played automatic games continuously as defence against closer examination of difficulties. Problem of learning difficulty was discussed, seriousness of problem stressed. Continued to play games which showed his ambition and inability to pursue something after initial failure. This he was able to admit; made some all-round improvement at school. Behaviour with other boys improved; made fewer bids for attention from teachers. Mother was also seen at clinic; it became clear there was similarity between her attitude and Roy's. Both superficially pleasant, but hide real feeling behind impenetrable façade of friendly and cooperative behaviour. Mother is rigid personality, unable to grasp another person's point of view as she talks and pursues her own thoughts all the time. Refused to accept psychologist's assessment of Roy's ability, fundamentally hostile and suspicious about treatment; continued to bring varying examples of boy's high intelligence. Insisted that he should go to superior secondary school; arranged for him to be coached for scholarship because she says he so much wants to get it; constantly and unnecessarily reassured psychiatrist that nothing at home prevented the boy from coming to the clinic. Roy's attendance, however, became irregular, then ceased. Treatment was considered satisfactory as far as the immediate symptom is concerned, but owing to exaggerated ambition, lack of confidence in boy and strong resistance in mother's attitude, no real change could be effected. Prognosis as far as later neurotic disturbance is concerned is doubtful.

Causative factors: mother's attitude which combined over-protectiveness with ambition disproportionate to boy's abilities; father's support for her in this attitude; lack of emotional sincerity and considerable mistrust and pretence in all family interrelationships; unfortunate intense focusing of parents' emotional life upon this one surviving child.

Case No. 69: Matthew. *Age:* 9 years, 9 months. I.Q. 122.

A pale-faced, attractive boy with high spirits and a sense of humour. Friendly, talks easily, adult in outlook.

Referral: by his mother on account of bed-wetting, laziness, backwardness, difficult and unmanageable behaviour at home.

Family background: elder of two boys in stable, middle-class home.

Mother: hard-working, anxious and domineering woman with high standards of conduct for the children. Neurotic; always suffered from repetitive anxiety dreams. Only child of eccentric father who did not conceal disappointment that she was a girl. She now wears mannish clothes. Hostile towards her mother. Intense relationship with Matthew whom she identifies with her father—i.e. gifted, but never really worked. Expresses hostility towards Matthew, cannot tolerate aggressive or masculine behaviour in him, fearing she is weaker than he; sarcastically ridicules him; he provokes her to be sadistic until she hits him. Regards his failures as her own shortcomings. Over-anxious, restrictive and hypercritical with him; gives weekly recital at Clinic of his misdeeds and failures.

Father: conscientious, effeminate, charming, and musical. Suffers from psychosomatic complaints. Defective vision caused by accident in youth. The mother dominates him; he will go to great lengths to avoid friction with her. Matthew has reduced him to tears. During the war, he was Major in Army; no overseas service because of poor vision. Now business man in the city, returns home late each evening. Demanding and ambitious for Matthew; deals with boy's outbreaks by moral appeals to his better nature. Matthew provokes father to beat him.

Maternal grandfather: alcoholic professional man who died in mental hospital of senile dementia. Formerly lived with family for 6 months when Matthew was 5; mother found him difficult and troublesome.

Maternal grandmother: aged 61; lives with family; suffers from arthritis. Matthew plays her up.

During Matthew's early years, family had no settled home. Now live under good middle-class though crowded conditions. Many tensions in household and not enough scope for a high-spirited boy.

History: pregnancy and confinement normal. Active baby; suffered from pyloric stenosis for which medically treated. Breast-fed for 3 weeks; screamed and cried so much that mother gave him bottle. Severe feeding difficulties; had to be forced to eat. Chewed sheets and pram straps; everything went into his mouth. Pyloric stenosis cured by 8 months. Walked at 18 months, talked at 2 years. Habit-training rigid; clean at 3. Bed-wetting began when family had no settled home and father was absent. Sleep restless. From early age provoked mother by pulling faces and making noises when she was out of reach. Children deliberately allowed to see parents naked. At 3, had dysentery three times; at 4½ whooping-cough and mumps; at 5, tonsils and adenoids removed; numerous colds. From 6–7 experienced air-raids with family; not particularly afraid. More frightened of doodle-bugs, cried and felt sick. After this was evacuated. Feeding difficulties have persisted since infancy; bed-wetting always acute.

School record and intelligence: began school at 4½, has always done badly. At 8, transferred to local grammar school. Is lazy and disobedient, always in detention. Teacher says, though of high intelligence, fails to concentrate, cannot settle down, makes no progress. He is mischievous, defiant and disobedient. Exceptionally good at music. Dislikes school.

In intelligence test, I.Q. 122. Good verbal comprehension and reasoning powers, failed in memory tests. Little surplus energy; attention impaired by anxiety.

Personality and behaviour: mother describes him as disobedient and incorrigibly rude, excessively lazy; apathetic about school failures, brazen about bed-wetting. Popular with outsiders, much liked by little girls. Good at cross-country running and games, but tends to hurt himself in games, especially football. Has fine singing voice, wants to join choir. Keen on religion, reads the Bible and goes to Bible classes. Dreams a great deal; worried about father's finances.

Clinical summary: diagnosed as case of primary behaviour disorder with neurotic trends; taken on for treatment. Turbulent external behaviour found to cover number of fears and anxieties which were worked through; as these were discussed, bed-wetting became less frequent. Preoccupation with blood, hurting fantasies, constant provocation of mother to hurt him related to sado-masochistic fantasies. Pleasure in masturbation excitement was discussed and also his passive fantasies and wishes towards father, whom he sees as the weak figure in the household while the mother is dominant. Improvements in the home situation and in the mother's handling have been effected; responding satisfactory; treatment is progressing well and symptoms have been greatly relieved.

Causative factors: high standards in the home of over-anxious and over-critical parents; possibly a neurotic constitutional factor; personalities of a weak, gentle, loving father and strong, dominant mother, where the usual parental roles are reversed. Mother herself was unable to cooperate in treatment until she discussed her own difficult relations with the father. Outcome of case thought to be satisfactory.

Case No. 70: Ross. *Age:* 11 years, 3 months. I.Q. 93.
An active and alert boy who appears anxious and ill-at-ease.

Referral: by school medical officer on account of facial and bodily twitches, school failure and lack of confidence.

Family background: older of two boys in stable home of good, working-class standards.

Mother: a pale, dull, immature woman of poor intelligence; numerous fears, particularly of the dark. Only child, very dependent upon her mother. Self-abnegating, anxiously defers to husband. Little insight into Ross's problems; inconsistent in handling, finds him irritating and restless; upset by his tempers.

Father: stocky, earnest and ambitious; is intelligent and has some degree of insight. Five years in R.A.F. (ground staff). Has been fitter and electrician, now shares own mechanical and motor-repair business with a friend. Coaches Ross in school work, is fond of him, anxious for his welfare, but is becoming exasperated by his so-called stupidity. Though over-ambitious and pressing, understands the boy more than mother does.

Sibling: aged 2, mother's favourite, though she says both children were unwanted. He pesters Ross by destroying his toys and following him about, which makes Ross impatient. Ross is probably jealous of brother who sleeps with mother.

A paternal aunt is hypochondriacal and a high-grade mental defective. A paternal great-aunt suffered from chorea in childhood.

Until father returned from Forces, family had no settled home. Now live in good working-class house with no financial difficulties.

History: mother suffered from piles during pregnancy. Confinement difficult. Breast-fed for 3 months, then refused breast; bottle-fed. Feeding difficulties until he went to school; appetite now good. Walked and talked at 15 months. Habit-training difficult despite much scolding and smacking. Dry at night at 3, mother then being in hospital. At 5, twitching began; feeding difficulties ceased. Onset of twitches was gradual; were various and interchangeable; now multiple, and include grunting and sniffing. Slow in falling asleep; some sleep-walking, much dreaming. Fears ghosts. While teething, had chickenpox and bronchitis; bronchial pneumonia at 5, measles and whooping cough after starting school.

School record and intelligence: unhappy at school; on first day there, had bad fall, very frightened but refused to cry. Frequent changes of school owing to changes of home. Backward and confused in basic processes; finds arithmetic impossible; worries. Father coaching him for scholarship.

In intelligence test, I.Q. 93. Defeatist in attitude, gave up easily, admitted failures.

Personality and behaviour: at home, is very stubborn; obeys father, plays mother up. Makes little effort to do things, gives up easily. Openly disobedient; anxious, tense and fidgety. Tried to learn piano and violin, but quickly gave up in face of difficulties. Only ambition is to be a tractor driver.

Clinical summary: diagnosed as primary behaviour disorder with neurotic traits; taken on for long-term individual treatment with aim of resolving conflicts behind school fears and twitches, and to accompany him through a difficult period of change to larger school. Made satisfactory progress, adjusted well; symptoms disappeared. Basis of intellectual inhibition uncovered. Coaching arranged after treatment, which was concluded, and satisfactory progress was made in fundamental processes. Settled down well at school, now holds his place successfully. Follow-up shows that he is well adjusted at larger school; twitches have disappeared entirely. Prognosis thought to be good.

Causative factors: mother's personality; her weak-willed, very misguided handling; absence of father. School difficulties were related back to frequent changes of home and to neurotic disturbance.

Case No. 71: Gregory. Age: 10 years, 8 months. I.Q. 98.

An apathetic, retarded boy who is depressed and is preoccupied with fantasies.

Referral: by a private doctor on account of behaviour difficulties, encopresis, enuresis, day-dreaming, and backwardness at school.

Family background: second in family of 3 children from stable, middle-class home.

Mother: large, fat, intelligent woman who goes out to work, is over-tired and has no patience with the children. An only child whose mother never let her forget she was not a boy; strict, Protestant upbringing. Her mother engaged in public work, was excellent orator, and preferred this work to family life. Children forbidden to mix. Mother married at 22. Has always been anaemic; hysterectomy 2 years ago. During first 5 years of marriage, no sexual intercourse as she and husband lived in father's house, agreed to have no children until they had home of their own. Now over-anxious about her children; inconsistent towards Gregory; finds it difficult to support father's authority without being unjust to children; frequent quarrels with father over handling of them. Because of asthma, Gregory has had least strict handling.

Father: aged 54; businessman who travels to London daily. Suffers from nervous dyspepsia and eczema. Tall, thin, shy, quiet and absent-minded. Particular about tidiness and cleanliness, and complains of mother's and children's lax standards. Very demanding when ill. Had strict religious upbringing; now has many fears, tends to hide anger; is said never to have been naughty. Blames mother's nervous heredity for Gregory's behaviour, says he is insane, but that wife exaggerates the difficulties; leaves major responsibilities to her. Sulks rather than gives steady influence, repressive in attitude, seeks trivial causes for complaint; refuses to discipline children, saying that if he hit Gregory he might kill him. Fears sight of blood. Gregory twists him round his finger.

Maternal grandmother: self-opinionated woman; weighs 15 stone, suffers from arthritis. Mother has identified Gregory's 'turns' with grandmother's difficult outbursts, fears he will become the terrible person she is.

Mother admits there is some hereditary nervousness in her family. Maternal grandmother has been in mental hospital; 2 brothers are peculiar, one has attempted suicide. Maternal first cousin has 2 children with peculiarities similar to Gregory's.

Siblings: older brother had number of early difficulties but is now doing well in 'A' stream at school. Gregory jealous, and fights with him. Gregory is also jealous of younger sister whom mother describes as wilful but good as gold. Sister regards Gregory as babyish, jeers at him because he sucks his finger and wets. She does not get on well at school where she is babyish, whining and demanding.

The family lives in comfortable conditions without financial difficulties.

History: mother ill during pregnancy; vomited from 7th month. Confinement easy; disappointed baby was not girl. Breast-fed for 8 months; weaning easy. Later, acute finger-sucking developed. At 15 months, influenza, pneumonia and ear trouble; in hospital for 14 days, fretted all the time, failed to recognize mother on return. Walked at 14 months. Except for 2 words, did not talk until 3, then suddenly started soon after sister's birth. Habit-training strict: late in becoming dry and clean. Eats and sleeps well, though dreams a lot. At 6, severe nightmares, period of skin eruptions, enuresis and encopresis. Subsequently, asthma developed, cleared up when he was 9 but has now developed again. Whooping cough and tonsillectomy at 6. Except for asthma, health now good. Experienced doodle-bug raids in London; undisturbed by raids or blasting.

School record and intelligence: started school at 6, keen to go; frequently absent because of doodle-bug raids. Occasional lapses of pilfering and lying. Cannot concentrate; day-dreams. Gets attention by clowning and making other children laugh, is sent from class, so learns nothing. In present school, makes no progress, is in 'D' stream; reads little, poor in arithmetic, handwork good. Dislikes his teacher. Troublesome with other children, is sometimes bullied. Reports show he is dull but amiable, unassertive, passive, and overlooked by teachers.

In intelligence test, I.Q. 98; slow, discouraged and depressed; cried easily, appeared to lack drive. Answered with great effort, required encouragement to go further. Reading and spelling age is only 7 years, 8 months. No special handicaps revealed in tests.

Personality and behaviour: mother says that at home he gets sudden but short-lived enthusiasms—i.e. for chemistry. Slow in all movements; good with hands. Plays mainly with boys of own age, is physically daring. Is disobedient and irritable. Mother occasionally finds him weeping bitterly; at times is very infantile. Main interests are drawing and nature-study and gardening; likes to sew, darn and make dolls' clothes, and to help in house. Remembers incidents that occurred when he was 15 months.

Clinical summary: diagnosed as case of neurosis. Father found to be obsessional character, mother possibly hysterical with recurrent mood swings. Gregory taken on for psychiatric observation and for remedial teaching in the hope that improvement in school work would contribute to stability and confidence. Much time taken in building relationship with him and securing cooperation. Activities and simple experiments used as means to this end, developed into coaching; cooperation very fitful. Direct discussion of home and school problems attempted, particularly that of sibling rivalry; this usually aroused resistance. After some coaching, school work improved, Gregory seemed to be happier, was reported to be holding his own at school. Follow-up showed that he is getting on well with his brother, but still jealous of sister. Slight recurrence of enuresis, coinciding with period when he was more aggressive and ill-at-ease with mother, lasted 3 days; now normal. At end of treatment, reading age had improved 2 years, better adjustment all round at school. Case is being followed up further. Prognosis good.

Causative factors: possibly some constitutional element; intense sibling rivalry; early hospitalization and unfavourable reaction to this; father's and mother's personalities and their handling.

Case No. 72: Alexander. *Age:* 13 years, 2 months. I.Q. 108.

A stolid-looking boy, very correct and polite. Minimizes or denies his difficulties, and his brief, polite replies make conversation difficult. He feels different from other boys, worries about being thin, describes himself as skinny.

Referral: by his mother on account of multiple fears, asthma and sleep disturbance.

Family background: elder of 2 boys from stable, middle-class home.

Mother: friendly, intelligent woman, says she comes from placid family. Suffers much from effects of old back injury for which she has considerable treatment. Worried about Alexander's symptoms, says she has been weak with him through not knowing whether to be firm or lenient. On whole, deals well with him.

Father: aged 42: businessman who travels to London every day. Was mechanic in R.A.F. for 4 years; away from home for 1 year when Alexander was 9. Healthy, active, highly-strung; has many hobbies, good with hands. Was one of four children, lost chance of higher education through father's business failure. Now anxious that Alexander should do well. Shares hobbies with boys—woodwork with Alexander, gardening with younger boy. Strict with them, insists upon order and tidiness and firmer handling than mother gives. Jealous and resentful when, as occasionally happens, Alexander makes a fuss during a thunderstorm and wants to get into mother's bed. Mother lets boy get into her bed while she goes to the boy's. Alexander worries if father comes home late; has expressed fear of father killing him, yet he and father get on fairly well.

Sibling: aged 9. A healthy, active boy, at first apt to laugh at Alexander's fears, then becomes frightened. Was not circumcised, as Alexander was.

Family lives in comfortable middle-class circumstances.

History: mother's pregnancy good except when she suffered from strained back. Confinement easy. Breast-fed for 6 months, weaning unusually slow and difficult; slow feeder, easily upset, then refused food. No food fads now; occasional fears that someone will poison him. Talked at 1 year, walked at 18 months. Habit-training strict but easy; reliably dry at 1 year. Until 3 sucked hand. Sleep always disturbed, nervous and afraid of dark. As baby, had own room, slept with family during air-raids. Now has periods of sleeping with father or mother; symptoms then disappear, especially when he shares father's bed while mother goes to his. From 2-12 has had fears and asthma; afraid of ghosts, trains, accidents, and poison. Since atomic bomb explosions his fears of doctors, death, night, travelling, poison, bombs, murder, thunder, and lightning have become so severe that they interfere with normal life. Different symptoms come and go in waves; it is their acuteness rather than their nature that varies. From 8–12 experienced air-raids in London; was sleepless and nervous. At 5, had whooping cough; at 13, cervical adenitis during which he lost weight and had difficulty in swallowing. Has never asked sex questions, was embarrassed by brother's naïve questions. Mother had told him of expected baby.

School record and intelligence: began school when nearly 6. Because of asthma, went to small private school; was slow, shy and afraid. At 7 changed school because of air-raids. At 8, another private school; frightened of headmaster. Yet another private school from 11–12; made good progress. Now goes to senior school, enjoys it, mixes fairly well with other boys at school. Free from symptoms and more boyish in behaviour than at home. Progress is average.

In intelligence test, I.Q. 108. Guarded response. Says he 'likes school better'.

Personality and behaviour: mother describes him as highly strung and nervous, but he joins in wild games out of doors. Fearful and timid at home, over-particular about cleanliness; tidy, takes long time dressing and undressing, carefully folding clothes. Undemonstrative; sensitive and uncommunicative; shy about expressing feelings. No interest in girls. Fears and worries occur mainly at night; insists on saying prayers in evening, worried if these are wrong. Makes lampshades and d'oyleys, designs patterns, shows great perseverance and patience in doing these. For 2 years, collected moths and butterflies. Reads little, likes to play games, such as ludo, with mother and brother. Dislikes films; unable to finish books because he dreams about them. Drawings consist only of stereotyped patterns.

Clinical summary: diagnosed as suffering from neurosis; taken on for observational period. Serious nature of boy's long-standing illness has been pointed out to mother, and attempt made to help her deal with it more adequately. Her own anxiety has been relieved, so was able to accept advice and deal with symptoms in

more helpful way. Question of further intensive treatment for
the boy at age of 16 or 17 was discussed with both parents.
Without this, prognosis for adult life thought to be poor. This
is a case requiring full psycho-analysis, but since it is improbable
that this will be practicable, every attempt is being made to
alleviate the present difficult situation and to help the boy into
normal adolescent development. Response satisfactory but limited
to symptomatic improvements.

Causative factors: these were not fully elucidated, but were thought
to be related to the mother's neurotic personality, her over-strict
training in the early years and later compliance with his symptoms, together with the father's repressively high standards for
the boy.

Case No. 73: Malcolm. *Age:* 13 years, 4 months. I.Q. 137.

A fair, rather fat boy who looked younger than his years.

Referral: by father on account of school difficulties, childish behaviour at home, dreaminess and nervousness.

Family background: eldest of three children from stable, middle-
class home.

Mother attractive, charming but shy; more mature than husband.
Fond of Malcolm, has good relationship with him; sees his problems more objectively than father. First 3 years of marriage unhappy; found husband hot-tempered and moody. Mother-in-law
neither liked nor welcomed her. Now ignores husband's tempers,
and they get on reasonably well. Before marriage, was nursery
teacher.

Father: civil servant; describes himself as self-satisfied, has few
friends; fond of home and family. Hardworking, likes ordering
and administrating. Was able to go to secondary school because
mother worked; in return, truanted, left at 15 without taking
exams. Is now unconsciously determined that Malcolm shall not
take matriculation, resents the boy being good at school, fears he
will surpass him in school achievements. Yet relationship with

boy is fundamentally good. The attitude of both parents prevents the boy from taking on responsibilities. They are concerned about him and willing to cooperate with the clinic.

Siblings: Father describes them as having lots of character and initiative while Malcolm dreams. The girl, aged 8, is especially lively, gets the better of Malcolm in disputes. There appear to be no major difficulties between the children. The younger boy is 4.

The family is Roman Catholic and lives in a comfortable, secure, middle-class home.

History: born 1 year after parents' marriage when mother was not happy. Breast-fed for 3 months; gained no weight, became bad-tempered, biting and refusing breast. Mother then lost milk; baby bottle-fed. Cried a lot during first months. At 1 year, still had dummy about which mother seemed ashamed. Walked and talked at 1 year, developed big appetite, always greedy. Lazy and passive baby; habit-training one long struggle; not clean or dry until 4. Soiled and wet, never asking to go to lavatory. No sleep problems. Played alone for hours; would sit passively wherever he was put. Has always day-dreamed. Loses pencils and pens, is clumsy and forgetful, unable to concentrate. Lefthanded, has difficulty in writing. Plays like a younger child, does not make friends and has always been unlike other children. Terrified of fighting or gangsterism in films. Health good. No separation from mother. At about 8½, very upset when maternal grandfather was killed in air-raid; showed morbid interest and asked many questions.

School record and intelligence: went to country school at 6; in first year was teacher's favourite. Then sent to Roman Catholic school in country town where he did not get on well. At 11, transferred to good private school; backward in spite of high intelligence. Is still backward, dislikes school.

In intelligence test, I.Q. 137. Mental age 17 years and 8 months, indicating very superior intelligence.

Personality and behaviour: parents describe him as difficult to get to know; lives in world of his own, always vague and dreamy;

clumsy and untidy. Cannot hold his own with other boys; nervous, especially at night. Unable to settle down to homework, which worries him; says he does not wish to grow up. Mother says he just moons about, harps upon morbidity; likes to play doll games with sister. Dislikes active games at school, uninterested in sports or swimming. Likes best to sit alone and read books about nature study. Has ideas but cannot do things—e.g. writing—feels he cannot be any good. Attitude is helpless and defeatist. Gets on better at mathematics.

Clinical summary: diagnosed as case of neurotic disturbance with gross learning inhibition; taken on for treatment. Parents were shown that their attitude did not allow the boy to take on responsibilities; they were asked to try to withdraw their interest from school situation. Boy made good progress in treatment; learning inhibition was found, on a superficial level, to be due to his feelings of impotence, but on deeper level to passive fantasies. Attempt made to show him how his inferiority influences his actions at school and at home towards father and siblings. Responded immediately with more active behaviour all round; behaviour improved in proportion to growing insight. Immediate success of this led to strengthening of self-respect and to further progress. No attempt could be made to change the underlying feminine indentification in his personality. Outcome thought to be satisfactory; follow-up shows that improvement has been maintained.

Causative factors: strict early handling of oral and anal demands; strict discipline from parents; father's personality; jealousy of father who constantly tells the boy how much better he himself is. The disturbance was thought probably to have originated about the age of 3–5 years. Mother's shyness and deference towards father together with her earlier depressed condition at time of Malcolm's birth were thought also to have contributed to his early disposition.

Case No. 74: Denny. *Age:* 12 years, 11 months. I.Q. 100.

A tall, slender, healthy boy who looks young for his age.

Referral: by School Medical Officer on account of fears, acute anxiety, temper outbursts, refusing to go to school, gastric upsets, poor appetite and enuresis.

Family background: second of three boys from stable home.

Mother: nervous, disturbed, middle-aged woman, impatient and easily exasperated by the boys but anxious to do her best for them. Garrulous and loud-voiced, grumbles at the boys; regarded by school teachers as interfering and tiresome. Uncooperative at clinic; thought to be in need of treatment. Derives satisfaction from Denny's illness, even fostering some symptoms.

Father: a skilled tradesman. Much preoccupied in trying to find an institution for his ill parents. Does not believe in doctors or clinics. Talks much to Denny, tells him the only cure lies within himself. Though concerned about the boy, does not support his treatment and has limited insight.

Siblings: brothers aged 14 and 6. Denny describes himself as the odd man out. Admires brothers; mother denies jealousy of younger one. Denny remembers this child's birth, refused to talk about it at the time. At clinic, expressed hostility towards him.

Family lives in new, comfortably furnished house in building estate. No financial difficulties.

History: pregnancy and confinement normal. Progress good. Walked and talked at normal age. Regarded as a nervous child; easily upset, cried wildly, especially when mother was pregnant with younger brother. Habit-training slow and difficult. Enuretic throughout childhood. Urticaria and fears for number of years; likes night-light. Even when sharing bed with brother, was wet: now has own bed. Can go to school only when protected by brother or friend. Dislikes other boys; remains in lavatory during play time. Health good though now has large, infected tonsils. Was not evacuated.

School record and intelligence: started school at 4½ so as to be with brother. Despite physical resistance and screaming, mother forced him to go. Showed many nervous reactions. Considerable absences through air-raids, his own and his mother's illnesses. Troubles became severe when moved to larger school where he did not get on well either at work or with other boys. Mother then tried him in four further schools. When he failed scholarship examination last year, about which he was intensely upset, mother decided to change school again, but first sought advice at clinic.

In intelligence test, I.Q. 100.

Personality and behaviour: at home, Denny is fearful and weepy; worries so much over school failures that mother thinks he is ambitious. Afraid of other boys unless under brother's protection; displays hysterical symptoms to avoid certain lessons. Unable to make friends because of underlying fears of boys and masters; afraid to go out lest he should meet some of the boys. Last year, took home-nursing examinations. Has belonged to Cadets, church choir, a boys' club, and ambulance classes, but has given up each in turn.

Clinical summary: diagnosed as primary behaviour disturbance with pronounced neurotic trends. Shows hysterical symptoms and considerable intellectual inhibition, inhibited in any subject requiring expression of aggression, e.g. metal work, science, physical training or games. Treatment strongly recommended and vacancy held open but mother sent boy only twice over long time and failed to come herself. She felt unable to cooperate; moved boy to new school. Mother and boy both thought to be very neurotic, and their disturbances interact with each other. He is a passive, effeminate boy who would have responded well to treatment since he was eager for help and very disturbed by his symptoms. Thought to be in great need of psychotherapy, but mother made insincere excuses or used treatment merely as threat to him. Her lack of cooperation made it impossible for treatment to proceed, and prognosis without it is thought to be poor.

Causative factors: mother's personality and disturbed relationship with boy; repression of intense sibling rivalry and of all feelings of aggression; exclusion by members of the family. He has been over-protected because of his hysterical symptoms, and his problems were accentuated by his experiences in the blitz.

423

Case No. 75: Angus. *Age:* 14 years, 7 months, I.Q. 138.

Angus is a shy, well-behaved, girlish-looking boy.

Referral: by his mother on account of school difficulties, lack of concentration, inability to mix with other boys, selfish and inconsiderate behaviour towards his mother.

Family background: only surviving child from good working-class home.

Mother: aged 43; intelligent and conscientious, tries to intellectualize her problems. Anxious and neurotic, still distressed about death, some years ago, of eldest son in air-raid. Nervous and over-anxious about Angus whom she treats as a young child. After bombing incident, went to work for first time for 3 years as secretary in military organization. Now does part-time work in social services in order to be able to send Angus to secondary school.

Father: aged 45; civil servant, not in Services. Casual, does not worry. Relationship between father and Angus is good.

Sibling: only brother was killed at 14½ when Angus was 10. He and Angus said to have been inseparable; when Angus talks about him, he almost cries, says he misses him, that brother was kind to him but now no one at home talks to him. He feels deprived of brother's support at home and at school.

No morbid heredity known in family. Mother's niece has been referred to psychiatrist on account of attacks of nervous behaviour.

Family lives in cottage with large garden. Angus has dog which he adores and talks about as a person.

History: pregnancy and birth normal. Baby suffered from sickness and diarrhoea from birth but doctors told mother he was all right. At 3 months, when mother had severe gastric 'flu, baby spent 2 weeks in Truby King Home; upset because of over-feeding. Walked at 1 year, talked at 15 months. Alert and intelligent toddler. At 18 months, bad attack of sickness. At 2, found to be suffering from mucous colitis; diet recommended. No habit-training problems. Sleeps well; has own room but likes to share mother's bed when father is on night duty. Appetite good, but mother watches his diet. At 10, he and brother were trapped by rubble and fallen timber in their room after a bomb fell. Mother heard Angus screaming, managed to rescue him. He seemed to be sick and suffering from slight concussion. Mother then went to look for brother, but police refused to allow her near. Boy was never found. Angus not told of brother's death for 2 days; he was inconsolable. Mother talked so much about this tragedy that clearly it is an unmastered traumatic experience for her. Angus and mother have no fears of the dark.

School record and intelligence: no problem at school until he was 10 when teacher then complained of him, saying he had no friends. Changed to present private secondary school upon mother's initiative after bombing incident. Progress poor; weak in mathematics and geography. Does not mix with other boys.

In intelligence test, I.Q. 138; very superior intelligence. Good knowledge of words, expresses himself clearly and accurately.

Personality and behaviour: described at home as being shy, well-behaved and obliging, never concentrates, likes to romp around with his dog like a younger child; has no hobbies. Clothes dirty and untidy; dislikes getting up in the morning. Seems to bear grudge towards the family. Sporadic outbursts of activity, i.e. going to club, learning to dance—but soon gives up. Spends much time over homework; likes science and reading. In algebra, problems which are easy to other boys, are difficult for him, and vice versa. Unable to draw maps. Wants to be veterinary surgeon. Has no friends.

Clinical summary: diagnosed as adolescence disturbance with pronounced neurotic trends; taken on for treatment. Quickly established good relationship to therapist, was able to discuss worries about homework, which were found to be related indirectly to masturbation worries. After a few months of treatment, became openly ambitious, revealed his relationship to girls where his fear of being inferior handicapped his activities. This, coupled with his fear of failure, was analysed; he improved greatly at school, came 5th instead of 19th in class, and became more manly. Follow-up showed great improvement, happy and successful at school, no further difficulties. Case closed as satisfactory, prognosis regarded as good.

Causative factors: passive, effeminate personality allied to puberty difficulties and enhanced by mother's tendency to keep up a neurotically intense relationship with him; mother's grief and disturbed personality; her wish that he should make up for her great disappointment in loss of elder son prolonged and intensified the difficulties.

Case No. 76: Rollo. *Age:* 13 years, 4 months. I.Q. 118.

Though small for his age, Rollo has a manly appearance and intelligent face. Voice not yet broken.

Referral: by school medical officer on account of school problems, a number of fears, obsessions, and queer habits which prevent him from leading a normal life.

Family background: Elder of 2 children from stable, lower-middle-class home.

Mother: tense, depressed woman with desperate and highly emotional attitude towards the boy's problems. Nervous breakdown when Rollo was 4½; in mental hospital for 6 months after a period when family had moved to new home. Now has intimate quarrel relationship with Rollo, but not with his sister. Has some insight into Rollo's condition but lacks enough conviction to act upon it. Never hits or punishes him, generally gives in; feels guilty about spoiling him and quarrels about it. Has provoked and over-protected him, which has contributed to his disturbance.

Father: sergeant in Army for 5 years. No overseas service, but away from home for irregular periods. Now works as Civil Servant. Happy-go-lucky, no belief in psychologist, thinks all Rollo needs is a good hiding, but never gives it. He and the boy got on well when first he returned from Army, but Rollo has now turned against him. Rollo has grown up in an atmosphere of quarrelling between mother and maternal grandmother, and between parents.

Maternal grandmother: lived with family until Rollo was 2; much conflict with her about his upbringing. He stayed with her while mother was in mental hospital.

Sibling: sister aged 3; pale child, inclined to whine; refused to be separated from mother. Rollo shows no interest in her, but during last weeks refuses to do anything for her and is jealous.

Family has had frequent changes of home.

History: mother had puerperal fever following Rollo's birth. Breast-fed for 5 months; cried a lot, and she gave in to him. No weaning difficulties. Habit-training easy; clean and dry at 2. Appetite poor; persistent food fads which are indulged; now fears mother is poisoning him. Sleep restless; developed fears of dark and poisoning. Was a whining, miserable, demanding child. At 2, family moved from maternal grandmother's house into flat. At $4\frac{1}{2}$ when mother had nervous breakdown, returned to grand-mother's for 6 months. When mother returned, her sister's illegitimate daughter lived with them, and because of poor heart condition, required much care. Mother was fond of this child who was later seized and removed by relatives. Early in the war, there were a number of evacuees in house. Rollo had chicken-pox, mumps, and scarlet fever in quick succession. Was 5 weeks in hospital at 9. Has always had acidosis; pulse rate very fast which doctor considers is self-induced. Given sex information when sister was born; mother evasive about subject, wanting to let school deal with it. Rollo now has number of touching rituals, washing and going to bed rituals; says one thing after another is wrong with him.

School record and intelligence: started school at 5, disliked it. Changed school each time family moved house. Happy in school he attended when he was 7. Reports excellent, passed scholarship examination to senior school at $10\frac{1}{2}$. Did not want to go to grammar school. 'Habits' began, then passed off before family moved to next village and mother became pregnant. Did well at grammar school; on basis of good reports, sent to select secondary school which he disliked, and now implores parents to let him leave. Likes only natural science; homework worries him. Unable to do any serious work.

In intelligence test, I.Q. 118. Nervous, needing much assurance; asked unnecessary questions, wanted instructions repeated, made excuses; though disturbed, made good response. Vocabulary score at Superior Adult II level.

Personality and behaviour: rude and disobedient to parents. Sensitive; never affectionate to mother, uncooperative in house. Number of obsessional rituals and avoidances; conscious of small size. When frustrated, has childish outbursts of temper. Interested in trains and cubic measurements. Good at sports; friendly and popular with village boys. Fears he will be ill and parents will send him away. Dramatically implores parents to let him leave school.

Clinical summary: diagnosed as suffering from obsessional neurosis, the present symptoms of which he has had for at least 6 months. Neurosis not yet fully established so that phases of compulsions, of touching objects or walking up and downstairs, alternate with phases of acute anxiety when the boy is terrified of getting ill and having to be operated upon. Taken on for individual treatment and the school situation fully investigated. Transfer was arranged immediately so that he could go as a boarder to a specially selected school which would help his social adjustment and where regular contact between teacher and psychiatrist could be maintained. Considerable improvement shown and boy has responded well to help with adolescent problems but full psycho-analysis recommended for the future.

As an example of severe neurotic symptoms and the extent to which they interfere with normal life is the following incident which occurred some time after treatment commenced:

New obsessional habit compels Rollo to walk twice past all old grey houses. On seeing such a house for the first time, he thinks this is where he will live when he goes to hell, goes back, passes the house for a second time in order to undo the thought. Once, having cycled with his cousin to the beach, the boys were late in returning and at 10.30 p.m. still had 11 miles to go. Rollo was tailing his cousin who passed a white spot on the road on the left-hand side. Rollo followed, then stopped immediately. It was bad to pass the spot from the left. Bad illnesses, such as appendicitis, infantile paralysis and lock jaw are 'left', while good illnesses like chickenpox and scarlet fever are 'right'. Right hands are given to girls because the right side is strong, and girls want men to be strong. Therefore right is good, and white spots must be passed from the right. Not only did Rollo want to return and re-pass the white spot, but he thought he ought to return 6 miles to where there had been an old grey house about which his cousin had remarked that it was a grey and lonely spot. Only by doing this did he feel that atonement for doing the bad thing would be complete. His cousin refused to comply, started to cry, saying he wanted food and bed. Rollo developed acute anxiety. The conflict was solved by a lorry driver who offered the boys a lift. The temptation was too strong for Rollo, who in typical obsessional fashion suddenly thought 'to hell with the old house and white spot', and rode home. (These old houses and white spots on the way formed a great obstacle to his coming to the clinic.) Treatment continues but prognosis thought to be doubtful as there is no possibility of full psycho-analysis. He is being given every help over present difficult situation, and both mother and school are being advised as to the handling of the boy during adolescence.

Causative factors: these were thought to be multiple and complex. Among them were mother's sado-masochistic attitude towards the boy; her personality, her illness and breakdown when he was 4½; the atmosphere of quarrelling in which he has been reared; father's absence and irregular visits home for 5 years; father's return when Rollo was 12½; increase in castration fears connected with puberty and struggles about masturbation. Rollo also influenced by simultaneous occurrence of mother's pregnancy and illegitimate cousin's exclusion from family in violent circumstances. Possible constitutional factors.

Case No. 77: Rupert. *Age:* 11 years, 9 months, I.Q. 96.

A strained, anxious looking boy who seems mildly depressed.

He tries to keep conversation at social level and to avoid mentioning his difficulties.

Referral: by a private doctor on account of enuresis, fears, inhibited behaviour and school failure.

Family background: elder of 2 children from good, middle-class home. Father works in Malaya, at home on leaves. Family formerly lived in Malaya where boys attended boarding schools. Mother has decided to remain in England and make a home for the children.

Mother: attractive, smartly-dressed woman, superficially pleasant but fundamentally hard. Dominating and intolerant when the boy fails to come up to her high standards of behaviour and attainment. At clinic, she gave little information about Rupert, was flippant, appeared to be bored, giggled and bit her nails. Was tense, resistive to treatment. She was at strict boarding school as a girl; education reached high standard. Has little sympathy for Rupert, considers his enuresis a social disgrace, criticizes and is ashamed of his symptoms. Tends to keep her children babies. Rupert appears to have no resentment towards her, though his relationship is somewhat sado-masochistic; he repeats this in play with his dog with whom he appears to have identified himself, handling the dog's training as severely as the mother handled his.

Father: engineer working for commercial firm in Malaya. Anxious, dominated by wife. When at home, distressed by Rupert's enuresis and lack of progress at school. While not as ambitious for the boy as the mother is, would like him to go to private school. Rupert has fantasies *about* father rather than any real relationship; wishes to take his place during his absence.

Sibling: sister, aged 10, with whom Rupert appears to be friendly. Mother had wanted a girl when Rupert was born and at present prefers the girl. Mother denies any jealousy on Rupert's part. He does not dare oppose or bicker with his sister, who scorns his wetting.

Family went to Malaya when Rupert was 3, remained there 8 years. Now live in secure, comfortable conditions in the country. When Rupert first went to Malaya, he was cared for from age 3 to 6 years by one ayah; since then had several until return home.

History: mother says Rupert was a placid baby and gave no trouble. Breast-fed; weaned at 6 months without difficulty. Good appetite. Habit-training early and rigid: dry by day at 2; never dry at night except for 6 months when 8½. Relapsed after going to boarding school in England. Sleeps heavily, no nightmares. Wets bed most nights; has done so increasingly while sister is at home. Nail-biter; fidgety; always looks pale, strained and worried. Had measles, German measles and mumps in Malaya. At 9, after going to boarding school, and on recommendation of school after bed-wetting had begun again, was circumcised. During Singapore riots, was in bus that was wrecked, and witnessed destruction of father's office.

School record and intelligence: attended 6 schools in Malaya, several of which were boarding schools. At present, is being coached by crammer for Common Entrance. Little interest in lessons and is slow. Parents have pressed him to improve school work.

In intelligence test, I.Q. 96; mental age 11 years 4 months; P.C.I. scores 499, indicating mental age of 9. Easily distracted or confused in the test, reasoned badly; memory good. Was cooperative and amiable, but slow, plodding and humourless.

Personality and behaviour: at home is described as a cautious, timid child, rigidly controlled, in many ways girlish, quiet and likes to help in the house, but mother despises his efforts. Mixes well with other children. No longer bites nails but picks at clothes, touches buttons; some perseveration trends. Seems to require much concentration before he can understand instructions. Mother says that neither she nor Rupert like kissing and cuddling. He likes swimming, games and his dog. Wants to be a farmer. Member of sea scouts, but does not get on as well as he might with boys there. Reads only books about birds. Talks in an unemotional, monotonous way which mother finds irritating.

Clinical summary: diagnosed as primary behaviour disturbance with neurotic trends; taken on for treatment. Slow in establishing relationship with therapist. Problems of intense castration anxiety, guilt in relation to sibling rivalry and feelings of rejection were discussed. After some treatment of mother, she became more permissive in attitude, decided not to send boy to boarding school. His overt symptoms lessened, which satisfied mother, who then ended his clinic visits. Treatment was terminated as incomplete, but thought to have been satisfactory within limits. Prognosis remains doubtful; passive-effeminate character structure remains unchanged. Mother's cooperation throughout was limited; some months later she sent him to public school.

Causative factors: rigid standards of the home; boy's unresolved castration anxiety which was aggravated by late circumcision; absence of father and generally unsettled background of the home; mother's personality, her somewhat sado-masochistic relationship with the boy, and her open preference for the girl entrenched his symptoms more deeply.

Case No. 78: Preston. *Age:* 14 years, 3 months. I.Q. 115.

A shy, inhibited boy who is generally frowning. His marked stammer increases when he talks to his younger brother.

Referral: by his mother, on the advice of his form master, on account of stammering, feeding disturbance, inhibited behaviour and other nervous symptoms.

Family background: elder of 2 boys whose father was killed. Mother goes out to work while elderly aunt keeps house.

Mother: aged 37, attractive woman of good intelligence; plucky and cheerful in face of her difficulties, and devoted to her sons. Tries to be impartial towards them, has close, intense relationship with Preston. Home was broken up in 1939 when father went abroad. Mother lacks companionship, since aunt is too old and dislikes the boys, whereas the boys are too young. Used to be a domestic servant.

432

Father: aged 39 when he died. Corporal in Regular Army, died in concentration camp abroad in 1945. Family had 2 postcards from him in 4 years, and did not know of his death for some time. Mother says he was a good father; said prayers with Preston while mother said them with younger boy. This appears to represent what was a regular division in the family. Preston's memory of father is dim. Mother says marriage was happy; she now badly misses the support of her husband.

Sibling: younger brother; boys get on well; Preston considered the cleverer, is jealous of brother. Both go to High School, both are Boy Scouts.

Family circumstances were good, but some financial difficulties since father's death.

History: 3 weeks premature after mother had been shocked by sudden death of grandmother. Both parents wanted a girl. Birth easy; breast-fed for 9 months; weaned easily. Walked and talked at normal time; clean and dry at 15 months without difficulty. Now has food fads. At 3, suddenly started night fears, insisted upon mother sitting near him while he went to sleep. Fears continued until 7, but had stopped before father went overseas. Stammer started a year later when Preston was evacuated with his brother to good foster-home where there was a girl of Preston's age. When mother visited them, he was shy and treated her as a stranger. Night terrors started again, but have now subsided. The home was unbroken until father went abroad. Preston's health good until mumps, aged 6; measles, aged 7.

School record and intelligence: began school at 4; would not separate from mother at first; later mixed well. At 7, changed school, but was soon evacuated; for 7 months went to school in country. At 11, took scholarship to local high school. Now in top half of form, said to be plodding but not brilliant worker. Brother at bottom of form.

In intelligence test, I.Q. 115. Results showed wide scatter, ranging from 10 years to Superior Adult II level. Best on verbal tests; good feeling for language, uncertain on reasoning tests. Favourite subjects English and Chemistry; dislikes French.

Personality and behaviour: mother says he is stodgy, obstinate and careful; seldom demonstrative. Tastes are serious, but at times shows sense of humour. Stammer increases when he has to go in for examinations or when in poor health. Has had elocution lessons, attended speech clinic, but has given this up because of worrying over exams. Wants to be civil engineer. Mother says that he took his father's departing injunction about being the man of the family and to stop depending upon his mother very seriously.

Clinical summary: diagnosed as primary behaviour disturbance with neurotic trends; taken on for treatment. Made good progress; gradually became able to express aggressive fantasies in drawings and to stand up for himself with younger brother. All-round symptomatic improvement except for stammer, which remained unchanged in short-term psychotherapy. Mother was satisfied with this degree of improvement and after summer holiday said she would not wish him to miss school any longer, and he failed to attend. Prognosis thought to be fair; follow-up showed that improvement was maintained.

Causative factors: reaction to sudden break-up of home at 7 when father went overseas, and the boy was evacuated, allied to death of father and intense sibling rivalry. The case was closed as satisfactory, but further treatment thought still advisable.

Case No. 79: Pierre. *Age:* 16 years, 2 months. I.Q. 109.

A fresh-complexioned, slender boy, whose voice is beginning to break. A downy moustache is appearing.

Referral: by school officer on account of school failure, inability to concentrate, religious difficulties and anxiety.

Family background: younger of 2 children from good, working-class home.

Mother: quiet, practical and intelligent; several minor obsessional symptoms. Fond of Pierre; has much insight into his needs and difficulties, and understands adolescent sexual conflicts and masturbation guilt.

434

Father: civil servant in large county town. Quiet; does not take full share in responsibility for children. Interested in Pierre, discussed his religious doubts and fears with him, but is now impatient and threatens to take him from school.

Sibling: sister aged 20. Boyish and noisy; training to be a domestic science teacher. Gets on well with Pierre.

Maternal grandmother: suffers from neurasthenia and minor depressions; threatens suicide. Used to live with family, disliked Pierre. Now lives some distance away, likes Pierre.

While not well off, the family has no serious financial strains.

History: mother is vague as to details of early history and development. Breast-fed for 4 months, but did not thrive and frequently soiled napkins, so mother changed to bottle-feeding. Walked and talked early, rigidly trained to be dry by 1 year. No feeding difficulties until recently when anxieties reached climax. Sleep also good until recently; now unable to sleep; reads Bible in bed. Since preoccupied with religious doubts, school work has deteriorated. Recently experienced what he calls religious conversion. Mother answered his questions about sex as father evaded doing so, gave him booklet on subject. Pierre told her of his nocturnal emissions and that he was masturbating until time of religious conversion which, mother suspects, has occurred simultaneously with a lapse into masturbation. Bowel trouble in early years; then measles, chickenpox and bronchitis. Health now good except for frequent colds.

School record and intelligence: began school at 5; progress good, above average in all subjects. For past 4 years, attended local high school for boys. 1st in class until this term, now in 'C' stream near bottom. Slow over homework, cannot concentrate. Copies long texts from Bible. General behaviour at school is good.

In intelligence test, I.Q. 109; conscientious, quiet, slow in response, poor sense of humour. In Raven Progressive Matrices, made score of 53, indicating mental age of 17–17½. Full of doubts and hesitation; some obsessional traits.

Personality and behaviour: at home, is quiet, slow, with no interest in games or outdoor activities. One close boy friend since infant school days. A year ago, had a girl friend for 7 months; now has girl friends only among those in choir, seeing them with group. After first exaltation of conversion, became morbid, went off food, was unable to sleep; talked of having committed the unforgivable sin. Discussed problem with local minister. Used to like astronomy and working with a telescope; now only interest is to be a missionary. Reads *Pilgrim's Progress* and the Bible, talks about a cage he could not escape. Has a dog, likes riding; good at P.T., handicrafts and woodwork. Used to be interested in jiu-jitsu: wanted to be P.T. instructor.

Clinical summary: diagnosed as obsessional neurosis in a passive-effeminate adolescent; taken on for individual treatment. Responded well, was helped over deeper psychological problems attached to religious worries. Passed matriculation, now has positive plans for future. Gained insight into sexual conflicts, particularly over masturbation. Basic obsessional character structure persists. Follow-up showed that he has girl-friend and leads full, normal social life. Has some conflicts over allowing himself worldly pleasures which he feels to be incompatible with the Christian life he should want to lead. He is making progress according to his abilities at school. Prognosis thought to be good.

Causative factors: family pattern of passive, neurotic behaviour, evident in personalities of mother, father and maternal grandmother; conscientious, repressive early discipline; restrictive and unenlightened attitude toward sexuality and religious crisis in adolescence.

Case No. 80: James. *Age:* 15 years, 7 months. I.Q. 129 plus.

Pale, under-sized, poorly-nourished boy with a round back and shoulders and tense, over-anxious expression. Movements are abrupt and quick. Little spontaneity in conversation.

Referral: by his mother on account of inhibited behaviour, school retardation and asthma.

Family background: eldest of 5 children from stable home.

Mother: aged 37; appears to be healthy woman, but during treatment found to be neurotic and full of deep anxieties. Little understanding of boy's difficulties; helps to create the situation which produces asthma, giving him much care and attention. Her relationship with him is intense; during father's absence, he slept with her.

Father: aged 39; skilled tradesman. In Army for 6 years, abroad for 2. A healthy, easy-going man. Mother says that since the war, he has been moody and impatient, especially with James's favourite brother, aged 3. Father is interested in James's aeroplane-making and stamp-collecting; plays with the boy when he is ill. Both parents foster boy's invalidism.

Siblings: 2 brothers and 2 sisters. Brother next to James is healthier and bigger, but sleep-walked and had nightmares in early years. James is jealous of him, but passive about his better school record and popularity. 11-year-old sister had asthma until a year ago. James, but not brother, gets on well with her. 3-year-old brother is bad-tempered and demanding; 5-months baby fretful over teething. Family atmosphere is not a happy one.

History: pregnancy and birth normal; breast-fed for 3 months. Habit-training lenient. Walked at 1 year, talked a little later. Sleep good, though much dreaming; shares room with brother. At 1 year, 4 months, first asthma attack, which lasted 2 days. Frequent attacks until 8. Between 8 and 9, during father's absence and during stay in camp, no attacks. Has had much treatment, is thought to be allergic to dogs and cats; no apparent organic cause, no high sensitivity to any food. X-ray revealed some deformity of chest. Since 14, attacks have increased; stays away from school longer than is necessary. Experienced air-raids during father's absence.

School record and intelligence: began school at 5; cried during first day. Work good. At 8, went to bigger school; mixed well, but inclined to be solitary. At 11, went to local high school; much absence because of asthma; dislikes homework, but does not find

437

P

work hard. Defeatist attitude towards extra work needed for school certificate exam. No reading or writing difficulties, though some crossed laterality. Good at drawing and arithmetic; 5th in class of 50.

In intelligence test, I.Q. 129; mental age 18 years, 11 months. Worried during test, gave up easily.

Personality and behaviour: at home, he is reliable, easy-going and full of common sense; good with his hands and seems to be happy. Fairly demonstrative, easily excitable; hesitant and unassuming in manner; prefers to lose at games. Always obedient; good cook. Likes to read mysteries, travel and aeroplane stories, cowboy and Indian tales, and his sister's books. Likes scouts, mathematics, engines, clocks and wireless. Dislikes essays or literature. Wants to be motor mechanic or engineer. Later on in treatment said he would like to be an office boy as being an engineer was too difficult.

Clinical summary: diagnosed as neurotic disturbance, with asthma being a psychosomatic illness. Found to be a passive, effeminate boy deriving much secondary gain from his symptoms; taken on for treatment with the aim of giving him relief from symptoms and some insight into his passive and jealous attitude towards his younger brother. He was willing to attend clinic so long as he could discuss dreams, but used these as a resistance, began to fail appointments as soon as other factors were discussed and insight increased. Unwilling to give up secondary gain from asthma; attacks now became associated with clinic visits instead of, as formerly, with going to church. Began to show some rivalry with brother, but finally adopted an even more passive attitude towards him and had no ambitions for future work. Mother developed some insight during treatment, and modified her attitude considerably. Treatment of mother in clinic increased James's resistance, and he himself decided to stop treatment. Follow-up showed that he had decided to leave school, had got a job on his own initiative as soon as he had given up treatment. No asthma attacks in 3 weeks following this, but prognosis thought to be poor. Treatment incomplete and outcome inconclusive.

Causative factors: passive-effeminate character development; re-pressed jealousy of brother; mother's neurotic personality, her attitude and over-protection; much secondary gain maintaining symptoms. Father's absence contributed a good deal. Outcome of case thought to be unsatisfactory.

Case No. 81: Joanna. *Age:* 4 years 5 months. I.Q. 102.

A sturdy, well-fed girl with a fretful, whiny manner and appearance.

Referral: by her mother who had first taken her to the Health Centre for advice on handling her tempers and feeding problems. Joanna will not mix with other children, constantly asks her mother to repeat phrases like 'I love you' until she says it in a specially affectionate manner.

Family background: elder of 2 children from good, middle-class home.

Mother: aged 28; stocky, expansive woman, impulsive and short-tempered; inconsistent in her handling of Joanna. Though volubly expresses desperation, is fundamentally happy-go-lucky and does not take Joanna's difficulties seriously.

Father: aged 25; in Services. Moody. First months of marriage were unhappy. Joanna is better when he is at home.

Maternal grandmother: aged 57; lives with family. Fussy and house-proud. Much conflict over handling of Joanna, though she, too, is inconsistent with the girl, and invariably goes contrary to the mother.

Grandfather: aged 50; easy-going. Joanna gets on well with him. In quarrels, he takes the mother's side.

Sibling: brother, aged 13 months. Joanna openly jealous when mother returned from hospital, gives baby sly digs, for which she is severely punished. Told he was bought at the hospital.

History: mother pregnant before marriage; had known father for 7 years and intended marrying. Unhappy during pregnancy because of husband's sullen, moody attitude and her mother's criticism of him. Though she had not wanted children, looked forward to having the baby, whose birth was normal. Breast-fed for 9 months; easily weaned.Walked and talked at 15 months. Habit-training harsh; potted from birth, clean within a few months. At 15 months, wetted and dirtied over house; was thrashed and napkins reintroduced; soiling ceased. At same time, feeding difficulties arose and still continue, though these disappeared when mother was in hospital and Joanna was in grandmother's care. Health good; at 2, mild attack of whooping-cough. No sleeping difficulties; sleeps alone, no fear of dark.

Personality and behaviour: described as very active and always in someone's way; likes to play with dolls or colour pictures. Constantly draws attention to herself, particularly when there are visitors, then deliberately does something naughty. Does same when mother nurses baby. Avoids other children; if taken to party, stands aloof. Bites nails, picks nose, not happy until mother takes her on her knee and reads to her after baby has gone to bed.

Main problems that have been acute since birth of baby: she rolls on floor when mother speaks harshly; demands constant repetition of 'I love you' (mother or grandmother usually complies with this request); continues to have feeding difficulties; refuses to mix with other children or adults; has severe temper.

Clinical summary: at Clinic, Joanna was shy and inhibited; slow and reluctant to make any effort in intelligence test; much delaying, many long pauses between question and answer which were filled in with chewing and sucking at lips, looking about room, sighing and wrinkling brows. Pretended ignorance in order not to have to speak; conversation was in monosyllables. I.Q. on this attempt was found to be 102 and is probably an underestimate.

Diagnosed as suffering from infantile neurosis.

In the psychiatric interview, Joanna showed definite obsessional tendencies; play activities severely disturbed. She wriggled, scraped her feet, made noises in her throat, did not settle down to any form of play. She and mother taken on for treatment. Mother's grave faults in handling were dealt with by Psychiatric Social Worker. Mother found to be stable and cooperative with a fundamentally good relationship to the child; responded well to treatment. After 5 months of individual treatment together with mother's regular visits to P.S.W., mother showed increased understanding of the causes of the problem. Joanna's overt behaviour difficulties and obsessional symptoms disappeared; she became happy, active, and did well at school. Some obsessional tendencies remain, however, since full psycho-analytical treatment was not available for her deeper disturbance. Prognosis after treatment thought to be good for latency period, but further difficulties are to be expected in puberty. Follow-up shows improvement maintained both at home and at school. Now has excellent relationship with mother.

Causative factors: jealousy and intense hostility towards younger brother; guilty feelings about this hostility, accentuated by alternately over-rigid and inconsistent handling from mother and grandparents; absence of father at this time.

Case No. 82: Laura. *Age:* 5 years, 6 months. I.Q. 100.

Slight, dark girl, with mild speech disturbance.

Referral: by speech therapist on account of speech difficulties, nightmares, temper tantrums, general nervousness, and severe fears.

Family background: fourth child in family of 5 girls (aged 11, 9, 7, 5, and 2) from stable Jewish home.

Mother: smart, brisk, motherly woman in her 30s. Before marriage was a milliner; continues this work to supplement income as family plans to emigrate to Canada. Earns about the same as husband. Fond of children, observes them well. Fairly good relationship with Laura, but irritated by her nervousness and unclear speech. Fears permanent stammer, so is cooperative in treatment.

Father: was an electrician before the war; in Services throughout the war. Demobilized 6 months ago, is now with engineering company. 9 years ago, broke back, was disabled for over a year.

Mother says this has left a permanent mark on his personality; he is jumpy and irritable since demobilization, dislikes children being noisy, and babies. Back trouble recurs. Mother gives impression of being tired of nursing him. His relationship with Laura is strained; shouts and smacks her when she is difficult, which she seems to expect, calmly disobeying him.

A maternal uncle stammers; maternal aunt suffered from chorea.

Family lives in bungalow in good financial circumstances, but under cramped conditions.

History: birth normal; breast-fed for 9 months; easily weaned. Walked at 15 months; first night terrors then appeared, which mother describes as delirious attacks. This occurred 6 months after night feeds were stopped, since when night terrors, accompanied by temperatures and screaming, occur at monthly intervals. Reliably dry at night at 1 year. Now has lavatory fears, dislikes any lavatory outside home. Talked clearly at 2, but after 3, speech deteriorated. At 3, whooping cough, then accident to head, causing broken artery, during mother's absence. Terrified when head was forcibly held down for stitching. Shortly afterwards there followed birth of baby. Following phases of night terrors, appetite is poor for 2 weeks, otherwise good. Between terror periods, sleeps well, shares bed with older sister; fights with her and other sisters, except baby, of whom she is fond and jealous. Older children say she is selfish; they cannot get on with her. Eldest sister had night terrors at 4½, associated with air-raids. Last one occurred 9 months before the onset of Laura's, who has not experienced air-raids.

School record and intelligence: began school at 3. Much absent during first year through chickenpox and measles. Now described as lazy but can do good work when she tries. Mixes well, fights with cousin, a year her junior, and of whom she is intensely jealous.

In intelligence test, I.Q. 100. Verbal comprehension her weakest point. Responded easily in spite of speech defect.

Personality and behaviour: always whining and complaining; terrified of doctors since traumatic incident at 3. Afraid of wild animals. Difficulties more pronounced since father's return at 4½; is rebellious and negativistic towards him. Destructive with toys; does not concentrate, is fidgety. Imagines people are against her, cringes when threatened. Is disobedient and impatient, flings things about when in a temper. Many accidents. Resents mother going out with father. Likes dolls, the baby, and drawing, but destroys books, puzzles, etc. belonging to other children, and is unpopular because of this and her general whining.

Clinical summary: diagnosed as primary behaviour disturbance with neurotic tendencies; taken on for individual treatment. Within a year made satisfactory progress; mother's cooperation excellent. Laura made great improvement at home in all relationships. Teacher reported great progress at school; main problems of jealousy, accident proneness, phobias and night terrors have cleared up. Speech is greatly improved. Treatment was terminated just before family left for Canada. Child now more independent of mother who is able to accept Laura's being a sensitive child with special needs, whereas the older girls are tougher and more self-sufficient.

Causative factors: jealousy of siblings, especially of baby which is related to her position in the family and long period as being the baby; intense wish to be a boy; strained relationship with father following long separation from him; early trauma and several illnesses and accidents led to a specially dependent and demanding relationship with mother, which prepared the way for her later difficulties and general immaturity. Birth of baby, homecoming of father in a disturbed unsettled condition, led to the appearance of her symptoms.

Case No. 83: Gertrude. *Age:* 8 years, 2 months. I.Q. 86.

A shy, frightened little girl.

Referral: by school medical officer on account of nervousness and fears. Gertrude has always been a nervous child, is afraid of doctors and nurses, has fears of death and of the dark.

Family background: younger of 2 children in stable, working-class family.

Mother: warm, forthcoming, garrulous woman. Started to train as an actress. Gives much information spontaneously; tends to over-dramatize herself. During war, had many evacuees, including 4 boys from London, which she enjoyed. Fond and proud of Gertrude.

Father: quiet unassertive man; 6 years in R.A.F.; no overseas service, home on leaves. Now runs village store. Adores and spoils Gertrude who can do what she likes with him. Never encourages her to dance and sing, though he himself plays the piano. Her difficulties have been more pronounced since his demobilization.

Sibling: brother, aged 11, who presents no problems. He was in a school that was bombed and 40 children killed. Was in hospital for 7 weeks with broken thigh when he was 8.

History: a planned baby. Both parents wanted a girl. Breast-fed; no weaning troubles. Appetite, sleep and health good. At 4, had an inoculation, did not appear to mind. At 5, scabies, week in hospital; no trouble, did not seem to mind leaving mother. Has had measles and whooping cough. Recent period of ringworm cured by X-ray. Exaggerated fear of doctors and nurses first noticed when she was $5\frac{1}{2}$ and had cut her hand. Not upset until taken to nurse, when she screamed and cried and asked if she would die. Was similarly terrified when ringworm was treated. Constantly refers to the Bible, especially to the Crucifixion. Fears the dark; during father's absence, slept with mother; refused to go to her own room on his return, so sleeps in brother's room. During the day, dislikes being alone in a room, though a cat or dog will serve for protection.

School record and intelligence: began school at 4; left home very early each morning as mother went to work. Made good progress, but hates sums. Likes school. Mother expresses surprise that Gertrude gets on well with girls as she is more used to boys.

In intelligence test, I.Q. 86; good vocabulary and verbal expression for this level; poor reasoning ability.

Personality and behaviour: mother says she is easy to manage but a tomboy. Bears no malice when corrected, occasionally sulks. Main interests are dressing-up, dancing and singing. Seems to be a happy, easy child who gets on well with everybody and has no problems other than her fears. These may have become more pronounced since the sudden death of a girl friend at school 6 months ago. Mother thought that Gertrude worried little at the time, but notices that she is constantly thinking she will die. At clinic, she clung to her mother, was fearful of strange places; talked willingly about her fears, said that her dog slept in her room to guard her, and that she takes a doll to bed. Feels safer if she sleeps with her brother, as she is afraid a man will come through the window and kill her. Says she has only nice dreams about being in a hospital; wants to be nurse. Brother has told her frightening tales about children being killed, so she and brother take a sword to bed to defend themselves against a man who will come to kill her.

Clinical summary: diagnosed as having a neurotic disturbance, probably anxiety hysteria, although it was not yet possible to ascertain what the phobic conditions are. Treatment was strongly recommended but mother, after some hesitation, declined this because she could not bring the girl regularly over a great distance. Given some advice on handling. Prognosis only fair; there is strong chance that girl will have severe neurotic disturbance in adolescence.

Causative factors: possible hereditary nervous disposition; dominating and histrionic personality of mother, who partly shares her nervous fears; absence of father for 6 years; acute sibling rivalry; sudden death of school friend.

Case No. 84: Ruby. *Age:* 7 years, 1 month. I.Q. 89.

A small girl with a solemn, anxious expression.

Referral: by School Medical Officer on account of enuresis, fears, difficult behaviour at home and at school, backwardness and refusal to talk at school.

Family background: elder of two children from stable home.

Mother: a dull, nervous woman who seems to find social contacts difficult and to expect criticism. The Headmistress of Ruby's school has found her unreliable. Fond of Ruby, does her limited best for her. Ruby clings to her mother.

Father: tractor driver; 5 years in Forces; demobilized 2 years ago. Pets and fusses over Ruby, but supports mother on points of discipline. Works long hours and leaves management of home and children to mother.

Sibling: brother, aged 4. He and Ruby quarrel constantly. Mother says he provokes the trouble and she is quick to respond.

Family circumstances are good rural working-class level, somewhat isolated from social life.

History: birth normal, weighed 5 lb. Breast-fed for 9 months. No weaning difficulties. Walked and talked before 18 months. No bowel training difficulties; has continued to bed-wet occasionally, also to wet knickers. Appetite poor, faddy about food. Slow in going to sleep, but sleeps well. Always been clean and healthy; no severe illnesses apart from measles and colds. A fear of dogs has persisted for some years.

School record and intelligence: mother has to take her to school; wept inconsolably during first week. Bad mixer, refuses to talk to teacher. No interest in lessons; shows extreme distrust and nervousness when teachers speak to her. Retarded in all subjects; cannot read, recognizes only a few letters. Inhibited in playground and rather solitary.

In intelligence test, I.Q. 89. Shy and frightened, offered only minimal verbal response. Too timid to volunteer information unless asked for it and gave monosyllabic replies.

Personality and behaviour: mother says child never settles for more than 10 minutes at anything. Never speaks to strange adults, refuses to join group play; plays only with one younger child. Easily frightened, clings to mother; seldom smiles or laughs. Particular about toys, keeps them wrapped up. Best subjects are dancing

446

and rhythmic work. Says she likes dramatic work although her speech is spoiled by nervousness.

Clinical summary: diagnosed as case of primary behaviour disturbance with neurotic trends; seen for period of observation at the clinic and treatment strongly recommended. Prognosis with treatment was considered to have been good, but the father was opposed to her attending the clinic and declined to allow her to attend any longer when she showed some superficial improvements. The prognosis is thought to be only fair, depending on the child's ability to achieve satisfaction outside the home, and she will probably have considerable neurotic difficulties in adolescence. Outcome inconclusive.

Causative factors: not fully elucidated. These were thought to be largely dependent upon the mother's isolated and nervous personality, her over-intense relationship with the girl whose dependence upon the mother was thus increased; the mother's attitude to the girl and the latter's intense sibling rivalry.

Case No. 85: Jean. *Age:* 9 years, 9 months. I.Q. 103.

A plain, spindly girl with straight hair. Slight facial disfigurement owing to an accident as a baby.

Referral: by school medical officer on account of sleep-walking, excessive reserve, moodiness and fears.

Family background: youngest of 3 surviving children of family of 4. Parents are separated; girls are with foster-mother; 17-year-old boy lives with grandmother.

Mother: large, coarse uninformed woman, reserved and undemonstrative. Foster-mother of girls dislikes her, reporting that she takes little interest in the children, has only visited them twice during last year, never remembers their birthdays, deceives them as to her movements. Mother is said to have uncontrolled temper, has impatiently smacked the girls' faces. They are upset after her visits. Tells them of physical quarrels with father which frightened her and she had to stand up to him and defend them.

She hopes to have marriage annulled, having discovered that father did not marry her in his own name. Works with Services canteen, hopes to go abroad soon.

Father: carpenter; has been away from family for some time, is now in Guernsey. Has violent temper; was brutally treated during unhappy childhood. On several occasions, interfered with 2 of his daughters before they left home. Girls afraid of him, and mother refuses to let them be alone with him. He takes little responsibility and makes no arrangements for them. Fretted and fussed over Jean as a baby, then suddenly started smacking her; later ignored her. Has always been much away from home.

Siblings: 9 months ago, eldest girl died suddenly, aged 15, from cerebral haemorrhage. Second girl, aged 14, goes out to work. Brother, aged 17, lives with grandmother. Much jealousy between 2 sisters; Jean, being submissive, tends to be bullied, fails to stand up for herself and gently weeps. The 2 older girls were billeted with a semi-invalid and her daughter under the evacuation scheme 8 years ago. Jean joined them 5 years later.

History: born at time when parents' marriage was disturbed and unhappy; constant fights during pregnancy. Grandmother then lived with family and gave much help. Birth normal; breast-fed for 12 months; no weaning difficulties. Clean early; mother trained her by smacking. Between 2 and 3, began wetting; was beaten continuously in manner bordering on cruelty. Before this there were sleeping, feeding and bladder disturbances. By $3\frac{1}{2}$, when family broke up, had developed lavatory fears and obstinacy. Until 4, lived in London with mother, then was billeted with her father in Wales. Jean continued to wet knickers, was nervy, bit nails and sucked lips continuously; had nightmares. Greatly upset over death of favourite dog. Then was sent to grandmother for a year, and at 6, joined sisters. Has abnormally large appetite, but remains very thin; is clean and healthy. Showed little emotion when sister died, but has been moody and depressed since. Nightmares continue; steals food from larder. Reads in an obsessional manner.

School record and intelligence: started school at 6 from foster-home, going straight to junior school instead of infants. Made average progress; is industrious, well-behaved, seems normal and happy. Worries a lot; when teacher wanted her to take scholarship exam a year under age, foster-mother forbade it as Jean was so frightened, nervy and moody.

In intelligence test, I.Q. 103; quiet, cooperated well. Serious, unhappy face. Thinks and speaks clearly. No special abilities or disabilities.

Personality and behaviour: at clinic, Jean was inhibited and over-polite, extremely obedient, never answered back. At home, helps with a desperate urgency as though frightened to refuse; worries, is solitary, dreamy and absent-minded. Has no friends of her own age, plays only with younger children, then she is dominating and wants her own way. Bites nails to the quick; is constantly washing her hands in an obsessional way, and going to the lavatory. Reserved, shows little affection, makes no spontaneous remarks. Likes best to be left alone to read or to do her stereotyped drawings and modelling.

Clinical summary: diagnosed as suffering from neurotic disturbance; taken on for treatment for a year. Made slow but satisfactory progress; sleeping, feeding and bladder disturbances cleared up. Definite obsessional trends, however, in her character structure remain, and further psycho-analytical treatment is recommended for the future. Prognosis thought to be good as far as symptoms are concerned; fairly good chance that emotional development will now go forward more rapidly.

Causative factors: unsatisfactory and unloving parent-figures; disturbed marital relationship of parents; early break-up of the home; her unhappy evacuation experience; mother's over-rigid and harsh training in early years; death of sister.

Case No. 86: Elspeth. *Age:* 9 years, 4 months. I.Q. 133.

A tall, fair girl who looks tense, discontented and unhappy.

Referral: by mother on account of obstinacy, disobedience and school failure.

Family background: elder daughter of parents who are both schoolteachers.

Mother: tall, handsome but severe-looking woman, with a discontented expression. Highly intelligent, but tense, dominating and self-opinionated; lacks insight into her own part in Elspeth's difficulties. She is excessively proud of her mastery of several languages, wide reading in child psychology and general education. She and her husband have high standards and great ambitions for Elspeth, who very much resents her parents' profession and exasperates them by refusing to take any interest in her lessons. Mother is emphatic and authoritative in her dealings with the girl, who defies her and is deliberately uncooperative.

Father: artist and teacher of languages. Psychiatrist observed him to be an obsessional type with constant fear of poverty and a disgruntled attitude to life. Leaves management and control of girls to wife; is inconsistent with Elspeth, ignores her uncooperative ways until these affect him, then loses his temper, literally shakes her, sometimes bruising and hurting her. Mother takes child's side; resents father's being more interested in his work than in the children's welfare.

Sibling: younger sister; already more competent than Elspeth in some respects, i.e. can carry things about without breaking them. Elspeth is jealous, teases and torments her.

Family has always had stable, comfortable middle-class home without any real financial difficulties.

History: mother wanted a girl. Breast-fed with difficulty for 10 months. Vomiting after meals, caused, mother says, by acidosis. Truby King rearing methods rigidly adhered to. During first 2 years, mother was ill, had an operation. Habit-training difficult; smacked by mother. Clean and dry at $2\frac{1}{2}$. At this time, family went to France where father had a job. Elspeth learned to speak French. From earliest years, has history of being clumsy, of hurting herself, banging into things, demanding attention and

450

bandages. Feeding difficulties have existed since 2½. Light sleeper; wakes up at about 5.30 a.m., goes downstairs to read, puts on kettle, calls to mother when it boils as though to get her attention and get her up earlier than is necessary. Has attacks of 'acidosis' with temperature; mother worries, so Elspeth has to stay in bed for a few days. Health is otherwise good.

School record and intelligence: began school at nearly 4. Mother upset when Elspeth was kept down at end of year. Teachers agreed that she should do better. Mother coached her in holidays; can now read; unable to spell or to do sums. Below average in all subjects.

In intelligence test, I.Q. 133. When retested at end of 6 months' treatment, was 139. Kept up lively conversation during test, revealing wide vocabulary, but was on the defensive and ill-at-ease; made little effort to succeed. On meeting difficulties, adopted blasé air, criticized herself, talked a lot but never once smiled.

Personality and behaviour: at home, is uncooperative. Endeavours to be tough and tomboyish, but fails. Discontented, lacks initiative, behaves in silly way, has frequent temper tantrums. Mother complains about her bad table manners.

Clinical summary: found to have neurotic character disturbance of unusual intensity; emotional difficulties are intensified by special home background; unable to make use of her high abilities. From the outset it seemed unlikely that she could be satisfactorily treated while at home. Attempts were made to find progressive boarding school, but individual treatment was begun because without it she could not succeed at any school. Elspeth, mother, and father were seen regularly over a period of 6 months. In short time, it was easy to understand the mother's irritation and complaints, because the child behaved in the same provocative, defiant way at the clinic. She acted out her conflicts, refused to admit there was anything wrong with her, nagged at the psychiatrist continually, wanted to be forced to do things, reacted to every small frustration as though it were a major one; had attacks of rage if she were kept waiting, or saw the psychiatrist with another child; once hit the psychiatrist with a whip, frequently swore; rarely talked naturally or openly, defended herself against unpleasant topics by denial or running away or turning the emotion into its opposite. Interpretation of her defence mechanisms used against the recognition of her main conflicts (which had caused the difficult behaviour and learning inhibition) had to be administered so that she was taken by surprise; otherwise she would shut her ears, climb out of the window or scream until it was impossible to hear one's voice. Her relationships were all disturbed by intense hostility, constantly 'staged' situations where she must be frustrated; and showed intense desire to get objects (or certain kinds of behaviour) from people, if necessary by bribery or force. Intense hostility and provocation to mother was thought to be due to her conflicting dependence and strong desire to get away from her. Pathological side of her development was her failure to sublimate energies linked with her wish to be a tomboy or to find outlets in other ways; this resulted in her learning inhibition. Intensity of defence mechanisms against her wish to be a boy caused a character disturbance, which, with suitable handling, may have been of a passing nature but which, if the way to sublimation was not opened, would probably have led to permanent perverse distortion in her personality. Treatment, which was carried on by ingenious methods, was very successful, and opened the way to normal development in puberty. A change of school and removal from home at her own wish helped her to achieve better sublimations. As a result of continued psychiatric supervision, she was able to adapt satisfactorily in school life, aided by an exceptionally capable and understanding headmistress. She improved in all directions; caught up with level of her age-group in a short time, was greatly liked by teachers, and has begun to develop her exceptional ability. Since she has great energy and originality, the prognosis is very good and she promises to become an unusually interesting and courageous personality.

Causative factors: emotional difficulties in both parents as a result of which they had specially ambitious expectations from the child (and placed over-emphasis upon success); mother's character structure and early illness led to disturbed relationship with

Elspeth from the beginning; she then became disappointed in her, expecting her to conform to rigid and impossible standards. The marital relationship, in which the mother plays the dominant part, is a most unequal one, and this has led to Elspeth finding difficulty in accepting her own feminine rôle.

Case No. 87: Penelope. *Age:* 10 years, 8 months. I.Q. 100.

A quiet, poised girl who gives the impression of being old-fashioned but not unduly shy.

Referral: by a private doctor for various illnesses without physical origin.

Family background: only child of broken marriage. Father deserted mother, and as they are Irish Roman Catholics, there is no question of divorce.

Mother: tense, excitable, talkative; intelligent and full of vitality. Her childhood was ailing and unhappy. At times she is much depressed by Penelope's illness; when told by the doctor that this was without organic origin, was unaccountably depressed and incredulous. Treats child as invalid, forbids her to lead a normal life, or go to school or mix with other children. Does dressmaking to supplement father's allowance for her and the child.

Father: in Regular Army until a year ago; now an unskilled labourer. Alcoholic, repeatedly unfaithful, never lived with family for long. Went overseas when Penelope was 3, returned for a few weeks, then left to take up work in London. No legal separation. Mother's attitude to sex is disturbed: sex relationship always unsatisfactory; there were quarrels each time father came home.

Maternal grandmother: family has always lived with her. She dislikes the father, supports mother against him. Mother's sister lives in house at present; is different from mother in temperament and interests. There is history of temperamental instability in the mother's family.

House is small and clean, but cluttered up with furniture, ornaments, and mother's dressmaking paraphernalia, leaving little room for movement.

History: mother sick throughout pregnancy; ill-treated by husband. Birth normal; breast-fed for 4½ months. A tiny, irritable baby, always crying, crying every night until 3. As family then lived in lodgings this exasperated the mother. Early sleeping and feeding difficulties. Habit-training rigid; excessively clean at 18 months, when feeding difficulties became more pronounced. For long time, shared mother's bed; now has own bed in mother's room. Sleep restless, has nightmares; refuses to go upstairs without mother. Periods of crying and picking herself until sore. At 8, whooping cough for 4 months. Returned to school for 3 weeks, then had mumps. Again 3 weeks at school, then had measles. Continuous colds, remained underweight; heart enlarged. Medically advised for malnutrition; seaside holiday recommended. Mother feared child was TB; on doctor's advice, kept child in bed for 3 months, then took house by the sea, pushed child around in pushchair for 6 months; then kept the child in bed for a further 5 months before consulting another specialist, who said child should not be in bed, that she had displaced heart and should run wild by the sea for a year. Mother has continued to take her from doctor to seaside and back, or to school for a few weeks at a time. She keeps constant record of child's weight, which appears to decrease each time she is moved. Penelope has been taken to 13 doctors in all, none of whom found anything wrong. County educational authorities have now visited mother because Penelope is not at school. Mother refuses to send her, fearing infection, so child is taught by governess; likes this and does not appear to be backward.

In intelligence test, I.Q. 100; response rather slow. Comprehension good. Better on verbal than on practical tests. Cooperative but not forthcoming.

Personality and behaviour: a solitary, good, obedient child, patient when ill; affectionate. Does not get on well with other children, is passive and shows no initiative towards them; likes only one friend. Gave up singing and dancing because of fear of other children. Never expected to help in house; spends time playing with kitten and dolls, and reading. Has a swing and see-saw, likes riding and jumping. Envies boys their more active pursuits; mother reiterates that she should have been a boy.

Clinical summary: diagnosed as suffering from severe neurotic disturbance; taken on for long-term individual treatment. It was also recommended that she should resume normal life and go to school. Made good progress, symptoms were alleviated. Follow-up shows that she is attending school regularly, has friends, and that her personality and appearance have become more normal, even sometimes rough and tomboyish.

Causative factors: mother's hysterical personality and rejection of normal marital life; over-protection and solicitude for child which covered her underlying ambivalence and rejection; over-strict training and discipline of the child; child's forced withdrawal from normal life. Predisposing or contributory conditions were probably the long series of childhood illnesses, the desertion by the father, and possibly early constitutional factors.

Case No. 88: Daphne. *Age:* 12 years, 11 months. I.Q. 88.

A tall, sallow girl, quiet, with a diffident, apathetic manner. Talks little about herself.

Referral: by a psychiatrist on account of organic pains with hysterical elements, tiredness and fainting turns.

Family background: youngest child in stable home.

Mother: elderly, harassed woman; seems to be underfed and over-worked, weary and over-anxious. Has constant headaches. Stolid and unresponsive, without insight, is unobservant and has a poor memory for details. She finds Daphne's behaviour aggravating, shows no sympathy for her and disregards her complaints. She made no effort to hide her hostility, repeatedly expressed her preference for the boy.

Father: skilled labourer; quiet, dominated by mother. Has great interest in Daphne, takes her cycling with him. Relationship between parents is deeply disturbed; sexual relations broken off since Daphne was 3.

Siblings: eldest sister is 26; married 7 years ago, was deserted shortly afterwards. Developed hysterical paraplegia last year, but this has cleared up. Two of mother's sisters have pains in arms without swelling or visible symptoms. Brother, now 17, was enuretic until 7; is now most helpful and reliable of children. Daphne does not get on well with her brother or sister, is jealous and constantly finds grievances against them. Mother prevents children from open squabbling. Two children have died—the second child at 2 months; the third at 11, when Daphne was 5 months.

Family lives in working-class home in quiet street under poor conditions.

History: birth normal; breast-fed for 9 months. Only difficulties when older girl died, Daphne then being 5 months, and mother very upset. No weaning difficulties. Appetite poor; fussy eater now. Habit-training easy; clean and dry between 2 and 3. At 2½, mother was in hospital for operation and treatment of gastric ulcers. Daphne was cared for by eldest sister, then 13; difficult at first, but soon settled down. Had measles 4 times; pneumonia before going to school and mumps shortly afterwards. Tonsils removed. Now healthy, but poor posture. Began menstruating 4 months ago, but has been given no information about it. Walks and talks in sleep, has nightmares. Mother sleeps in bedroom with 2 girls, father shares room with boy. Daphne took great interest in sister's marital disharmony; upset when marriage was broken up as she got on well with her brother-in-law and liked being made much of by him. Her present difficulties started 17 months ago; period of indecision; began dropping things, unable to do drill with hands over head; developed pains, lost use of right arm; talked of nothing to live for and drowning. Many slight accidents, likes to wear big bandages. Fairly frequent fainting fits, especially at beginning of menstrual periods.

School record and intelligence: backward at school; bad memory, cannot concentrate. Slow, tired, languid, lethargic; no interest in anything she does. Behaviour good; teachers in present senior school consider her idle, ask if she is malingering or not. Backward in English, arithmetic and history; prefers domestic subjects.

In intelligence test, I.Q. 88. Slow response with wide scatter from 8 years to average adult level. Cooperation was limp and unenthusiastic. Little serious effort made.

Personality and behaviour: at home, prefers to play with younger children, is herself childish; always complaining; quarrels with brother and sister; thinks everyone is against her. Loses things, especially money, breaks things and has many minor accidents. Is described as lazy, untidy, floppy, and nurses grievances against people. Has some friends of her own age, but sees little of them and is not a good mixer. Reads little, has no interest in films or radio. Likes handicraft, though not good at it, playing with dolls and talking to them.

Clinical summary: diagnosed as primary behaviour disturbance with hysterical tendencies. Attended clinic in an activity group with 2 or 3 dull girls over a considerable period. Seemed to make friends fairly easily, but relationships remained superficial. Displayed little affect; effort poorly sustained in activities. Went through phase of hurting herself and wearing bandages, but latterly made no reference to aches and pains unless asked. Still complains of painful elbow. Prognosis thought to be poor and intensive psycho-analytic treatment recommended but little practical hope for this. Supervision continues.

Causative factors: constitutional inadequacy and rigid neurotic family pattern; neurotic personality of mother; disturbed family relationships, including disturbed sexual relation between parents and between elder sister and her husband; mother's repressive handling of the girl.

Case No. 89: Janice. *Age:* 12 years, 3 months. I.Q. 138.

Pretty, friendly, red-haired girl with a noticeable facial paralysis. Very sincere; talks of symptoms like an adult, tried hard to hide real feelings.

Referral: by a friend of her parents on account of enuresis, not mixing, and feeling different from other girls.

Family background: elder of 2 children from happy, stable home.

Mother: charming, educated woman whose relationship to Janice is close and friendly. Nervous manner, said she had breakdown when Janice was 9½ because her family suddenly resented her marriage on account of her huband being Jewish, while she is not. Spent some time in nursing-home.

Father: professional man. Brusque, hurried manner, but charming, friendly, and popular. Worried about Janice, but minimizes her difficulties. Preoccupied with her symptoms and has not yet got over her severe illness when she was paralysed for a year. Massaged her thigh every night for 2 years; worried about her facial paralysis; fears bed-wetting will prevent her from taking up profession. Idea underlying this is that child cannot marry so must have a profession. Janice is attached to her father, though argumentative with him.

Sibling: brother, aged 9. Considered clever. No difficulties at school. As small child, Janice mothered him and was kind. Mother thinks this masked jealousy.

Maternal grandparents have lived with the family for some time. Grandmother died recently. Grandfather, aged 80, is now a great trial.

Standards of home are of secure, upper middle-class level.

History: pregnancy and birth normal; bottle-fed by Truby King methods. At 5 months, feeding difficulties began, baby refusing solids. At 1 month, had nannie who remained with her until she was 5; became attached to her. Habit-training not difficult except that she was not dry at night. Nannie tried scolding her, and was reprimanded by mother. Between 2 and 4, temper tantrums. At 5, became dry for a year. Nannie left, but has kept in touch since. Mother remembers that Nannie preferred the boy. Between 6 and 7, religious phase; Bible and correspondence course from synagogue. Children have been given option of both religions;

458

at present Janice is Jewish with father, but not professing. Between 8 and 9, had difficulty in making contact or friends with other children. At 9½, mother's breakdown occurred; tension in the home. At 10, Janice developed encephalomyelitis; was in hospital, partially paralysed, for a year. Father undertook massaging of her legs, thighs and back, and continued this for 2 years. After hospital period, she was irritable and aggressive when forbidden to do things, would have outbursts and refuse to obey.

School record and intelligence: began school at 5, liked it and did well. From 7-9 had private governess in country, returned to school until hospital interruption at 10. Despite year's absence, progress good; is 2 years below average of class. Does not get on well with other girls. Work is good, though slow, steady and conscientious. Janice has never been in trouble or broken a rule; has no particular friends, rarely invites children home. She is only day-girl in her form. Being Jewish in a non-Jewish school, elects to attend chapel. Has some histrionic gifts; elocution best subject.

In intelligence test, I.Q. 138, indicating very superior intelligence. High verbal facility.

Personality and behaviour: an adult, quiet child with a great deal of intellectual ambition who is satisfied only with the best. She plans a university training; is rather too serious and conscientious about her work. Sensible, reliable, tidy and punctual with an adult sense of humour, but she has babyish outbreaks when she becomes angry and flounces about. Bossy with her brother and other children at home, and likes to organize them, but at school she is very quiet. Thinks people are against her although teachers say girls like her. Reserved and modest, became very self-conscious after her illness since she cannot run about and play games; does homework instead. Her physical disability and her high intellectual ability have made her into a highly individual personality.

Clinical summary: diagnosed as suffering from a neurotic character disturbance; taken on for long-term individual treatment. Made satisfactory progress; prognosis thought to be good. Treatment supplemented by environmental changes. Her feeling of being different from other children was related both to her religion and illness. She protested against the massage and exercise at school which show up her disability. Analysed her bed-wetting and her relationship to her brother; showed no emotion about her enuresis although she realized it is a handicap. Her inability to make friends is probably due to her unconscious feelings about herself. The follow-up shows that Janice is perfectly happy, has friends, made many other improvements and is top of her form. The bed-wetting has decreased.

Causative factors: mother's neurotic personality and breakdown; her rigid methods of habit-training; the girl's prolonged illness and facial disfigurement which she tries to hide; the father's over-preoccupation with her symptoms and his long-continued physical stimulation; Janice's dissatisfaction with being a girl.

Case No. 90: Dorothy. *Age:* 11 years, 11 months. I.Q. 94.

Tall, slim, attractive girl with sensitive face; reserved and on the defensive; looks unhappy. Seemed friendly, but was inhibited and unable to speak freely about her difficulties.

Referral: by her mother on account of hysterical symptoms, sleeping and feeding disturbances, aggressive behaviour at home, apathy and jealousy.

Family background: second child in family of 3 girls from united, stable home, though all members of family have open and expressive aggression.

Mother: aged 35; vivacious and attractive Welshwoman; healthy, warm and kind-hearted; possessive and over-anxious. Has sympathy and understanding for Dorothy's moods, but has also developed minor quarrel relationship with her, and is easily hurt by the girl's behaviour and rudeness. Dorothy is greedy, dependent and provocative towards mother, who blames herself for having given the children too much, making them dependent upon her. Regards food as special link with her children, is inclined to over-feed them. Standards rigid; insists on many immaterial points. Talks cheerfully and vigorously, even humorously, about difficult scenes at home. Convinced that Dorothy should have been a boy.

Father: private in Army for 5 years, only home on leaves. Now has own nurseries, which he manages well. On strict diet because of gastric trouble. Good with children, though openly disappointed not to have had a son. Dorothy very attached to him and on the whole behaves well with him, though at times is as rude to him as to the mother. During family rows, he withdraws into a book (generally a murder story).

Siblings: elder girl, aged 12, is training to be a cook. Nervous and hysterical during air-raids. She and Dorothy have always quarrelled. Younger sister, aged 3, had still-born twin. Dorothy is now irritable and snappy with all the family and especially loses temper with the baby. She feels all the world is against her.
  Paternal aunt became insane, died after 10 years in a mental hospital. Much catarrh and asthma in father's family.

Family now lives in downstairs flat in modern estate which is comfortable, pleasantly but poorly furnished.

History: pregnancy and birth normal, baby weighed 10 lb. Breast-fed for 12 months; greedy, fussy about food. Easily bowel-trained; dry in day-time early; enuretic until 10; guilty and ashamed about this. Sleep disturbed; still calls out; temper tantrums in early years; used to cry at night to be taken to mother's bed. An irritable, moody child. A year ago, developed twitches and grimaces. Previous to this, was sent away while baby was born; felt rejected and hostile on return. Showed no undue nervous strain during doodle-bug raids. Appetite still greedy, much concerned about food. Health uneven, many periods of acidosis. At 3, victim of practical joke by other children; pushed into tub of water, was then ill with fever. At nearly 6, in bed 3–4 weeks with undiagnosed illness, attacks of vomiting and headaches. Family feared they would lose her. At this time, house was full of evacuees one of whom, aged 2½, was ill with bronchitis, so mother was very busy. At 7, chickenpox; at 9, chorea.

School record and intelligence: began school at 6; liked it and mixed well. Is now unhappy and bullied. Not backward in any subject; likes sums, sewing and games; dislikes history and geography.

In intelligence test, I.Q. 94; performance low average. Rather reserved and obstinate. Not forthcoming.

Personality and behaviour: at home, is resentful, so is bullied by other girls. Prefers boys of her own age or younger girls. Shows no feelings towards family except when hurt, then is aggressive. Never excited or enthusiastic, is easily hurt, cries at slightest provocation; cannot take criticism, makes accusations, threatens to kill herself, swears at her mother. Thinks everything and everyone is against her. Has always been a tomboy; wants to work on land or be a farmer. Careless about appearance and cleanliness. Likes to withdraw from family and lose herself in a book. Reads about witches and fairies with magic wands. Has a pleasant singing voice.

Clinical summary: diagnosed as primary behaviour disturbance with neurotic tendencies; taken on for treatment. Very inhibited and uncooperative at first, but became able to establish good relationship. Jealousy of sister and feelings of being rejected by family were discussed. The intensity of her instinctive urges was shown to her; in short time she changed her attitude towards food; also became aware of her inability to express aggression openly and understood that her feeling that all the world is against her is really a projection of her own feeling of guilt because of her hostility to others. Mother also responded well to treatment, her insight improved, and she became less anxious and possessive towards all the children. Prognosis thought to be very good, and outcome of the case is in every way satisfactory.

Causative factors: mother's possessiveness and the girls' dependence upon her; parents' disappointment that she is not a boy; jealousy and repressed hostility for siblings; her inability to succeed in masculine achievements.

Case No. 91: Patricia. *Age:* 13 years, 5 months. I.Q. 124.

Pleasant-faced girl with unusually mature facial expression. Embarrassed about coming to the clinic.

Referral: by mother on account of truanting and romancing.

Family background: older of 2 girls from stable, working-class home.

Mother: tearful, overworked, miserable-looking woman; tense and nervous, with highly emotional reaction to Patricia's romancing. Works extremely hard looking after the family and doing full-time domestic work in a local school so that she can buy good clothes for the girls. Refuses to let them do anything in the house; has a fixed idea that her children must never work as she has done. There is probably some degree of compulsion in the amount of work she does and the high standards she has to maintain. Because of long working hours, she sees little of Patricia.

Father: skilled labourer; more intelligent than mother; won scholarship at school. He and Patricia are good friends; he likes to talk with her when he returns from work.

Sibling: sister, aged 6, with whom Patricia gets on fairly well. She is bright and family is ambitious for her to win a scholarship.

History: mother was able to give little information about the child's early years. All development seems to have been normal. No difficulties arose until Patricia began telling romantic stories at school and passing notes to other girls containing swear words. She has told stories about her parents not being her real ones, about being an orphan, that she was going to hospital for an operation, that there had been triplets born in the local hospital and that her mother had died. When it was discovered that none of these fantastic stories was true, Patricia truanted.

School record and intelligence: dislikes school, feels out of things, has no friends. Finds science, geometry and algebra difficult. Popular with teachers; won several cups at sports. Won scholarship to high school: made average progress there. Since her home background is different from that of other girls, she is said to mix with girls above her station who give her ideas.

In intelligence test, I.Q. 124. 'Over-good' behaviour. Rather sensitive and embarrassed.

Personality and behaviour: mother maintains that she knows little of Patricia or of her interests. The girl is easy to manage, obedient, never cheeky or argumentative. Plays for pity and sympathy at times. Mother lacks contact with her, constantly reminds her of how much she herself has sacrificed to give her a good home. Patricia likes cinemas, is interested in her appearance and boys. Reads a lot, but cannot wash up or prepare meals.

Clinical summary: diagnosed as primary behaviour disturbance with neurotic trends in an adolescent girl. Her neurotic reaction to a difficult situation in reality was found to have existed for a considerable time; taken on for group treatment. Made good contact with therapist. Fears of other girls looking down on her were discussed; she became conscious of her school ambitions, her fear of being a social outcast, and her failure to identify with the social class of her parents. Difficulties in her relationship with her mother were worked over. Truanting continued until it was arranged for her to change to a more suitable school in accordance with her own wishes. She settled down well there; follow-up shows that she is happy and had made many friends. Prognosis thought to be good.

Causative factors: mainly mother's rigid and reserved personality and her strict and unsympathetic methods of handling the girl. This produced an attitude which made it difficult for an intelligent girl of working-class background to enter into and compete with social companions of her own age. She reacted to this situation with an outbreak of neurotic tendencies which had formerly been hidden.

Case No. 92: Pamela. *Age:* 12 years, 5 months. I.Q. 99.

A tall, thin girl who looks old for her age and wears glasses. She drags a stiff leg and flat foot along in a hopping fashion, never smiles, and has a discontented expression.

Referral: by her mother on account of fears, pains, disobedience and an unhappy disposition.

Family background: elder of two children from a stable home.

Mother: aged 36, but looks older. Thin, worn, depressed and apathetic woman. She made little contact with the psychiatrist, never smiled or offered personal remarks. Suffers from neurasthenia; has had much financial worry; is now bitter and aggressive towards people and has no friends. Little insight into Pamela's difficulties, is hurt by girl's apparent dislike of her. Admits shouting at the child, 'I wish you had never been born, you have brought nothing but trouble.' Her attitude is unconsciously ambivalent; she expressed no positive feelings for the girl, who says the mother has no love for her. Father expects mother to return to work soon, as younger child is now 3, but mother refuses to do this.

Father: aged 41; delivery man, formerly small tradesman. Foot severely crippled through infantile paralysis; easily tired. Friendlier and warmer person than mother but intolerant of noise, repressive, forbids children to bring anyone to the house. He and mother are unable to discuss their problems; constantly disagree over discipline, and he fails to support mother. Resented second baby as this prevented mother from going out to work; expressed disappointment by refusing to take family out, and has never done so since.

Sibling: brother 9 years younger than Pamela. She was promised a sister, and at the time of his birth, said she loathed him. Now appears to worship him but punches him on the sly.

In family history, tendency towards T.B. An aunt was born blind.

The family lives in three-bedroomed house which they have shared with lodger for 6 years. Mother regrets having this lodger, but needs the money. He is 10 years older than the father, likes the children, and takes mother out. This causes friction and jealousy with husband.

History: pregnancy difficult; vomiting and severe cramp until seventh month; three days in labour, breech birth. Breast-fed for 2 months with difficulty. Cried steadily until 6 months, so was coddled and spoiled. Developed food fads, which continue. Walked at 11 months, talked in long sentences at 2 years and 3 months. Habit-training strict: reliably clean and dry at 18 months. At 2, severely scalded in hot bath; was terrified. For months afterwards, screamed at bath time. Since small child, temper tantrums and horror of blood; fears going to lavatory, the dark, and going upstairs alone. Pronounced nail-biter and thumb-sucker. Between 6 and 7 would fall out of bed and be found sleeping under it. Then followed period of talking in sleep. Now is often awake for much of the night, has asked to share room with brother; refuses to go to bed without him. At 7, evacuated for 6 months: declared she loved the billet, but ran wild and refused to wash, and for this foster-mother finally threatened to send her home. At 2, had severe bronchitis; at 3½, whooping cough; at 4, German measles; and at 9, measles. At 4, ankle was broken when she was knocked down by a car. At 11, again broke ankle when climbing a tree; was severely shocked and 'her personality changed—she went all to pieces' after this incident. Has had much medical and orthopaedic treatment.

School record and intelligence: at 5, went to nearby convent, though not Roman Catholic. Liked it at first, but tried to dominate others and was soon disliked. Attended another school during evacuation period, then returned to convent. Now wants to become a Roman Catholic. Moderately good at lessons, but lazy; has special dislike of French and algebra. Best subjects are English, drawing and painting.

In intelligence test, I.Q. 99. A serious child, showed no unusual reactions.

Personality and behaviour: disagreeable at home; never smiles or laughs, furious when crossed, always unhappy and disobedient; thinks everyone is against her, says parents, especially mother, do not love her. Takes a lot of trouble over clothes, especially shoes: does not want to wash or do her hair. Sucks handkerchief. Children do not play with her as she must always have her own way. Mother says it is impossible to be nice to her. Will go to films four times a week: enjoys adventure and mystery stories. Dislikes housework, exaggerates its difficulty, but does not mind cooking at school. No plans for the future, has few interests beyond her likes and dislikes.

Clinical summary: diagnosed as suffering from neurotic disturbance with large hysterical element in her symptoms together with some genuine organic disability. Repeated self-injury appears to be identification with father's injury. At present is under regular supervision while on waiting-list for long-term individual treatment. Parents have not yet accepted this, and mother repeats whenever angered, 'It would be better to send her away.' Outcome inconclusive (incomplete).

Causative factors: thought to include mother's neurotic personality and unconscious hostility to the girl; disturbed mother-child relationship; repressive handling by both parents.

Case No. 93: Eva. *Age:* 12 years, 10 months. I.Q. 133.

Pale, unhappy-looking girl, immature and small for her age. Nervous and ill-at-ease at first, speaking in low voice, but soon became friendly and responsive. She is thin, flat-chested and flat-footed with faulty vision in left eye.

Referral: by Headmistress on account of school backwardness, difficult and attention-seeking behaviour, and frequency of micturition.

Family background: elder of two children from stable home.

Mother: smartly dressed woman in middle 30's; looks tired and hard, admits she is impatient because overwhelmed by household duties. Quick and impulsive, lacks self-control, is fearful of criticism. Openly prefers the boy. Anxious to conceal Eva's difficulties, blaming school. Eva constantly provokes mother who then nags her. Mother fails to appreciate the girl's good qualities, has no faith in her and the clinic's assessment of her abilities. Father supported her in this attitude.

Father: professional man in his 60s. Kindly but obstinate, afraid of and dominated by his wife. A tall, heavy, ponderous and slow-moving man, rigid in his views, self-opinionated, old-fashioned.

He and mother set high standard for Eva, are disappointed in her
school failure. Father has coached her, and was patient and persistent in this but very strict. He regards her as lazy and careless.
The parents' attitude to the clinic was uncooperative: father
terminated treatment so as to give Eva period of 'forced training
in concentration'.

Sibling: young brother. Deals with her jealousy by ignoring the
boy, prefers to play with her pets.

History: 8-months baby born after mother had fall. Confinement
easy; weighed 5 lb. Breast-fed for 1 month. Appetite poor, soon
developed food fads. Habit-training rigid from first months:
reliably clean and dry at 18 months. Mother's rigid ideas about
upbringing were interfered with by a maid who formed a strong
attachment to Eva as a baby, and who spoiled her. Eva loved the
maid. Because of this, maid was dismissed without any explanation being given to the child when she was 4. Intellectually precocious; walked and talked at 1 year—first word being 'rhino-
ceros'. Sleep good. No severe illnesses, though many heavy colds
and temperatures. Until 6 or 7 openly wished to be a tomboy.
This phase ended after showing sex curiosity at time of brother's
birth when she was told that a stork would bring the baby from
Holland. Eva was laughed at when she asked if the baby would
be Dutch. While mother was in nursing home, Eva was cared for
by father, shown lambs being suckled by way of preparation for
sight of mother feeding baby.

School record and intelligence: until 10, at private school, then transferred to local High School. Backward in most subjects, especially
arithmetic and reading. Shows most interest and promise in poetry
and art: work invariably depends upon her liking of teacher. She
is inattentive, destructive, plays the fool and gets into scrapes.
Difficult to make her concentrate. Hates geography, has great
difficulty in remembering shapes of maps; dislikes scripture and
mathematics.

In intelligence test, I.Q. 133; mental age 17. Vocabulary score
excellent for her age. Seemed immature, restless and insecure, unable to use her capacities to the full. Anxious and inhibited.

468

Personality and behaviour: symptom of frequency of micturition has existed for 2 or 3 years at home and at school. Though always playing the fool or seeking attention, never looks happy. Slothful in morning, refuses to work at home. Moody, passionate in affection, sensitive, easily hurt, lacking in self-confidence, needs encouragement. Though tomboyish, full of fantasies and day-dreams. Unliked by other children because she is quiet and un-friendly. Upset by sight of suffering: has many accidents. Reads a great deal: tastes are morbid, prefers ghost and pirate stories to girls' books. Likes pirate games, wants to be a pirate. Likes draw-ing scenes of early morning in the woods and witches. Mother says she is clumsy and unreliable: recently managed a holiday alone in France quite capably. Fond of animals.

Clinical summary: this intelligent girl was found to be suffering from a neurosis; taken on for individual treatment by the clinic psychiatrist. Responded at once but the parents, however, termi-nated treatment almost as soon as it had begun, saying they had decided that a treatment plan of their own would be better for her. Prognosis thought to be doubtful: neurosis may break out again as adolescence progresses.

Causative factors: mother's quarrelsome personality and open preference for the boy; unequal marital relationship in which mother is dominating personality; rigid training in early years from both parents; disturbed relationship between mother and daughter; deliberate attempts to mislead child—i.e. over dismissal of loved maid, and over sexual questions; an irrational attitude to sexual education in both parents.

Case No. 94: Juliet. *Age:* 12 years, 10 months. I.Q. 98.

An attractive, rather untidy girl, with strong North-country accent. Nails badly bitten.

Referral: by school medical officer on account of difficult be-haviour and quarrelling at school, following the family's move from north to south of England. Symptoms include aggressive behaviour, spiteful attacks on other girls at school, lack of friends,

469

untidiness, difficult behaviour at home, greediness and thumb-sucking, and nail-biting.

Family background: only child in stable middle-class home. Parents moved from north to south of England 2 years ago because of father's appointment to the staff of local school.

Mother: slightly deaf woman whose impassive expression covers extreme anxiety. Eyes filled with tears several times: father had warned P.S.W. that interview might upset her. Anxious to talk, relieved to share problems. Sets extremely high standards for Juliet. Both parents are over-strict, probably through fear of spoiling her. Mother unsure in handling. She describes father as very excitable and a worrier. Both he and Juliet are highly strung, easily upset in an emergency.

Father: came to clinic on his own asking for urgent appointment before informing wife of plans. Intelligent, outspoken but not authoritative; good insight into Juliet's difficulties. Concerned about her, anxious to be assured that help would be possible. He is more preoccupied than most fathers with upbringing of the child.

Family has always lived in secure home of middle-class standards.

History: pregnancy normal; birth difficult. Baby weighed 12 lb., and it was an hour before she breathed. Severe convulsions during first 3 days: survival was doubtful. No further fits: development proceeded normally. Bottle-fed. Habit-training rigid: clean at 9 months. As toddler, was destructive; sucked thumb continuously, constantly put things in mouth. At this time, family lived near 4 grandparents. At 3, stayed with grandmother while mother gave birth to still-born boy weighing 14 lb.; mother was very ill. Juliet has had no sleeping problems; appetite always greedy; has passion for fats; pilfered food. At 5, in hospital for 2 weeks as diphtheria suspect: not ill, sobbed all the time. Period in hospital was followed by nail-biting and continuation of thumb-sucking.

School record and intelligence: went to strict elementary school in north of England: complaints made about her lack of concentration.

Left-handed, but was trained to write with right hand. Two years ago, transferred to high school in south; work below standard, teased about her northern accent. Ambitious in relation to other girls: feels inferior. Work now fairly good: fourth in class for backward children. Best subjects are geography and biology. Standard of work depends on whether or not she likes the teacher. Ashamed of things she does wrong.

In intelligence test, I.Q. 98. Average performance. Looks anxious and tense. Excitable.

Personality and behaviour: untidy at home, destructive and aggressive to other children; spills things, makes mistakes, behaves in clumsy, foolish way which exasperates parents. Vague, wandering and forgetful; no temper. Lately has become sulky; upsets other children by self-righteousness and gloating. Childish: wants what other children have; affectionate, easily upset if reprimanded but soon forgets. Reads little, does nothing really well. Fond of animals, pressed flowers, and stamp-collecting, like her father. Wants to be a veterinary surgeon or teacher.

Clinical summary: diagnosed as case of neurotic disturbance: taken on for individual treatment with aim to alleviate her symptoms although no change in her underlying character formation could be attempted in weekly interviews. Aggressive behaviour was found to be a defence against her feelings of inferiority and fear of being 'different' focused on her northern accent. She was made aware of this and of her strong desire to be liked by other girls; symptoms disappeared as her insight increased. Prognosis thought to be fairly good. Treatment continues.

Causative factors: mother's general anxiety: her over-rigid, over-strict training in early years; girl's reaction to move from north to south of England and her attendance at a 'snob' school which brought to a head a number of difficulties established many years earlier in her relationships with other girls.

Case No. 95: Edith. *Age:* 13 years, 10 months. I.Q. 108.

A pleasant-looking, friendly girl who wears glasses.

Referral: by her mother on account of acute fears, anxiety over school work, inhibited behaviour and frequency of micturition.

Family background: only child in stable home. Twin was born dead and undeveloped.

Mother: small, bustling, wiry woman with forceful personality; flits fretfully about from topic to topic, is full of whims and fancies, of ideas of danger and fantasies of being attacked. Probably even more disturbed than the girl. She herself is an only child whose twin brother died in infancy. Over-protective towards Edith; while disparaging the girl's symptoms, definitely shares in them, and has prolonged them by her own anxiety. She declares Edith should have been a boy. Immature.

Father: a clerk. Did not wish to join Services but was called-up on D-day: abroad for 2 years, not yet demobilized. Mother has known him since she was 12, and they were childhood sweethearts, says he is gentle but excitable, terrified of spiders; has frequency of micturition, anxiety attacks before exams, and is prudish. He is always teasing Edith, who misses him intensely. His family is reported to have 'nerves'; are all the same about wanting to go to the lavatory, and are very tolerant towards physical ailments and interesting nervous symptoms.

Mother and Edith lived with maternal grandmother for 3 years, but now have their own house and live in comfortable middle-class circumstances. During father's absence, mother takes lodgers in the summer. Edith is mainly with adults.

History: pregnancy and birth normal: breast-fed. No weaning or feeding difficulties. Habit-training rigid; no napkins after 9 months. Wet bed after death of loved grandmother when 4. Appetite good. At 2, night terrors; at 4, developed fear of dark. While father is abroad, sleeps with mother: they go to sleep holding hands. At 8, mumps and measles; no accidents, operations or illnesses; is menstruating regularly. Has pronounced fear of accidents, doctors, crowds, spiders, the dark, tunnels and trains, and of men. Episodes of compulsive nail-biting: still has night terrors. First fear appeared after grandmother's death; the child was not supposed to know of this until 2 years later and her questions were answered in misleading fashion. Fear of death seems to have become elaborated and spread to other things. Fears have been worse since father went away. She was frightened during an air-raid, but tried to hide her fear from mother. Mother shares intimate knowledge of all her present fears and worries.

School record and intelligence: began school at 5; disliked it. At 7, transferred to another which she likes. Reports are good: is popular and form captain. Described as quiet, dependable, tense, nervous and easily upset. Attendance irregular owing to illness: worries about homework. Average in reading poor, but good in arithmetic and practical subjects.

In intelligence test, I.Q. 108. Easily upset and nervous: slow in reasoning: verbal lower than general ability.

Personality and behaviour: described as having a nice nature, being tender-hearted and considerate. Discreet, perhaps too sensible for her age, has never had time for childish things. Not greedy, but has never been denied anything. Lacks self-confidence, never thinks she can do anything; has much imagination and tears come easily. Likes to go to cinemas and to read school books; loves games, plays tennis, hockey and swims. For 2 years, took ballet lessons; now learns piano and practises regularly. Has only one special friend, a girl of her own age, and a dog to which she is devoted. Keen on figures and wants to work in an office.

Clinical summary: diagnosed as adolescent disturbance with pronounced neurotic tendencies; taken on for treatment in small group of adolescent girls where she slowly gained insight into her conflicts. Symptoms gradually cleared up, behaviour greatly improved. She became more independent of her mother. Follow-up reports show that she had made marked progress in all directions, was able to mix well, and fears were much diminished. The mother, who had forced the child to keep her attendance at the clinic a secret, and found it hard not to share in her treatment also, eventually described her as 'a changed child'.

Causative factors: neurotic personalities of parents; mother's tendency to share her own disturbed emotional life with the girl and to emphasize her fears; over-strictness in earlier training; absence of father; mother's over-dependence on girl to subdue her own nervousness; mother's anxiety and over-protectiveness; good deal of repression of sexual and other intimate matters in family life.

Case No. 96: Juanita. *Age:* 13 years, 2 months. I.Q. 107.

A vivacious, active girl who makes a quick and positive contact but becomes silent and ill-at-ease when asked about her difficulties.

Referral: by her mother on account of behaviour difficulties, lack of concentration, tempers and romancing.

Family background: illegitimate: adopted after death of parents.

Adoptive mother: middle-aged, rigid, conventional person with limited insight; average intelligence. Married for 5 years before her own girl was born. At 22 months, this child was killed when with parents in a car accident. Juanita was adopted 4 months later. Mother has a passion for tidiness: is equally rigid with father and child about this. She complains of Juanita's moods and change-ability, treats her as a very young child, still washing her; complains of her dirtiness and untidiness; is easily disturbed and obsessed by child's behaviour difficulties. Responds to her tempers by punishments and deprivations. Has told Juanita that she would not have adopted her had she known how difficult she would be.

Adoptive father: served in 1914–18 war; since demobilization has remained in clerical work attached to neighbouring service head-quarters. In late fifties, heavily built, stolid and pleasant. Fond of but impatient with Juanita, self-conscious when questioned. Rather passively devoted to wife whose opinions he gives more readily than his own. He and wife strive to be better than their neighbours: have high standards, but little idea of the needs of an adolescent girl. Particular about Juanita's friends. Very obedient to wife's repressive ideas of tidiness, etc. in the house.

Family lives in small, comfortable villa in country village.

History: nothing known of parents except that mother was only 19 when Juanita was born. At 4½ months, adopted through Adoption Society. Bottle-fed. No feeding difficulties: eats well now. Habit-training rigid: clean and dry at 10 months and had no napkins night or day. Has always slept heavily, difficult to wake; talks in sleep. Restless child, always difficult to manage; has tempers at home, grizzles in public. Three years ago was told by another child that she was adopted: since then, has been more difficult. Health fairly good: has had measles, tonsilitis, mild bladder infection. Has been menstruating for some months: discussed this with teacher, but refused to talk to mother about it.

School record and intelligence: at 5, went to local village school: met rough type of child and did not get on well. Transferred to convent school: dislikes the nuns, does not concentrate or conform to rules. Romances, tells lies, creates difficulties with attention-seeking behaviour.

In intelligence test, I.Q. 107. Good verbal ability: responsive but inclined to give up easily. Uncritical of her performance.

Personality and behaviour: envious of other children, always thinking they have something better than she has; boasts she does not care and is negativistic. Likes to play with much younger children or to follow dominating ones. Obstinate and disobedient, constantly shows off, must be centre of attention. Dislikes criticism; when thwarted, has temper tantrums, stamps and screams. Untidy at home, rarely shows affection for anyone. Enjoys drawing and dancing: for a time took ballet lessons which she now regrets having given up. Likes playing with dolls and sewing for them; also likes reading or games. Ambitions are to be film star, mannequin, clothes-designer on one hand; on other to work in a stable, learn horse-riding, be a naturalist. Likes the radio: favourite programmes are Dick Barton and the William stories. Mother says she loves dressing up and buying new clothes, but is careless and untidy with them. Tends to find wild and noisy friends.

Clinical summary: diagnosed as adolescent disturbance with neurotic tendencies of a clearly hysterical type. Taken on for treatment with a group of adolescent girls, attended for 6 months and made good progress. Prognosis thought to be fair, depending upon some adjustments in the rather incompatible situation of a vivacious, active girl of hysterical character adopted by elderly parents in a rigid home where she is treated as a small child.

Causative factors: early change in mother-relationship; adoptive mother's strict and rigid training and girl's rebellion against this following discovery of deception about her adoption; considerable sexual repression in the home; possibly constitutional nervous instability.

Case No. 97: Theresa. *Age:* 14 years, 5 months. I.Q. 85.

A heavy, unattractive girl with greasy skin and worried expression.

Referral: by Headmistress on account of asthma, backwardness, enuresis, feeding disturbances, and nervousness.

Family background: middle child in family of three surviving children from stable home.

Mother: aged 42: large, breathless, affable woman of pyknic type, obviously hysterical. Easily tearful. Suffers from urticaria and continual heavy chest colds. Relationship with Theresa is intense and ambivalent. She is fussing and over-solicitous, yet openly rejecting. Insists on the child always going about with her, admonishes her in public. Admits her inadequacies, blames symptoms on physical complaints. Goes out to work to avoid monotony and 'because Theresa costs so much'.

Father: aged 50: storekeeper. Mother describes him as being exactly like Theresa, conscientious and worrying. Has had asthma since boyhood, now has duodenal ulcers. Gets on moderately well with daughters, but not with son. A maternal and a paternal aunt have asthma. Paternal grandmother lived with family for 15 years, died 3 years ago aged 89.

Siblings: brother aged 17, sister aged 12. Father does not get on with his son, but girls are quite friendly with him.

Family lives in comfortable middle-class circumstances.

History: mother had repeated colds, influenza, and whooping-cough during pregnancy. Birth easy: baby weighed 7½ lb. Both parents wanted girl to take place of first-born child, a girl, who had died at 4 months of whooping-cough. Breast-fed for 1 year; good baby, slept most of the time; never cried, never naughty. Mother denies having early difficulties. Habit-training rigid; clean at 7 months. Hated sticky hands, could keep frocks clean for a week. Sleeps well: originally shared bed with sister, but since 9, when enuresis and asthma started, has had separate bed. At 7, tonsils and adenoids removed: reacted badly to operation and for some time afterwards could not eat or drink. Asthma and chest colds developed. At 2 or 3, had sunstroke. Apart from asthma, health fairly good.

School record and intelligence: began school at 5: always happy there; much absent because of illness. Progress fair in relation to limited capacities.

In intelligence test, I.Q. 85. Listless and disinterested; only limited reasoning capacity, poor memory.

Clinical summary: diagnosed as a case of primary behaviour disturbance with neurotic trends in a dull girl. Theresa is due to leave school soon. She will be helped to find a job away from home in the hope that this will increase her independence and relieve her symptoms, which are largely dependent upon the mother's handling of her and her attitude of expecting the girl to be inadequate. The case is being followed up, and the question of treatment will be reconsidered when the girl has been settled in a job. Outcome inconclusive.

Causative factors: subtly rejecting home background; mother's neurotic personality and disappointment in her dull, nervous child; reaction to faulty and repressive handling by both parents. Some constitutional inadequacy and acceptance of psychogenic illness as family pattern.

Case No. 98: Ruth. *Age:* 13 years, 0 months. I.Q. 100.

A tall, attractive girl, well-built, clear-complexioned with a frank expression. Looks older than her age, and seems unhappy.

Referral: by her headmistress, who is her mother's employer, on account of extreme disobedience and defiance at home, sleep disturbance, train sickness, tempers, 'romancing' and lying.

Family background: illegitimate child of woman who was double bigamist. Lives with step-mother since her father's death a few years ago.

Mother: aged 30 when she married Ruth's father, who was 21, but said she was 20. Posed as hospital nurse and niece of famous author. Paternal grandmother says she spent all her husband's savings and ruined the family. At time of court appearance, Ruth was 6 months old. Mother was sentenced to 2 years' imprisonment for false pretences: has not been seen or heard of since. Had several other children before her 'marriage'.

Father: genial, easy-going: owned several businesses until joining R.A.F. Sent abroad during the war, where he was killed, aged 31. Had married step-mother a year earlier. Ruth greatly upset by news of his death, as she was devoted to him. Rarely mentions him now, but always in a light tone and present tense.

Ruth has idolized her own mother although she had heard rumours that mother had abandoned her. Family had kept the truth from her. Ruth in turn has been at pains to hide her secret fears of resembling her mother.

Step-mother: friendly, pleasant and intelligent, but unstable. Has illegitimate son of 16. She wants to help Ruth because she feels her efforts to make her good have failed. Her attempts to do so have been inconsistent and impulsive. Both she and Ruth are hot-tempered and changeable: atmosphere has been one of nagging, recrimination and blame. Ruth's difficulties are largely confined to her relationship with her step-mother.

There have been many changes of home; at times living with relatives or in furnished rooms and invariably in a quarrelling atmosphere. Now Ruth, her step-mother and step-mother's son share a bungalow with a friend who is a businesswoman. Ruth and the step-mother's son quarrel: Ruth is both jealous and fond of him. Step-mother works, has fairly heavy financial burdens.

478

History: little known about early life. Lived for first 3 or 4 years with foster-mother; father visited her occasionally. When 2, boy was born in foster-family: Ruth was neglected and became difficult. Between 3 and 4, father removed her; for next 5 years lived with father's brother and his wife. After a year, baby girl was born, Ruth again jealous. She was a restless, frightened child particularly afraid of bathing. Many food fads: talked in sleep. She was so restless that private doctor prescribed bromide. At 8, father joined the household, met step-mother, married her early in war. After a few leaves together, father went overseas. Step-mother took Ruth to live in house of friend with 2 girls of 8 and 10. Constant difficulties between Ruth and step-mother. A year later, father was killed. Before marriage, step-mother was a police-woman. A year ago, Ruth was involved in a sex episode with a man of 60 who lives next door. Since then she has become especially difficult, behaves in precocious fashion; at school was discovered passing notes full of detailed prescription for sex-play with soldiers in the park. Has been menstruating for 2 months. Health good. At 10, mumps and tonsillectomy.

School record and intelligence: began school at 5: hated it, had screaming fits. After a year, moved to another school, liked it better. Many bad reports complaining of daydreaming and in-attention. Then moved to present school where she especially hates one form-master. Reports are good, she is popular with mistresses. No difficulties, work good. Described as courteous and willing and a girl who loves to take responsibility. Best subject hygiene. Likes elocution, music and drawing.

In intelligence test, I.Q. 100. Manner was suspicious, behaviour slightly boastful and exhibitionistic. Wide scatter in results.

Personality and behaviour: at home, Ruth is sulky, untidy and dirty, takes every advantage of people's kindness, lies shamelessly and cries when she is found out. Moody and unsociable, has invented a brother called Adrian with whom she has imaginary conversations. She is a great tomboy and prefers to play with boys, usually younger than herself. Excessively modest, prudish and self-conscious about her body, but casual about clothes and appearance. Rude to her step-mother, deceitful, quarrelsome

479

and flares up easily; constantly forgets or falsifies what she has said. Likes playing school and camping with guides. Never helps in the house, but has job where she does domestic work for 2 hours on Saturday mornings to earn pocket money. No girl friends: extremely good with small children. Wants to learn hairdressing. Step-mother complains that she is mad about film stars. Likes only murder and sexy love-stories.

Clinical summary: diagnosed as suffering from a neurotic disturbance; taken on for weekly treatment with a group of adolescent girls. Talked freely about her difficult relationship with her step-mother and her general unhappiness. The psychiatrist discussed with her individually the true story of her mother's life: the girl wept a great deal, then became very affectionate and attached to the psychiatrist. Made steady and considerable improvement, but was very guilty about her step-mother's complaints. Step-mother apparently used the clinic as a threat, and forced her to come. She began to arrive looking sullen and hostile, was very anxious for extra attention, jealous of other girls. In competition, always wanted to be leader. Step-mother did not support the girl's treatment, said that there was no improvement at all. Ruth at length admitted that she no longer wanted to attend because of her step-mother's interference. It was recommended that she should attend boarding school. Prognosis thought to be poor while she remains at home and case will be followed up. Treatment incomplete and outcome inconclusive but girl shows considerable relief from her symptoms.

Causative factors: these were thought to lie in her extremely unsettled home background; the loss of and mystery about her mother; repeated changes of home and persons to care for her; loss of father; step-mother's unstable personality and an intense sado-masochistic relationship with the girl.

Note: Ruth's case is interesting because she is one of the few neurotic children who showed in such degree the background of broken home life allied to gross environmental disturbances and frequent changes of parent-substitute, etc., such as were commonly seen amongst delinquent children. She is also an example of a child who has been deliberately misled on matters important to herself, and kept in ignorance of the truth about her own mother. She has reacted to this with, on the one hand, depression, and on the other, outbursts of romancing, the invention of imaginary companions, writing sexual notes, and having various deceptive and secret activities of her own. (See Healy, 1915.)

Case No. 99: Jane. *Age:* 15 years, 7 months. I.Q. 105.

A tall girl with lank, greasy hair and a spotty though pleasant face. She wore her shabby clothes carelessly; was friendly but reserved, and took care to keep the conversation to unemotional topics.

Referral: by Headmistress on account of depression, tearfulness and fears.

Family background: eldest of four children from stable home.

Mother: intelligent, but weary and harassed. Fond of children, anxious for their welfare. Marital relationship very disturbed, and she is now considering separation. She is worn out by father's constant nagging: loses patience with the children because of fatigue.

Father: skilled tradesman; until recently was often away on jobs for long periods. A disappointed man, not happy in his work and without hobbies. He wants the easiest way out of everything. Mother feels he is fond of the family but fails to realize how his continuous quarrelling and nagging are wrecking the home. He is especially unsympathetic towards Jane, compares her adversely with her 8-year-old sister, who is his favourite and of whom Jane is jealous, He insists that Jane should mind the younger children. Her favourite is the 4-year-old boy who she feels is sensitive like herself.

Family lives in small working-class house, poorly furnished but tidy. Father earns regular wages, but there have been some financial struggles.

History: pregnancy and birth normal; breast-fed for 3 months. Mother blames father's nagging for loss of milk; had difficulty in finding right food. Walked and talked at 11 months. Good appetite as toddler, slept well. Habit-training easy. At 4, showed talent for dancing, and from 4–8, while she was an only child, learned dancing and danced in pantomimes. Between 6 and 8, bad periods of constipation, and first fears of dying and unhappiness appeared. At $7\frac{1}{2}$, when sister was born, feared mother would die, lost appetite, could not sleep. Now, when depressed, suffers from insomnia and loss of appetite: also has night terrors, is tearful, afraid of illness and dying. Before 14, had measles, whooping-cough and chicken pox. Last year, appendicectomy: was 3 weeks in hospital, and was very upset when woman in bed next to her died. Had just begun menstruating, was embarrassed and resentful about it. Mother had reluctantly given her some sex information, but finds subject of sex distasteful. Since then, Jane has been depressed and her fears have increased.

School record and intelligence: has always done well until recently; now says she cannot concentrate; has special difficulties with geography and biology; feels dismal about prospects in School Certificate Examination.

In intelligence test, I.Q. 105; showed much indecision and lack of confidence, and although vocabulary was good, verbal expression was extremely inhibited.

Personality and behaviour: Jane has friends at home and at school but is not a very sociable girl; began to bring friends home, but because father criticized them stopped doing so. Careless and untidy with clothes and possessions; is easily reduced to tears, and father tells her not to be so soft. When he nags, she does not answer back. She wants to be a teacher, her choice of work with children of 7 or 8, or with adults—not with people of her own age. Belongs to girls' club, but says she does not like children of her own age. Finds difficulty in playing games, though plays tennis. Dislikes and fights with boys. Belongs to school dramatic society. Her plans for the future are vague: she does not want to leave school. 'Doesn't know what she wants.'

Clinical summary: diagnosed as suffering from a neurotic disturbance; taken on for individual treatment. She made a good relationship with her therapist, was seen over a long period, and made very satisfactory progress. All her symptoms have entirely cleared up. Situation at home has improved, and the follow-up shows that Jane's work at school has recovered and she has regained standards normal for her age and ability.

Causative factors: disturbed and over-intense relationship with father; deeply repressed sibling jealousy (which seems to have been especially intense, and to have become hidden at the birth of next baby, after she had been an only child for so long); very disturbed marital situation; prolonged absence of father; possibly some constitutional elements are also present.

Case No. 100: Frances. *Age:* 15 years, 11 months. I.Q. 103.

A plump, young-looking girl with untidy hair who has no interest in how she wears her clothes.

Referral: by school medical officer on account of chronic stomach pains without physical cause.

Family background: only child from stable home. Parents are Welsh, now live in England and have renounced Roman Catholic faith.

Mother: stout, grey-haired, aggressive woman, unstable and impulsive. Her appearance is over-powering, she has domineering tendencies, is ready to attack as a means of defence. Seems guilty that the child's trouble should have other than physical cause: herself. Neurotic; has nervous headaches; irrational about all matters of sex education, shielding Frances from all knowledge of it. Expresses open disappointment in husband. Her aggressiveness masks insecurity and anxiety, especially as she shoulders many financial family worries. Considers Frances needs special care; antagonistic to clinic and to Frances having treatment. Ambitious, but disappointed in Frances, consoling herself by saying that it is not as bad as if Frances were a boy, for boys must have careers. Suffers from abdominal pains similar to those of Frances.

Father: a small man whom Frances resembles in size and appearance. Owned a farm in Wales, is now a lorry-driver. Left farm because of family quarrels, now feels his subordinate position. He is not ambitious, longing only to return to Wales. Easy-going with Frances, pleased that she is interested in the farm in which lie all his interests. Persistent friction between parents about their differing ambitions for themselves and for Frances: marital relationship is not happy. Paternal grandmother is said to be unpleasant, difficult and dominating.

Family live in cottage on a farm, and is of working-class level.

History: birth and development normal. Parents can recall no early difficulties. At 7, came to England. Appetite always good; no sleep disturbances. Began menstruating 2 years ago, periods regular, but severe pain, goes pale when pains begin. Many doctors have been consulted about her pains; 4 thought her appendix caused the trouble: twice X-rayed. Saw 2 further private doctors. Mother seemed to enjoy these thorough medical examinations. In all, Frances has seen 8 or 9 doctors, and been to 2 hospitals since the onset of the pains 2 years ago. While never robust, has had no operations, accidents or serious illnesses.

School record and intelligence: did not go to school until she was 7½, after she had come to England. Has been to 9 different schools because of family's moving about. Now in local high school in the upper fourth modern class. Teacher says she is retarded in work by about 1 year, but tries hard and is delightful to teach. Quiet and well-behaved. Best subjects are art and biology.

In intelligence test, I.Q. 103. Responses very slow and tentative; failed badly on all tests of mathematical reasoning. Immature, lacks confidence.

Personality and behaviour: although father has renounced Roman Catholic faith and mother has become strongly anti-Catholic, Frances is rather pious and likes to go to various Sunday schools. Gets on well with other children, has plenty of friends at school where she is a tomboy. Has mainly masculine interests: wants to be a farmer, belongs to a Young Farmers' Club, keeps her own chickens, and breeds dogs. Goes in for cattle and poultry-keeping competitions, is good with her hands, likes planning farm affairs with her father. Sensitive about her small size, says she does not want to be 16 next month. Sensitive and imaginative, inclined to take over other people's worries; is unselfish, not at all self-centred or sophisticated, and emotionally younger than her years. Helps willingly at home, has a happy disposition. No indoor interests: likes active games but is not good at them: likes gymnasium but has given it up. Likes reading adventure or detective stories, going to cowboy films, or doing outdoor jobs involving hammering, making things or taking care of animals. Recently, has developed exaggerated modesty, scorns being at all feminine, scoffs at girls who show interest in glamour or film stars. Has always wanted to be a boy: likes fancy-dress parties where she can dress up as a boy.

Clinical summary: diagnosed as a case of neurotic disturbance with pains of psychogenic origin; taken on for treatment with group of girls for 10 months. Made satisfactory progress: symptoms improved, but she is still a very inhibited, immature girl. Mother is unable to change her attitude, remains ignorant and full of doubts and inhibitions over sex matters, which she refuses to discuss with anybody. She hides her own and Frances's visits to the clinic as she fears people will think she is a criminal. Girl's adjustment to group improved. Prognosis thought to be fair, depending on the circumstances in which Frances finds herself. Under adverse conditions, she may develop an hysterical neurosis. Group treatment continues.

Causative factors: mother's unstable personality and ambivalence towards Frances's sex; disturbed parental relationship in which the mother is the dominating personality; mother's repressive handling; irrational attitude to sex matters and preoccupation with her own similar psychogenic symptoms.

APPENDIX 1: TABLES OF RESULTS

The following tables present in condensed form a summary of the results obtained by systematically observing and comparing the incidence of a number of important variables in these two well-studied groups of children. The statistical technique which has been used in making this comparison is a simple and straightforward test to determine the goodness of fit of the actual data observed to the theoretically expected normal distribution. This test was devised by Karl Pearson and involves the calculation of χ^2 (chi square):

$$\chi^2 = \epsilon \left(\frac{(f_0 - f)^2}{f} \right)$$

where f_0 = the observed or actual frequencies
f = the theoretical frequencies.

The calculation of chi square[1] provides a means of assessing the probability of obtaining a fit, due to chance, as poor as or worse than the one obtained. If this probability is small the likelihood that the disparities between the observed and actual data are ascribable to chance is small. The larger the chi square the greater the probability of a true divergence of the observed entities from the expected results. If p, the probability that χ^2 will not exceed any specified value, lies between .1 and .9, there can be no reason to doubt the hypothesis to be tested. If the chi-square test demonstrates that the disparity between the actual and the expected frequencies is too large to be due to chance (if p is less than the selected fiducial limit of .01 or .05), the hypothesis may be said to be false, i.e. that it fails to account for the whole of the observed facts. In accordance with the usual procedure, p of .05 or less was taken as indicative of a significant deviation from expectancy. This means that there are only 5 chances in 100 that the given (or a greater) value could have arisen by chance or is due to fluctuations of sampling. The 5 per cent level (indicated throughout in the body of the tables by one asterisk*) is reached by χ^2 in excess of 3.841, and the 1 per cent level (indicated by two asterisks**) is reached by χ^2 in excess of 6.635.

Tetrachoric correlations were calculated to show in another form how big the difference is. Reliable coefficients could not be calculated in a direct manner but the use of the correlation coefficients in relating the variables of the present investigation had the advantage that the information as to direction (positive or negative) could be provided in addition to the probability of distribution differences shown by the chi-square

[1] Following Fisher and using Yates' correction for continuity. See Fisher (1941) especially sections 21:01 and 21:02.

test. These positive or negative correlations are occasionally referred to in the main body of the text but for reasons of space they have been omitted from this condensed presentation of the tables of results. Detailed reference to them may be had, however, by consulting the author's unpublished thesis in the University of London Library (Bennett, 1951).

NOTE

For easier reference the following tables are not included in this Appendix, but appear at the appropriate places in the text:

Table 2 AGE DISTRIBUTION OF PRELIMINARY GROUPS

Age in years and months	I. Delinquents			II. Neurotics		
	Boys	Girls	Totals	Boys	Girls	Totals
4.0–5.11	0	0	0	7	4	11
6.0–7.11	9	5	14	11	4	15
8.0–9.11	17	3	20	19	7	26
10.0–11.11	13	4	17	10	5	15
12.0–13.11	18	5	23	9	9	18
14.0–15.11	5	9	14	3	9	12
16.0–17.11	3	2	5	1	1	2
18.0–19.11	0	1	1	0	1	1
Totals	65	29	94	60	40	100

Combined Total = 194†

† Three neurotic boys whose intelligence tests results were in some way unreliable or incomplete are included here but not in *Tables 3* and *4*.

Table 3   DISTRIBUTION OF STANFORD-BINET I.Q.s
IN THE PRELIMINARY GROUPS

I.Q.	I. *Delinquents*				II. *Neurotics*		
	Boys	Girls	Totals		Boys	Girls	Totals
50–69	8	5	13		0	0	0
70–89	16	12	28		9	4	13
90–109	25	10	35		25	21	46
110–129	11	2	13		16	5	21
130–149	5	0	5		5	9	14
150–169	0	0	0		2	1	3
Totals	65	29	94		57	40	97

Combined Total = 191

Table 4   TABLE SHOWING MEAN AGE AND MEAN I.Q.
OF PRELIMINARY GROUPS

	I. *Delinquents*				II. *Neurotics*		
	Mean age in years and months	Mean I.Q.	No. of Cases		Mean age in years and months	Mean I.Q.	No. of Cases
Girls	12.1	85	29		11.2	112	40
Boys	11.0	95	65		9.6	107	57
Totals	11.4	93	94		10.3	109	97

Combined Total = 191

Table 5   CHARACTERISTICS OF DELINQUENT BEHAVIOUR

	Delin-quent	Neu-rotic	χ^2
1. Stealing, pilfering, forgery, and embezzlement	43	3	61.20**
2. Lying	32	4	31.60**
3. Truanting	22	2	19.80**
4. Wandering, running away from school or home, staying out late at night	31	3	15.80**
5. Aggressive and destructive behaviour (Malicious damage, housebreaking, much fighting)	24	4	17.90**
6. Quarrelsome, tormenting, provocative behaviour	40	12	29.20**
7. Extreme disobedience and defiance	34	14	14.50**
8. Unmanageable, 'beyond control'	11	0	10.20**
9. Openly hostile to parents and teachers, 'up against authority'	17	3	10.60**
10. Open cruelty to animals or to younger children	9	0	7.81**
11. Incorrigible, impervious to punishment, does not respond to ordinary discipline	6	0	4.43*
12. Member of tough or aggressive gang	6	0	4.43*
13. Verbal aggressiveness, cheeky, insolent, rude, swearing and bad language	18	5	8.13**

Table 6   CHARACTERISTICS OF NEUROTIC BEHAVIOUR

	Neu-rotic	Delin-quent	χ^2
1. Fears and phobias	30	11	13.4**
2. Over-anxious behaviour, tense, worries a lot	25	7	13.3**
3. Described as 'nervous', 'highly strung', 'over-sensitive'	23	8	9.16**
4. Tearful, cries easily, easily upset	23	5	14.3**
5. Pavor nocturnis, frequent nightmares, bad dreams	22	10	5.56*
6. Babyish behaviour, clings to mother, extremely dependent	20	7	7.31**
7. Watches other children, cannot join in, fight back, etc.	15	3	8.20**
8. Passive, submissive, no initiative or ambition	18	5	8.13**
9. Subdued and inhibited behaviour, over-quiet, over-serious, etc.	20	4	12.30**
10. Cannot express emotion or real feelings	14	2	9.00**
11. Timid, hesitant, cautious behaviour, indecision	11	1	7.67**
12. Awkward, ill-at-ease, clumsy, self-conscious, has accidents, etc.	19	6	7.68**
13. Feels inferior, gives up easily, pessimistic, defeatist	20	4	12.30**
14. Depression	9	2	3.68
15. Fears of death, suicidal ideas	7	0	5.53*
16. Obsessional symptoms, (e.g. rituals, compulsions, etc.)	11	4	2.82
17. Obsessional traits and reaction formations (e.g. over-clean, over-modest, etc.)	21	1	21.00**
18. Hysterical symptoms	7	3	1.0

Table 7   SOCIAL RELATIONS

	Delin-quent	Neu-rotic	χ^2
1. Well-behaved, good and 'biddable'	1	28	32.8 **
Cf. Extreme disobedience and defiance	34	14	14.50**
2. Uncooperative and unhelpful in the house	7	4	0.41
3. No friends, unsociable, does not mix, etc.	20	29	2.56
4. Exhibitionistic:			
(a) Boastful, shows off, etc.	17	6	5.65*
(b) Plays the fool, or clowns, etc.	5	6	0.00
5. Envy, jealousy, searching other people's belongings	9	18	5.07*
6. Easily led, follows dominating child	4	2	0.18
7. Prefers companionship of younger children	8	9	0.00
8. Chooses bad companions	5	1	1.60
9. Gets bullied, teased, victimized, etc.	9	10	0.00
10. Bullies, victimizes other children	3	2	0.00
11. Dislikes meeting people, refuses to speak to strangers	0	5	3.37
12. Solitary, seclusive, 'feels different', etc.	4	12	3.65
13. 'Crushes', many intense friendships or enmities	2	2	0.00
14. Difficult behaviour towards siblings or other children	27	24	0.16
15. Shy, blushes easily, withdrawn, reserved, retiring	4	11	2.82

Table 8   SCHOOL DIFFICULTIES

	Delinquent	Neurotic	χ^2
16. Retardation in school subjects	30	25 (n=48)	0.34
17. Learning difficulties in special subjects	0	8 (n=48)	6.99**
18. Cannot concentrate, inattentive, poor memory, etc.	15	21 (n=48)	1.44
19. Intense dislike of school or teachers, refusing to go to school	7	12 (n=47)	1.33
20. Does not fit in with school routine	6	5 (n=47)	0.01
21. Difficult and unsettled behaviour in school	21	12 (n=47)	1.65

Table 9   DAY-DREAMING AND FANTASY

	Delinquent	Neurotic	χ^2
22. Fantasies, over-vivid imagination, day-dreams, etc.	14	26	5.04*
23. Fantasy companions	2	1	0.00
24. Romancing	8	6	0.08

Table 10   DIRTY AND UNTIDY BEHAVIOUR

	Delinquent	Neurotic	χ^2
25. Untidy, careless about clothes, appearance, etc.	7	6	0.00
26. Dirty, dirty habits, will not wash	6	7	0.00
27. Playing with faeces or urine, eating or smearing faeces	5	0	3.37

Table 11   PERSISTENT HABITS

	Delinquent	Neurotic	χ^2
28. Tics, twitching, grimacing, etc.	6	9	0.31
29. Thumb-sucking, sucking lips, etc.	4	6	0.11
30. Nail-biting	8	8	0.00
31. Other bodily habits	7	13	1.56

Table 12   SEXUAL BEHAVIOUR

	Delinquent	Neurotic	χ^2
32. Exaggerated masturbation	5	2	0.61
33. Precocious sex games, offences	10	3	3.18
34. Imitation of opposite sex (Totals)	2	23	21.30**
(a) Girlish behaviour in boys(n=30)	1	14	12.80**
(b) Boyish behaviour in girls (n=20)	1	9	6.50*

Table 13   'TOUGH-GUY' ATTITUDES

	Delinquent	Neurotic	χ^2
35. 'Don't care' attitude, bravado, acts 'tough guy', pretends unconcern	13	4	4.54*
36. Affectionless, callous, hard, shows no affectionate feelings	11	1	9.00**
37. Uncommunicative, evasive, denies difficulties	17	4	8.68**

Table 14   THE 'ANTISOCIAL GRUDGE'

	Delinquent	Neurotic	χ^2
38. Whining, complaining, self-pitying behaviour	4	10	2.08
39. Blames and accuses others, resentful and bitter, bears a grudge, nurses his grievances	3	8	1.63
40. Martyr attitude, sullen and sulky, thinks others are against him	9	13	0.52
41. Revengeful, spiteful tell-tale, gossiping	11	2	5.66*
42. Ringleader for trouble, mischievous, incites others, is blamed or 'scapegoated'	16	1	15.40**

Table 15   DEFECTIVE SUPER-EGO FORMATION

	Delinquent	Neurotic	χ^2
43. No sense of guilt or shame, plausible	18	0	24.00**
44. Does not own up, repent or make good his misdeeds, no remorse or regret	18	0	24.00**
45. Impulsive, wilful, poor control over impulses	14	0	14.90**
46. Shows no concern for the consequences of his behaviour, heedless of advice or warning	14	0	14.90**
47. Cannot bear frustration or thwarting, resents criticism or correction	15	4	6.50*
48. Mistrustful of adults and fearful of authority, cringes and flinches easily	17	7	4.88*
49. Cannot wait, must have immediate satisfaction of impulses, impatient	9	2	3.68
50. Greedy, demanding, dissatisfied, insatiable, gluttonous	15	7	2.86
51. Greedy, demanding and extravagant attitude towards money and material goods	7	0	6.38*

Table 16   OTHER 'DIFFICULT' BEHAVIOUR

	Delinquent	Neurotic	χ^2
52. Temper outbursts			
(a) temper tantrums, screaming attacks and outbursts of rage	19	15	0.40
(b) bad-tempered, irritable, easily becomes angry and resentful	24	17	1.49
53. Stubborn, obstinate, negative behaviour	14	8	1.46
54. Unreliable, irresponsible at school or at work, cannot be trusted, cannot keep jobs	7	1	3.40
55. Restless and discontented, easily impatient and bored, changeable	16	11	0.81
56. Lacks persistence, does what takes his fancy only, gives up if criticized, incapable of sustained effort	9	2	3.68
57. Lazy and idle	11	5	1.86
58. Selfish, inconsiderate for others' feelings or property, cannot share or take turns	8	4	0.85
59. Moody	7	6	0.00
60. Unemotional, apathetic, lethargic	0	8	6.99**
61. Absent-minded and forgetful	4	6	1.00
62. Fidgety, irritating habits	5	1	1.60
63. Religious doubts and difficulties, worries about 'unforgivable sin'	1	6	2.46
64. Self-punishment, hurting self and getting hurt, provoking punishment	10	6	0.67
65. Unhappy, seldom smiles, often dejected and miserable	14	15	0.00
66. Feels unwanted, rejected, disliked	9	7	0.00

Table 17   QUEER HABITS AND 'ODD' BEHAVIOUR

	Delinquent	Neurotic	χ^2
65. Queer habits, odd behaviour, bizarre ideas	5	4	0.00
66. 'Old for his age', unchildlike, does not play, etc.	4	9	1.41
67. Humourless, rarely smiles, never makes jokes, etc.	9	11	0.06
68. Morbid interests	0	5	3.37

Table 18   NEUROTIC DISORDERS OF ORGAN FUNCTION

	Delinquent	Neurotic	χ^2
69. Feeding disturbances	19	21	0.04
70. Sleep disturbances	14	21	1.58
71. Speech disturbances	2	9	3.68
72. Disturbances in bladder control	10	18	2.43
73. Disturbances in bowel control	8	3	1.63
74. Disturbances in the alimentary system	1	4	0.84

Table 19   LABILITY OF NERVOUS SYSTEM AND ALLERGY

	Delinquent	Neurotic	χ^2
75. Headaches and temperatures	1	5	1.60
76. Sick turns with vomiting or train-sickness	0	2	0.51
77. Fainting turns	0	1	0.00
78. Asthma	0	6	4.43*
79. Urticaria	1	1	0.00

DELINQUENT AND NEUROTIC CHILDREN

Table 20   SOCIAL LEVEL OF THE HOME

	Delinquent	Neurotic	χ^2
A. Working class	36	27	2.75
B. Middle class	14	23	2.75

Table 21   GROSS ENVIRONMENTAL DISTURBANCES

	Delinquent	Neurotic	χ^2
(a) Unsettled home, frequent moves	31	13	11.70**
(b) Overcrowding	17	4	8.68**
(c) Periods spent in foster-homes	12	2	6.72**
(d) Absence with friends and relatives	20	10	3.86**
(e) Evacuation	7	5	0.09
(f) Travel abroad	5	4	0.00
(g) Hospitalization	17	14	0.19
(h) Air-raid experience	7	12	1.04
(i) 'Vicious homes'	1	0	0.02

Table 22   PERIODS SPENT IN INSTITUTIONS

	Delinquent	Neurotic	χ^2
Periods spent in institutions, etc.	12	2	6.72**

Table 23 UNFAVOURABLE CONDITIONS IN FAMILY HISTORY

	Delinquent (n = 41)†	Neurotic (n = 49)†
Alcoholism	6	2
Epilepsy	1	0
Psychosis	4	5
Temperamental instability	4	2
Suicide or attempted suicide	4	0
Mental defect	2	0
Criminality	7	1
Neurotic conditions	10	21

† See footnote to *Table 24.*

Table 24   POSSIBLE HEREDITARY FACTORS

	Delinquent (n = 41)†	Neurotic (n = 49)†	χ^2
Miscellaneous conditions	20	8	9.51**
Neurotic conditions	10	21	2.60

† The data about family history were unknown or incomplete in the case of one neurotic child and nine delinquent children. These were cases where the child was adopted, his parents were unknown, or both parents were dead.

DELINQUENT AND NEUROTIC CHILDREN

Table 25   FAMILY STRUCTURE

	Delinquent	Neurotic	χ^2
Stable home	17	37	14.50**
Parents separated, divorced, deserted	15	3	8.20**
Mother or father dead (or unknown)	12	3	1.69
Irregular unions	3	3	0.18
Prolonged absence of mother or father	33	22	4.04*
True parentage concealed from child	13	4	4.54*
Child of stable marriage	17	38	16.20**
Child step-, foster-, or adopted	17	9	2.55
Illegitimate child	10	5	1.25
Position in family			
(i) First child	22	25	0.16
(ii) Last child	6	4	0.11
(iii) Only child	13	11	0.54
Size of family			
(i) Family three children or less	33	43	4.44*
(ii) Family four children or more	17	7	4.44*
'Broken family'	22	11	4.52*
'Stable family'	28	39	4.52*

Table 26 PARENTAL ILLNESS OR DEFORMITY: SEX DIFFERENCES

	Delinquent			Neurotic		
	Girls (n=18)	Boys (n=27)	Total (n=45)	Girls (n=19)	Boys (n=28)	Total (n=47)
Illness of mother	6	9	15	4	6	10
Deformity of mother	1	2	3	0	0	0
Illness of father	5	7	12	4	4	8
Deformity of father	1	1	2	2	3	5

Table 27 CHRONIC ILLNESS OR DEFORMITY OF PARENTS

	Delinquent	Neurotic	χ^2
Chronic illness of mother	15	10	0.85
Chronic illness of father	12 (n=45)	8 (n=47)	0.75
Chronic illness of mother or father	27 (n=95)	18 (n=97)	2.08
Deformity of mother	3	0	1.37
Deformity of father	2 (n=45)	5 (n=47)	0.53
Chronic illness or deformity of either parent	30 (n=95)	18 (n=97)	3.67

Table 28 PERSONALITY OF CHILD'S PARENTS

	Delinquent	Neurotic	χ^2
Mother's Personality			
Normal	25	27	0.04
Antisocial or morally unstable	16	3	9.36**
Neurotic	8	20	9.51**
Psychotic	1	0	0.02
Father's Personality			
Normal	35	42	1.49
Antisocial or morally unstable	14	1	12.1**
Neurotic	0	7	5.29*
Psychotic	1 (n=45)	0 (n=47)	0.02
Neurotic personality of mother or father	8	27	13.47**
Antisocial personality of mother or father	30	4	22.98**
Psychotic personality of mother or father	2 (n=95)	0 (n=97)	0.03

Table 29   ABSENCE OR DEATH OF PARENTS

| | Delinquent | | | Neurotic | | |
	Girls (n=20)	Boys (n=30)	Total	Girls (n=20)	Boys (n=30)	Total
Mother dead	1	3	4	0	1	1
Father dead	2	2	4	1	2	3
Both parents dead	0	1	1	0	0	0
Mother absent	3	10	13	2	8	10
Father absent	14	19	33	5	14	19
Both parents absent	3	10	13	2	6	8
One or both parents quite unknown	2	3	5	1	1	2

Table 30   INTERRUPTED MOTHER-CHILD RELATIONSHIP

Relationship interrupted at age of	Delinquent	Neurotic	χ^2
Years			
0–1	14	5	4.16*
1–2	17	1	15.20**
2–5	16	6	4.72*
5–7	15	4 (n=48)	6.03*
7–11	9 (n=45)	3 (n=43)	2.16
11+	4 (n=23)	0 (n=23)	2.46
Total no. of cases experiencing interrupted mother-child relationship	36	11	23.12**

Table 31   INTERRUPTED FATHER-CHILD RELATIONSHIP

Relationship interrupted at age of	Delinquent	Neurotic	χ^2
Years			
0–1	16	4	7.56**
1–2	23	4	16.40**
2–5	29	8	17.20**
5–7	26	5 (n=48)	17.70**
7–11	25	1 (n=45) (n=43)	27.40**
11+	9	2 (n=23) (n=23)	4.30*
Total no. of cases experiencing interrupted father-child relationship	40	11	31.37**

Table 32   DISTURBED EMOTIONAL RELATIONSHIPS WITHIN THE
FAMILY

	Delinquent	Neurotic	χ^2
Disturbed mother-child relationship	42	31	5.07*
Disturbed father-child relationship	35 (n=45)	15 (n=47)	17.70**
Disturbed mother-father relationship	26 (n=45)	15 (n=47)	5.22*
Disturbed sibling relationship	20 (n=38)	20 (n=40)	0.00

Table 33   PHYSICAL CONDITIONS

Physical Conditions	Delinquent	Neurotic	χ^2
Undergrown	6	12	1.69
Overgrown	8	10	0.68
Chronic illnesses in the past	23	33	3.29
Chronic illnesses in the present	0	3	1.37
Special defects (i) Hearing	3	1	0.26
(ii) Vision	7	4	0.41
(iii) Speech	1	5	1.60
(iv) Disability or disfigurement	4	6	0.11
Totals (one or more special defect)	14	14	0.00
Accidents and injuries	10	7	0.28
Many operations	9	13	0.52

Table 34   DURATION OF BREAST-FEEDING

Period of breast-feeding (in months)	Delinquent (n=38)	Neurotic (n=42)	χ^2 (2 × k table)
0	19	8 ⎫	
0–1	6	3 ⎪	
2–3	6	6 ⎬	16.273**
4–6	2	13 ⎪	
7–12	5	12 ⎭	

Table 35   DURATION OF BREAST-FEEDING: NEW SOUTH WALES CASES

Period Breast-fed (in months)	Totals (n=99)	Behavioural Difficulties (n=28)	Delinquent (n=41)	Neurotic (n=30)	χ^2 (2 × k table)
0	17	7	7	3 ⎫	
0–1	12	5	7	0 ⎪	
2–3	12	4	8	0 ⎪	
4–6	13	4	3	6 ⎬	14.4*
7–9	34	5	11	18 ⎪	
10–12	10	2	5	3 ⎪	
13–18	1	1	0	0 ⎭	

R*

Table 36

COMPARISON OF STUDIES ON BREAST-FEEDING

Period Breast-fed (in months)	English Clinic Cases			Goldman Childers & Hamil		N.S.W. Clinic Cases			
	Delinquent (n=99) %	Neurotic (n=42) %	Total (n=80) %	Normals (n=100) %	Maladjusted (n=469) %	Delinquent (n=469) %	Neurotic (n=30) %	Behavioural Difficulties (n=28) %	Total (n=99) %
0	50	19	34	10	24	17	10	25	17
1–5	37	31	31	34	22	42	13	39	32
6–10	10	43	31	} 56	25	29	77	32	44
11–24	3	7	4		29	12	0	4	6

Table 37   DIFFICULTIES IN EARLY HABIT-TRAINING

	Delinquent	Neurotic	χ^2
(a) *Sleep Disturbances at the age of*			
Years			
0–2	5 ⎤	3 ⎤ (n=49)	0.40
2–5	11 ⎟ (n=41)	10 ⎦	0.22
5–7	12 ⎟	12 (n=47)	0.02
7–11	13 ⎦	14 (m=43)	0.02
11+	7 (n=18)	11 (n=22)	0.15
Total cases of sleep disturbance	20 (n=41)	27 (n=49)	0.66
(b) *Feeding Disturbances at the age of*			
Years			
0–2	15 ⎤	23 ⎤ (n=47)	0.73
2–5	15 ⎟ (n=45)	15 ⎦	0.10
5–7	13 ⎟	9 (n=45)	1.13
7–11	13 ⎦	8 (n=41)	1.17
11+	8 (n=18)	11 (n=22)	0.00
Total cases of feeding disturbances	21 (n=40)	34 (n=47)	2.85
(c) *Difficulties in Bladder control at the age of*			
Years			
0–2	18 ⎤	27 ⎤ (n=49)	0.54
2–5	19 ⎬ (n=40)	20 ⎦	0.17
5–7	12 ⎦	17 (n=47)	0.14
7–11	11 (n=41)	14 (n=43)	0.11
11+	2 (n=17)	5 (n=22)	0.21
Total cases having difficulties in establishing bladder control	24 (n=40)	29 (n=49)	0.19
(d) *Difficulties in Bowel Control at the age of*			
Years			
0–2	14 ⎤	22 ⎤ n=49	1.35
2–5	15 ⎬ n=40	10 ⎦	2.40
5–7	6 ⎦	3 (n=47)	0.93
7–11	5 (n=41)	3 (n=43)	0.19
11+	1 (n=17)	0 (n=22)	0.02
Total cases having difficulty in establishing bowel control	18 (n=40)	23 (n=49)	0.00

Table 38   'INFANTILE WANDERINGS'

Frequent changes of home or maternal care	Delinquent	Neurotic	χ^2
(a) Before aet. 1 year	15	3	8.20**
(b) Before aet. 2 years	20	4	12.3**
(c) Before aet. 5 years	24	4	17.9**

Table 39   DISCIPLINE IN THE HOME

Type of Discipline	Delinquent	Neurotic	χ^2
Normal	4	14	5.49*
Over-strict	7	19	6.29*
Over-lenient	3	3	0.18
Inconsistent	36	14	17.60**

Table 40   EARLIER DIFFICULT BEHAVIOUR

Difficulties at the age of	Delinquent	Neurotic	χ^2
Years			
0–2	21	34	5.82*
2–5	32	38	1.19
5–7	36	36 (n=48)	0.05
7–11	29 (n=45)	33 (n=43)	2.24
11+	16 (n=23)	20 (n=23)	3.19
Total number of cases showing earlier difficult behaviour	48	48	0.26

Table 41   TRAUMATIC EXPERIENCES

Trauma at the age of	Delinquent	Neurotic	χ^2
Years			
0–2	14	8	1.46
2–5	20	22	0.37
5–7	19	14 (n=48)	0.51
7–11	14 (n=45)	14 (n=43)	0.01
11+	8 (n=23)	3 (n=23)	1.91
Total cases having had traumatic experience at various times	37	41	0.52

Table 42   TRAUMATIC EXPERIENCES IN BOYS AND GIRLS

Traumatic Experiences	Girls (n=20)	Boys (n=30)	χ^2
Delinquent	19	18	5.93*
Neurotic	17	24	0.01

Table 43   INTERESTS AND ACHIEVEMENTS

Level of attainment	Delinquent	Neurotic	χ^2
(a) School attainments			
above average	0	4	2.34
average	21	19	0.04
below average	29	25	0.36
(b) Reading interests			
above average	5	8	0.35
average	26	24	0.04
below average	19	16	0.18
(c) Interests and achievements			
above average	7	14	2.17
average	28	28	0.04
below average	15	8	2.03

Table 46   CLUSTERS OF FACTORS AFFECTING
DELINQUENT CHILDREN

No. of Factors	Factors	Delinquent	Neurotic	χ^2
3	3 4 10	34	7	25.00**
	4 7 10	34	8	
4	3 4 7 10	31	6	24.71**
	2 3 4 10	30	4	
5	2 3 4 7 10	28	4	20.62**
	3 4 7 8 10	25	3	
6	2 3 4 7 9 10	17	2	12.57**
	2 3 4 7 8 10	23	3	18.75**
7	2 3 4 5 7 8 10	15	0	12.05**
	2 3 4 7 8 9 10	15	1	
	1 2 3 4 7 8 10	15	2	
	2 3 4 5 7 8 9 10	12	0	11.46**
	1 2 3 4 5 7 8 10	11	0	10.20**
	1 2 3 4 7 8 9 10	11	1	9.00**
9	All except 6 & 11	9	0	7.81**
	9 & 11	8	0	6.99**
	5 & 11	8	0	
	1 & 11	8	0	

Table 47   CLUSTERS OF FACTORS AFFECTING
NEUROTIC CHILDREN

No. of Factors	Factors	Neurotic	Delinquent	χ^2
3	13 18 19	22	3	17.24**
4	12 13 14 16	12	0	11.46**
	12 13 14 19	12	0	
	13 16 19 20	12	0	
	13 16 18 19	12	2	6.72**
	12 13 14 18	11	0	10.20**
5	12 13 14 16 19	9	0	7.81**
	12 13 14 18 19	9	0	
	12 13 14 16 18	8	0	6.99**
	12 13 14 16 20	8	0	
6	12 13 14 16 18 20	7	0	5.53*
	12 13 14 16 19 20	6	0	4.43*
	12 13 14 16 18 19	6	0	

APPENDIX II: BIBLIOGRAPHY

This bibliography has been arranged chronologically to illustrate the development of the literature over the past sixty years. Titles of journals are abbreviated according to the usage of the *World List of Scientific Periodicals*. S.P. stands for *Selected Papers*; C.P. for *Collected Papers*.

1880. DOSTOEVSKY, F. M. *The Brothers Karamazov*. English trans. by Constance Garnett. London: Heinemann, 1912.

1890. HALL, G. STANLEY. 'Children's Lies.' *Amer. J. Psychol.*, Jan., pp. 59–70.

1893a. FREUD, S. 'On the Psychical Mechanisms of Hysterical Phenomena.' C.P., Vol. I, p. 24.

1893b. FREUD, S. 'Some Points in a Comparative Study of Organic and Hysterical Paralysis.' C.P., Vol. I, p. 42.

1894. FREUD, S. 'The Justification for Detaching from Neurasthenia a Particular Syndrome: the Anxiety-Neurosis.' C.P., Vol. I, p. 76.

1895a. FREUD, S. 'A Reply to Criticisms on the Anxiety-Neurosis.' C.P., Vol. I, p. 107.

1895b. FREUD, S. 'Obsessions and Phobias; their Psychical Mechanisms and their Aetiology.' C.P., Vol. I, p. 128.

1896. FREUD, S. 'The Aetiology of Hysteria.' C.P., Vol. I, p. 183.

1898. FREUD, S. 'Sexuality in the Aetiology of the Neuroses.' C.P., Vol. I, p. 220.

1900. FREUD, S. *Traumdeutung*. Leipsig and Wien.

1905 FREUD, S. *Three Contributions to a Theory of Sexuality*. Vienna: Deuticke, 1905. First English edition (trans. James Strachey) under the title *Three Essays on the Theory of Sexuality*. London: Imago, 1949.

1905a. FREUD, S. 'My Views on the Part Played by Sexuality in the Aetiology of the Neuroses.' C.P., Vol. I, p. 272.

1905b. FREUD, S. 'Fragment of an Analysis of a Case of Hysteria.' C.P., Vol. III, p. 13.

1907. FREUD, S. 'Obsessive Acts and Religious Practices.' C.P., Vol. II, p. 25.

1908a. FREUD, S. 'Hysterical Phantasies and their Relation to Bisexuality.' C.P., Vol. II, p. 51.

1908b. FREUD, S. 'Character and Anal Erotism.' C.P., Vol. II, p. 45.

1908c. FREUD, S. 'On the Sexual Theories of Children.' C.P., Vol. II, p. 59.

1908. MCDOUGALL, W. *An Introduction to Social Psychology*. London: Methuen.

1909a. FREUD, S. 'General Remarks on Hysterical Attacks.' C.P., Vol. II, p. 100.

1909b. FREUD, S. 'Analysis of a Phobia in a Five-year-old Boy.' C.P., Vol. III, p. 147.

1909c. FREUD, S. 'Notes upon a Case of Obsessional Neurosis.' C.P., Vol. III, p. 296.

1913. FREUD, S. *The Interpretation of Dreams*. English translation by A. A. Brill. London: Macmillan.

1913a. FREUD, S. 'Infantile Mental Life: Two Lies Told by Children.' C.P., Vol. II, p. 144.

1913. HUG-HELLMUTH, H. von. *Aus dem Seelenleben des Kindes*. Vienna: Deuticke.

1914. FREUD, S. 'On Narcissism: An Introduction.' C.P., Vol. IV, p. 30.

1915a. FREUD, S. 'Instincts and their Vicissitudes.' C.P., Vol. IV, p. 60.

1915b. FREUD, S. 'Repression.' C.P., Vol. IV, p. 84.

1915c. FREUD, S. 'The Unconscious.' C.P., Vol. IV, p. 98.

1915d. FREUD, S. 'Some Character-Types met with in Psycho-Analytic Work.' C.P., Vol. IV, p. 318.

1915. GODDARD, H. H. *The Criminal Imbecile*. New York: Macmillan.

1915a. HEALY, W. *The Individual Delinquent*. 1st ed. London: Heinemann.

1915b. HEALY, W. and HEALY, M. T. *Pathological Lying, Accusation and Swindling*. London: Heinemann.

1917. FREUD, S. 'Mourning and Melancholia.' C.P., Vol. IV, p. 152.

1917. HEALY, W. *Mental Conflicts and Misconduct*. London: Kegan Paul, Trench, Trubner & Co.

1918. FREUD, S. 'From the History of an Infantile Neurosis.' C.P., Vol. III, p. 473.

1918. GLUECK, B. 'A Study of Admissions to Sing Sing.' Ment. Hyg., Vol. II, No. 1, pp. 84–139.

1918. LOMBROSO, C. *Crime, its Causes and Remedies*. English translation by Henry P. Horton. Boston: Little, Brown.

1919. FREUD, S. 'A Child is being Beaten. A contribution to the Study of the Origin of Sexual Perversions.' C.P., Vol. II, p. 172.

1919. GORING, C. *The English Convict*. Abridged ed. London: H.M.S.O.

1919. WHITE, W. A. *The Mental Hygiene of Childhood*. London: Heinemann.

1921. FLUGEL, J. C. *The Psycho-Analytic Study of the Family*. London: Hogarth.

1921a. HUG-HELLMUTH, H. von. 'On the Technique of Child Analysis.' *Int. J. Psycho-Anal.*, Vol. II.

1921b. HUG-HELLMUTH, H. von. 'Von Mittleren Kinde.' *Imago*, Vol. VII.

1922. FREUD, S. *Beyond the Pleasure Principle.* English translation by C. J. M. Hubback. London: Hogarth.

1922. LAWRENCE, D. H. *Sons and Lovers.* London: Duckworth.

1923. FREUD, A. 'The Relation of Beating Phantasies to a Daydream. *Int. J. Psycho-Anal.*, Vol. IV.

1923. FREUD, S. *The Ego and the Id* International Psychoanalytic Library Series, 1927.

1923. KLEIN, M. 'The Development of a Child.' *Int. J. Psycho-Anal.*, Vol. IV.

1923. WHITE, W. A. *Insanity and the Criminal Law.* New York: Macmillan.

1924. ABRAHAM, K. 'The Influence of Oral Erotism on Character Formation.'

1924 FREUD, S. 'The Passing of the Oedipus Complex.' C.P., Vol. II, p. 296.

1924. GLOVER, E. 'The Significance of the Mouth in Psycho-Analysis.' *Brit. J. med. Psychol.*, Vol. 4.

1924. KLEIN, M. 'The Role of the School in the Libidinal Development of the Child.' *Int. J. Psycho-Anal.*, Vol. V.

1924. SEARL, M. N. 'Some Analytical Observations from a Child's Behaviour.' *Int. J. Psycho-Anal.*, Vol. V.

1925. AICHHORN, A. *Verwahrloste Jugend.* Vienna. English translation, London: Putnam, 1936.

1925 BURT, C. *The Young Delinquent.* 4th ed. London: 1944.

1925a. BURT, C. *The Psychology of the Young Criminal.* Howard League pamphlets No. 4, new series.

1925. FREUD, S. 'Psycho-Analysis and Delinquency.' C.P. Vol. V, p. 98.

1925. GLOVER, E. 'Notes on Oral Character Formation.' *Int. J. Psycho-Anal.*, Vol. VI.

1925. HEALY, W. and BRONNER, A. F. *Delinquents and Criminals: Their Making and Unmaking. Studies in Two American Cities.* New York: Macmillan.

1925. REICH, W. *Der triebhafte Charakter.* Vienna: Internationaler Psychoanalytischer Verlag.

1925. STEKEL, W. *Peculiarities of Behaviour.* London: Williams & Norgate.

1925. WHITE, W. A. *Essays in Psychopathology.* New York and Washington: Macmillan.

1926. GLOVER, E. 'The Neurotic Character.' *Int. J. Psycho-Anal.*, Vol. VII.

1926. WHITE, W. A. *Mechanisms of Character Formation.* New York: Macmillan.

1927. ABRAHAM, K. 'Notes on the Psychoanalytic Investigation and treatment of Manic-Depressive Insanity and Allied Conditions' (1911). S.P. p. 137. London: Hogarth.

1927. ABRAHAM, K. 'The First Pre-genital Stage of the Libido.' *Int. Z.* (*ärtzl.*) *Psychoanal.*, 1916. S.P., p. 248. London: Hogarth.

1927. ABRAHAM, K. 'A Short Study of the Development of the Libido viewed in the Light of Mental Disorders.' (1924). S.P., p. 418. London: Hogarth.

1927. ABRAHAM, K. 'Character Formation on the Genital Level of the Libido.' (1925). S.P., p. 407. London: Hogarth.

1927. FREUD, A. *The Psycho-Analytic Treatment of Children.* London: Imago, 1946.

1927. GLOVER, E. 'On Child Analysis.' Contribution to symposium. *Int. J. Psycho-Anal.*, Vol. VIII.

1927. KLEIN, M. 'On Child Analysis.' Contribution to symposium. *Int. J. Psycho-Anal.*, Vol. VIII.

1927. MALINOWSKI, B. *Sex and Repression in Savage Society.* New York: Harcourt.

1928. FREUD, A. *Introduction to the Technique of Child Analysis.* New York: Nervous and Mental Diseases Publishing Co.

1928. GORDON, R. G. *Autolycus: or the Future of Miscreant Youth.* London and New York: Kegan Paul, Trench, Trubner & Co.

1928. THOMAS, W. I. & D. S. *The Child in America: Behavior Problems and Programs.* Ch. II. New York: Knopf.

1929. FERENCZI, S. 'The Unwelcome Child and his Death Instinct.' *Int. J. Psycho-Anal.*, Vol. IX, July.

1929. HEALY, W. & BRONNER, A. F. *Reconstructing Behavior in Youth: Problem Children in Foster Homes.* New York: Knopf.

1929. ISAACS, S. *The Nursery Years.* London: Routledge.

1929. KARPMAN, B. 'The Problem of Psychopathies.' *State Hospital Quart.*

1929. SHAW, C. R. *Delinquency Areas.* University of Chicago Press.

1929. STEKEL, W. *Sadism and Masochism.* New York: Liveright.

1930. ALEXANDER, F. 'The Neurotic Character.' *Int. J. Psycho-Anal.*, Vol. XI.

1930. BARTEMEIER, L. H. 'The Neurotic Character as a New Psychoanalytic Concept.' *Amer. J. Orthopsychiat.*, Vol. I, p. 512.

1930. MENNINGER, K. A. *The Human Mind.* New York and London: Knopf.

1930. SHAW, C. R. *The Jack Roller: a Delinquent Boy's Own Story.* University of Chicago Press.

1931. ALEXANDER, F. & STAUB, H. *The Criminal, the Judge and the Public: a Psychological Analysis.* English translation by G. Zilboorg. New York: Macmillan.

1931. FERENCZI, S. 'Child Analysis in the Analysis of Adults.' *Int. J. Psycho-Anal.*, Vol. XII.

1931. FREUD, A. 'Psychoanalysis of the Child.' In Carl Murchison (Ed.) *Handbook of Psychology.*

1931. MEAD, M. *Growing Up in New Guinea.* London: Routledge; New York: Morrow, 1930.

1931. MURCHISON, C. (Ed.) *Handbook of Child Psychology.* Worcester, Mass.: Clark University Press.

1931. PRESTON, G. H., & SHEPLER, W. M. 'A Study of the Problems of Normal Children.' *Amer. J. Orthopsychiat.*, Vol. 1.

1932. CHILDERS, A. T. & HAMIL, B. M. 'Emotional Problems in Children as related to the Duration of Breast-feeding in Infancy.' *Amer. J. Orthopsychiat.*, Vol. II, p. 134.

1932. KLEIN, M. *The Psycho-Analysis of Children.* London: Hogarth.

1932a. LEVY, D. M. *Studies in Sibling Rivalry.* American Orthopsychiatric Association.

1932b. LEVY, D. M. 'On the Problem of Delinquency.' *Amer. J. Orthopsychiat.*, Vol. II, p. 197.

1932. MCDOUGALL, W. *Character and Conduct of Life.* London: Methuen.

1932. PRESTON, G. H. & ANTIN, R. 'A Study of Children of Psychotic Parents.' *Amer. J. Orthopsychiat.*, Vol. II, p. 231.

1932. TIEBOUT, H. M. & KIRKPATRICK, M. E. 'Psychiatric Factors in Stealing.' *Amer. J. Orthopsychiat.*, Vol. II, p. 114.

1933. ACKERLEY, S. S. 'Rebellion and its Relation to Delinquency and Neurosis in 60 Adolescents.' *Amer. J. Orthopsychiat.*, Vol. III, p. 147.

1933. BIDDLE, S. 'The Use of Transference in Dealing with Delinquents.' *Amer. J. Orthopsychiat.*, Vol. III, p. 14.

1933. BUHLER, CHARLOTTE. 'Social Behavior of Children.' In C. Murchison (Ed.) *Handbook of Child Psychology.* Worcester, Mass.: Clark University Press.

1933. CHESHIRE, R., SAFFIR, M. & THURSTONE, R. R. *Computing Diagrams for the Tetrachoric Correlation Coefficient.* Illinois: University of Chicago Press.

1933. FREUD, S. *New Introductory Lectures in Psycho-Analysis.* London: Hogarth.

1933. GLOVER, E. *War, Sadism, and Pacifism.* London: Allen & Unwin.

1933a. ISAACS, S. *Social Development in Young Children: a Study in Beginnings.* London: Routledge.

1933b. ISAACS, S. *Intellectual Growth of the Child.* London: Routledge.

1933. KARPMAN, B. *Case Studies in the Psychopathology of Crime.* Vol. I. Washington, D.C.: Medical Science Press.

1933. MENNINGER, K. A. 'Psycho-analytic Aspects of Suicide.' *Int. J. Psycho-Anal.*, Vol. XIV, Pt. 3, p. 376.

1933. SCHMIDEBERG, M. 'The Psycho-analytic Treatment of Asocial Children.' *New Era*, Vol. XIV.

1933. WHITE, W. A. *Forty Years of Psychiatry.* New York & Washington: Nervous and Mental Diseases Monographs Series (No. 57).

1934. ALEXANDER, F. 'Evaluation of Statistical and Analytical Methods in Psychiatry and Psychology.' *Amer. J. Orthopsychiat.*, Vol. IV, p. 43.

1934. FENICHEL, O. *Outline of Clinical Psychoanalysis.* New York: Norton.

1934. GLUECK, S. & GLUECK, E. T. *One Thousand Juvenile Delinquents.* Cambridge, Mass.: Harvard University Press.

1934. GOODMAN, S. E. & MICHAELS, J. E. 'Incidence Intercorrelation of Enureses and other Neuropathic Traits in so-called Normal Children.' *Amer. J. Orthopsychiat.*, Vol. IV, p. 79.

1934. HEALY, W. 'Psychoanalysis of Older Offenders.' *Amer. J. Orthopsychiat.*, Vol. IV, p. 25.

1934. LEVY, D. M. 'Experiments on the Sucking Reflex and Social Behavior of Dogs.' *Amer. J. Orthopsychiat.*, Vol. IV, p. 203

1934. NEWELL, H. W. 'The Psychodynamics of Maternal Rejection.' *Amer. J. Orthopsychiat.*, Vol. IV, p. 387.

1935. ALEXANDER, F. & HEALY, W. *The Roots of Crime: Psychoanalytic Studies.* New York & London: Knopf.

1935. BURT, C. *The Subnormal Mind.* Oxford University Press.

1935. HORNEY, K. 'Personality Changes in Female Adolescents.' *Amer. J. Orthopsychiat.*, Vol. V, p. 19.

1935. MAKARENKO, A. "Педагогическая поэма." Moscow: Foreign Languages Publishing House, p. 607.

1935. MEAD, M. *Sex and Temperament in three Primitive Societies.* New York: Morrow; London: Routledge.

1935. SCHMIDEBERG, M. 'The Psycho-analysis of Asocial Children and Adolescents.' *Int. J. Psycho-Anal.*, Vol. XVI, p. 22.

1935. SILVERMAN, B. 'The Behavior of Children from Broken Homes.' *Amer. J. Orthopsychiat.*, Vol. V, p. 11.

1935. STODDARD, G. D. & WELLMAN, B. L. *Child Psychology.* New York: Macmillan.

1936. AICHHORN, A. *Wayward Youth.* (English translation). London: Putnam.

1936. FREUD, A. *The Ego and the Mechanisms of Defence.* London: Hogarth.

1936. FREUD, S. *Inhibitions, Symptoms, and Anxiety.* Trans. Alix Strachey. London: Hogarth.

1936. HEALY, W. & BRONNER, A. *New Light on Delinquency and its Treatment.* New Haven: Yale University Press.

1936. LEVY, D. M. 'Hostility Patterns in Sibling Rivalry Experiments.' *Amer. J. Orthopsychiat.*, Vol. VI, p. 183.

1936. LOWREY, L. G. 'The Family as a Builder of Personality.' *Amer. J. Orthopsychiat.*, Vol. VI, p. 117.

1936. MAKARENKO, A. *The Road to Life.* Trans. Stephen Garry. London: Lindsay Drummond.

1936. MENNINGER, K, A. *Man against Himself.* New York: Harcourt.

1936. NEWELL, H. W. 'A Further Study of Maternal Rejection' *Amer J. Orthopsychiat.*, Vol. VI, p. 576.

1936. SCHILDER, P. 'The Analysis of Ideologies as a Psychotherapeutic Method, especially in Group Treatment.' *Amer. J. Psychiat.*, Vol. 93, No. 3.

1937. BENDER, L. & BLAU, A. 'The Reaction of Children to Sexual Relations with Adults.' *Amer. J. Orthopsychiat.*, Vol. VII, p. 200.

1937. BENDER, L. & SCHILDER, P. 'Suicidal Preoccupations and Attempts in Children.' *Amer. J. Orthopsychiat.*, Vol. VII, p. 225.

1937. KANNER, L. *Child Psychiatry.* Baltimore: Thomas.

1937. KARPMAN, B. 'Crime and Adolescence.' *Ment. Hyg.*, Vol. II.

1937. LEVY, D. M. 'Primary Affect Hunger.' *Amer. J. Psychiat.*, Vol. 94, p. 643.

1937. LIPPMAN, H. S. 'The Neurotic Delinquent.' *Amer. J. Orthopsychiat.*, Vol. VII, p. 114.

1937. PLANT, J. S. *Personality and the Cultural Pattern.* New York: Commonwealth Fund.

1937. POWDERMACKER, F., LEVES, H. T. & TOURAINE, G. ' Psychopathology and Treatment of Delinquent Girls.' *Amer. J. Orthopsychiat.*, Vol. VII, p. 57.

1937. WILE, I. S. 'Further Considerations on Suicide.' *Amer. J. Orthopsychiat.*, Vol. VII, p. 235.

1937. WITTELS, F. 'The Criminal Psychopath in the Psychoanalytic System.' *Psychoanal. Rev.*, Vol. XXIV.

1937. ZILBOORG, G. 'Considerations on Suicide with Particular Reference to that of the Young.' *Amer. J. Orthopsychiat.*, Vol. VII, p. 15.

1938. ALEXANDER, F. 'Notes and Comments.' *Ment. Hyg.*, Vol. 22, p. 163.

1938. FISHER, R. A. & YATES, F. *Statistical Tables.* Edinburgh: Oliver & Boyd.

1938. MACDONALD, M. W. 'Criminally Aggressive Behavior in Passive Effeminate Boys.' *Amer. J. Orthopsychiat.*, Vol. VIII, p. 70.

1938. MICHAELS, J. C. 'The Incidence of Enuresis and Age of Cessation in 100 Delinquents and 100 Sibling Controls.' *Amer. J. Orthopsychiat.*, Vol. VIII, p. 460.

1938. MOWRER, O. H. & MOWRER, W. M. 'Enuresis—a Method for its Study and Treatment.' *Amer. J. Orthopsychiat.*, Vol. VIII, p. 436.

1938. PRESCOTT, D. A. *Emotion and the Educative Process.* New York: American Council for Education.

1938. SHAW, C. *Brothers in Crime*, University of Chicago Press.

1939. BENEDICT, R. 'Sex in Primitive Society.' *Amer. J. Orthopsychiat.*, Vol. IX, p. 570.

1939. EAST, N. & HUBERT, W. H. DE B. *Home Office Report on the Psychological Treatment of Crime.* London: H.M.S.O.

1939. FROSCH, J. & BROMBERG, W. 'The Sex Offender—a Psychiatric Study.' *Amer. J. Orthopsychiat.*, Vol. IX, p. 761.

1939. GERARD, M. 'Enuresis—a Study in Etiology.' *Amer. J. Orthopsychiat.*, Vol. IX, p. 48.

1939. HENDERSON, D. K. *Psychopathic States.* New York: Norton.

1939. KARDINER, A. *The Individual and his Society: the Psychodynamics of Primitive Social Organisation.* Foreword by R. Linton. New York: Columbia University Press.

1939. KARPMAN, B. 'The Delinquent as a Type and Personality.' *J. crim. Psychopathol.*, Vol. I, No. 1.

1939. LEVY, D. M. 'Sibling Rivalry Studies in Primitive Groups.' *Amer. J. Orthopsychiat.*, Vol. IX, p. 205.

1939. MENAKER, E. 'The Neurotic Stealing Symptom.' *Amer. J. Orthopsychiat.*, Vol. IX, p. 368.

1939. MICHAELS, J. C. & GOODMAN, S. B. 'The Incidence of Enuresis and Age of Cessation in 1,000 Neuro-Psychiatric Patients: with a Discussion on the relation between Enuresis and Delinquency.' *Amer. J. Orthopsychiat.*, Vol. IX, p. 59.

1939. SHASKAN, D. 'One Hundred Sex Offenders.' *Amer. J. Orthopsychiat.*, Vol. IX, p. 565.

1939. SLAVSON, R. In 'Proceedings of the 1939 Symposium.' *Amer. J. Orthopsychiat.*, Vol. IX, p. 226.

1939. WORTIS, J. 'Sex Taboos, Sex Offenders, and the Law.' *Amer. J. Orthopsychiat.*, Vol. IX, p. 554.

1940. BOWLBY, J. 'Influence of Early Environment in Development of Neurosis and Neurotic Character.' *Int. J. Psycho-Anal.*, Vol. 21.

1940. BURT, C. 'The Incidence of Neurotic Symptoms among Evacuated Schoolchildren.' *Brit. J. educ. Psychol.*, Vol. X, No. 8.

1940. CANTNOR, N. 'Dynamics of Delinquency. *Amer. J. Orthopsychiat.*, Vol. X, p. 789.

1940a. LOWREY, L. G. 'Treatment and What Happened After, by Healy and Bronner.' *Amer. J. Orthopsychiat.*, Vol. X, p. 172.

1940b. LOWREY, L. G. 'Personality Distortions and Early Institutional Care.' *Amer. J. Orthopsychiat.*, Vol. X, p. 576.

1940. MANNHEIM, H. *Social Aspects of Crime in England between the Wars.* London: Allen & Unwin.

1940. MICHAELS, J. C. 'A Psycho-biologic Interpretation of Delinquency.' *Amer. J. Orthopsychiat.*, Vol. IX, p. 501.

1940. RECKLESS, W. *Criminal Behavior.* New York & London: McGraw Hill.

1940. RIEMER, M. D. 'Runaway Children.' *Amer. J. Orthopsychiat.*, Vol. X, p.522.

1940. YARNELL, H. 'Fire-setting in Children.' *Amer. J. Orthopsychiat.*, Vol. X, p. 272.

1941. BENDER, L. & PASTER, S. 'Homosexual Trends in Children.' *Amer. J. Orthopsychiat.*, Vol. XI, p. 730.

1941. FISHER, R. A. *Statistical Methods for Research Workers.* (8th ed.) Edinburgh: Oliver & Boyd.

1941. HEALY, W. & ALPER, B. S. *Criminal Youth and the Borstal System.* New York: Commonwealth Fund.

1941. KARPMAN, B. 'Symptomatic and Idiopathic Psychology.' *J. crim. Psychopathol.*, Vol. II, Reviewed by L. G. Lowrey in Karpman, 1948a.

1941. KASANIN, J. & HANDSCHIN, S. 'Psychodynamic Factors in Illegitimacy.' *Amer. J. Orthopsychiat.*, Vol. XI, p. 66.

1941. LANDER, J. 'Traumatic Factors in the Background of 116 Delinquent Boys.' *Amer. J. Orthopsychiat.*, Vol. XI, p. 150.

1941. LEWINSKY, H. 'The Nature of Shyness.' *Brit. J. Psychol.*, Vol. 32.

1941. LOWREY, L. G. 'Runaways and Nomads.' *Amer. J. Orthopsychiat.* Vol. XI, p. 775.

1941. MICHAELS, J. G. 'Parallels between Persistent Enuresis and Delinquency in the Psychopathic Personality.' *Amer. J. Orthopsychiat.*, Vol. XI, p. 260.

1941. TOPPING, R. 'Case Studies of Aggressive Delinquents.' *Amer. J. Orthopsychiat.*, Vol. XI, p. 485.

1941. WAGGONER, R. W. & BOYD, D. A. 'Juvenile Aberrant Sexual Behavior.' *Amer. J. Orthopsychiat.*, Vol. XI, p. 275.

1942. BURLINGHAM, D. & FREUD, A. *Young Children in Wartime: A Year's Work in a Residential War Nursery.* London: Allen & Unwin.

1942. CARR-SAUNDERS, A. M., MANNHEIM, H., & RHODES, E. C. *Young Offenders: an Enquiry into Juvenile Delinquency.* Cambridge University Press.

1942. MANNHEIM, H. Certain chapters in CARR-SAUNDERS, MANNHEIM & RHODES (1942) above.

1942. ROSENHEIM, F. 'Character Study of a Rejected Child.' *Amer. J. Orthopsychiat.*, Vol. XII, p. 487.

1942. SHAW, C. R. & MCKAY, H. D. *Juvenile Delinquency and Urban Areas.* University of Chicago Press.

1942. WATSON, J. A. F. *The Child and the Magistrate.* London: Cape.

1943. BENDER, L. 'Aggression in Childhood.' In 'Round Table Discussion.' *Amer. J. Orthopsychiat.*, Vol. XIV, p. 384.

1943. BURLINGHAM, D. & FREUD, A. *Infants without Families.* London: Allen & Unwin; New York: International Universities Press.

1943. FRIEDLANDER, K. 'Delinquency Research.' *New Era*, May.

1943. GOLDFARB, W. 'Infant Rearing and Problem Behavior.' *Amer. J. Orthopsychiat.*, Vol. XIII, No. 2, p. 249.

1943. LEVY, D. M. *Maternal Overprotection.* New York: Columbia University Press.

1943. LIPPMAN, H. S. 'Treatment of Aggression: Psychoanalytic.' *Amer J. Orthopsychiat.*, Vol. XIII, No. 2, p. 415.

1943. MULLINS, C. *Crime and Psychology.* London: Methuen.

1943a. SLAVSON, S. R. 'Treatment of Aggression Through Group Therapy.' *Amer. J. Orthopsychiat.*, Vol. XIII, No. 2, p. 419.

1943b. SLAVSON, S. R. 'Group Therapy.' In 'Round Table Discussion.' *Amer. J. Orthopsychiat.*, Vol. XIII, p. 648.

1943c. SLAVSON, S. R. *An Introduction to Group Therapy.* New York: Commonwealth.

1943. TOPPING, R. 'Treatment of the Pseudo-social Boy.' *Amer. J. Orthopsychiat.*, Vol. XIII, p. 353.

1944. BANISTER, H. & RAVDEN, M. 'The Problem Child and his Environment.' *Brit. J. Psychol.* (General Section), Vol. XXXIV, Pt. 2.

1944. BOWLBY, J. *Forty-four Juvenile Thieves.* London: Baillière.

1944. GLOVER, E. *The Diagnosis and Treatment of Delinquency, being a Clinical Report of the Work of the Institute for the Scientific Treatment of Delinquency during the five years, 1937-41.* I.S.T.D. Pamphlet No. 1. London: I.S.T.D.

1944. GOLDFARB, W. 'Effects of Early Institutional Care on the Adolescent Personality: Rorschach Data.' *Amer. J. Orthopsychiat.*, Vol. XIV, p. 441.

1944. GREENACRE, P. 'Infant Reactions to Restraint.' *Amer. J. Orthopsychiat.*, Vol. XIV, p. 204.

1944. HORSLEY GANTT, W. *Experimental Basis for Neurotic Behavior.* London & New York: Harper.

1944. LEVY, D. M. 'On the Problems of Movement Restraint.' *Amer. J. Psychiat.*, Vol. XIV, p. 644.

1944. LINDNER, R. *A Rebel without a Cause.* New York: Grune & Stratton.

1944. MILNER, M. 'A Suicidal Symptom in a Child of Three.' *Int. J. Psycho-Anal.*, Vol. XXV, p. 53.

1945. BANISTER, H. & RAVDEN, M. 'The Environment of the Child.' *Brit. J. Psychol.* (General Section), Vol. XXXV, Pt. 3, p. 82.

1945. FENICHEL, O. *The Psychoanalytic Theory of Neurosis.* New York: Norton.

1945. FRIEDLANDER, K. 'Formation of the Antisocial Character.' *Psychoanal. Study Child*, Vol. I, p. 189.

1945. GOLDFARB, W. 'Psychological Privation in Infancy and Subsequent Adjustment.' *Amer. J. Orthopsychiat.*, Vol. XV, p. 167.

1945. GOLDMAN, G. S. & BERGMAN, M. S. 'A Psychiatric and Rorschach Study of Adult Male Enuresis.' *Amer. J. Orthopsychiat.*, Vol. XV, p. 160.

1945. GREENACRE, P. 'Conscience in the Psychopath.' *Amer. J. Orthopsychiat.*, Vol. XV, p. 495.

1945. HARTMANN, H. & KRIS, E. 'The Genetic Approach in Psychoanalysis,' *Psychoanal. Study Child*, Vol. I.

1945. MULLINS, C. *Why Crime?* London: Methuen.

1945. PAVENSTEDT, E. & ANDERSEN, I. 'The Uncompromising Demand of a Three-Year-Old for her own Mother.' *Psychoanal. Study Child*, Vol. I, p. 211.

1945. SPITZ, R. A. 'Hospitalism: an Inquiry into the Genesis of Psychiatric Conditions in Early Childhood.' *Psychoanal. Study Child*, Vol. I, p. 53.

1946. ANDRIOLA, J. S. 'The Truancy Syndrome.' *Amer. J. Orthopsychiat.*, Vol. XVI, p. 174.

1946a. FRIEDLANDER, K. 'Psychoanalytic Orientation in Child Guidance Work in Great Britain.' *Psychoanal. Study Child*, Vol. II, p. 343.

1946b. FRIEDLANDER, K. 'Some Notes on the Organization of a Child Guidance Service.' In *Child Guidance: a Psycho-Analytic Approach.* London: New Education Fellowship.

1946. HARTMANN, H., KRIS, E. & LOEWENSTEIN, R. M. 'Comments on the Formation of Psychic Structure.' *Psychoanal. Study Child*, Vol. II, p. 11.

1946a. SPITZ, R. A. 'Hospitalism: a Follow-up Report.' *Psychoanal. Study Child*, Vol. II, p. 113.

1946b. SPITZ, R. A. 'Anaclitic Depression.' *Psychoanal. Study Child*, Vol. II, p. 313.

1946. VOLLMER, H. 'Jealousy in Children.' *Amer. J. Orthopsychiat.*, Vol. XVI, p. 660.

1947. DEUTSCH, H. *The Psychology of Women. A Psycho-analytic Interpretation.* Vols. I & II. London: Research Books.

1947. FRIEDLANDER, K. *The Psycho-Analytical Approach to Juvenile Delinquency.* London: Kegan Paul.

DELINQUENT AND NEUROTIC CHILDREN

1947a. FRIEDLANDER, K. *Annual Report of a Child Guidance Service* (private papers).

1947. GARRETT, H. E. *Statistics in Psychology and Education.* New York & London: Longmans.

1947. GLOVER, E. 'The Investigation and Treatment of Delinquency.' *Brit. med. J.*, 29 March, 1957.

1947. GOLDFARB, W. 'Variations in Adolescent Adjustment of Institutionally Reared Children.' *Amer. J. Orthopsychiat.*, Vol. XVII, No. 3.

1947. GOODMAN, W. L. 'Makarenko's Sense of the Mean.' *New Era,* Vol. 28, No. 1.

1947. KARPMAN, B. 'Passive Parasitic Psychopathy.' *Psychoanal. Rev.,* Vol. 24.

1947. SCHMIDL, F. 'The Rorschach Test in Juvenile Delinquency Research.' *Amer. J. Orthopsychiat.*, Vol. XVII, p. 151.

1947. SLAVSON, S. R. (Ed.). *The Practice of Group Therapy.* London: Pushkin Press; New York: International Universities Press.

1948. BAZELEY, E. T. *Homer Lane and the Little Commonwealth.* London: New Education Book Club.

1948. FLUGEL, J. C. (Ed.). *Proceedings of the International Congress on Mental Health* (4 vols.) London: Lewis.

1948a. FRIEDLANDER, K. 'The Significance of the Home in Emotional Growth.' *New Era,* Vol. 29, No. 3.

1948b. FRIEDLANDER, K. 'On the Modification of Instincts.' *Yearb. Psychoanal.*, Vol. IV, p. 74.

1948a. GOLDMAN, F. 'Breast Feeding and Character Formation.' *J. Personality,* Vol. 17, No. 1.

1948b. GOLDMAN, F. 'The Etiology of the Oral Character in Psychoanalytic Theory.' (unpublished).

1948. GREENACRE, P. 'Anatomical Structure of Superego Development.' *Amer. J. Orthopsychiat.*, Vol. XVIII, p. 459.

1948a. HAUSER, R. 'Planning for Mental Health: Organization, Training, Propaganda.' *Proceedings of the International Congress on Mental Health,* Vol. IV, p. 240.

1948b. HAUSER, R. 'A Philosophy for Children's Communities.' *New Era,* Vol. 29, No. 8.

1948. HEALY, W. & BRONNER, A. F. 'The Child Guidance Clinic: Birth and Growth of an Idea.' In Lowrey, L. G. & Sloane, V. (Eds.), *Orthopsychiatry 1923-48: Retrospect and Prospect.* Wisconsin: Banta. Pp. 14, or-45.

1948a. KARPMAN, B. 'Milestones in the Advancement of Knowledge in the Psychopathology of Delinquency and Crime.' In Lowrey & Sloane (Eds.) *Orthopsychiatry 1932-48.* Wisconsin: Banta. Pp. 100-89.

1948b. KARPMAN, B. 'Conscience in the Psychopath: another Version.' *Amer. J. Orthopsychiat.*, Vol. XVIII, p. 455.

1948. KRIS, E. 'On Psychoanalysis and Education.' *Amer. J. Orthopsychiat.*, Vol. XVIII, p. 622.

1948. MANNHEIM, H. *Juvenile Delinquency in an English Middletown.* London: Kegan Paul.

1948. MEAD, M. *From the South Seas: a Study of Adolescence and Sex in Primitive Societies.* New York: Morrow.

1948. MERRILL, M. A. *Problems of Child Delinquency.* London: Harrap.

1948. MOWRER, O. H. 'Learning Theory and the Neurotic Paradox.' *Amer. J. Orthopsychiat.*, Vol. XVIII, p. 571.

1948. RAPAPORT, D. 'The Psychologist in the Clinical Setting.' Round Table, 1947. *Amer. J. Orthopsychiat.*, Vol. XVIII, p. 495.

1949. BOWLBY, J. 'The Field for Future Research.' In *Why Delinquency? The Case for Operational Research.* Report of a Conference on the Scientific Study of Juvenile Delinquency. London: N.A.M.H.

1949. BURT, C. 'Recent Discussions on Juvenile Delinquency'. *Brit. J. educ. Psychol.*, Vol. XIX, Pt. I, p. 32.

1949. FREUD, A. 'Certain Types and Stages of Social Maladjustment.' In K. R. Eissler (Ed.) *Searchlights on Delinquency: New Psycho-Analytic Studies.* London: Imago, p. 193.

1949a. FRIEDLANDER, K. 'Latent Delinquency and Ego Development.' In K. R. Eissler (Ed.) *Searchlights on Delinquency.* London: Imago, p. 205.

1949b. FRIEDLANDER, K. 'Neurosis and Home Background: a Preliminary Report.' *Psychoanal. Study Child,* Vol. III–IV, p. 423.

1949. GLOVER, E. 'Outline of the Investigation and Treatment of Delinquency in Great Britain: 1912–48.' In K. R. Eissler (Ed.) *Searchlights on Delinquency.* London: Imago, p. 433.

1949. GOLDFARB, W. 'Rorschach Test Differences between Family-Reared, Institution-Reared, and Schizophrenic Children.' *Amer. J. Orthopsychiat.*, Vol. XIX, No. 4.

1949. HEALY, W. 'Psychiatry and Delinquency: Critical Evaluations.' *Amer. J. Orthopsychiat.*, Vol. XIX, No. 2, p. 317.

1949. HOFFER, W. 'Deceiving the Deceiver.' In K. R. Eissler (Ed.) *Searchlights on Delinquency.* Part III. London: Imago, p. 150.

1949. MANNHEIM, H. 'The Limits of Present Knowledge.' In *Why Delinquency? The Case for Operational Research.* Report of a Conference on the Scientific Study of Juvenile Delinquency. London: N.A.M.H., p. 10.

1949. MEAD, M. *Male and Female: a Study of the Sexes in a Changing World.* New York: Morrow. London: Gollanz, 1950.

1949. ROSE, D. E. 'Social Factors in Delinquency.' *Austral. J. Psychol.*, Vol. I, No. 1, p. 1.

1949. SIMEY, T. S. 'The Field for Future Research.' In *Why Delinquency? The Case for Operational Research.* Report of a Conference on the Scientific Study of Delinquency. London: N.A.M.H.

1949. WILLOCK, H. D. *Mass Observation: a Report on Juvenile Delinquency.* London: Falcon Press.

1950. ADORNO, R. W., FRENKEL-BRUNSWIK, E., LEVINSON, D. J. & SANFORD, R. N. *The Authoritarian Personality.* New York: Harper.

1950. BENNETT, IVY. A Comparative Study of Delinquent and Neurotic Children. Unpublished Ph.D. thesis. London University Library.

1950. COLLIS, A. & POOLE, V. *These Our Children.* London: Gollancz.

1950. COMFORT, A. *Authority and Delinquency in the Modern State.* London: Routledge & Kegan Paul.

1950. ESCALONA, S. K. 'Approaches to a Dynamic Theory of Development.' Round Table, 1949. *Amer. J. Orthopsychiat.*, Vol. XX, p. 157.

1950. SEARS, R. R. & WISE, G. W. 'The Relation of Cup-Feeding in Infancy to Thumb-Sucking and the Oral Drive.' *Amer. J. Orthopsychiat.*, Vol. XX, No. 1, p. 123.

1950. STOTT, D. H. *Delinquency and Human Nature.* Dunfermline: Carnegie United Kingdom Trust.

1951. BENNETT, IVY & HELLMAN, ILSE. 'Psychoanalytic Material related to Observations in Early Development.' *Psychoanal. Study Child.*, Vol. VI, p. 307.

1951. BOWLBY, J. *Maternal Care and Mental Health.* Geneva: W.H.O.

1951. FREUD, A. 'The Contribution of Psychoanalysis to Genetic Psychology.' *Amer. J. Orthopsychiat.*, Vol. XXI, No. 3, p. 476.

1952. GLOVER, E. 'Research Methods in Psycho-Analysis.' *Int. J. Psycho-Anal.*, Vol. XXXIII, No. 4.

1953. BURLINGHAM, DOROTHY. 'Notes on Problems of Motor Restraint during Illness.' In R. M. Loewenstein (Ed.) *Drives, Affects, and Behaviour.* New York: International Universities Press.

1953. GLOVER, E. *Psycho-Analysis and Child Psychiatry.* London: Imago.

INDEX

INDEX

habits:
  difficulties in early training, 180-2
  persistent, 88-90
  queer, 109-10
Hall, Stanley, 86
Hamil, on breast-feeding, 173, 174, 178
Handschin, on illegitimacy, 140
Hauser, R., 9
headaches, 114
health and physical conditions, 170-2
Healy, 4-5, 8, 10, 12, 13, 15-16, 18, 21, 22,
  56, 86, 100, 105, 115, 117, 120, 124,
  137, 154, 160, 172, 176, 185, 190, 212,
  214, 215, 217
  Chicago and Boston study of, 132
  on 'antisocial grudge', 99
  on Borstals, cit., 133
  on broken homes, cit., 138
  on defective family life, cit., 156
  on environment, 115
  on heredity, 135
  on parentage, cit., 138-9
  on psychiatry, 29
  on sex behaviour, 90, 91
  on 'tough guys', 98
Henderson, 26, 91
heredity, 13, 120, 135-7, 212
Hirsch, on enuresis, 111
Hoffer, 9, 107
homes (home), see also family, foster homes:
  absence from, 125-6, 127
  broken, 125, 137-40, 143, 144, 211, 212
  change of ('infantile wanderings'), 182-5
  middle-class (categories of), 122-3
  overcrowded, 124, 125, 127
  psycho-analysis and, 206-7
  social level of, 122-3, 212
  stable, 125, 140, 143, 144, 211-2, 227
  unsettled, 124, 125, 127, 128
  'vicious', 13, 124, 127
  working class (categories of), 122-3
homosexuality (inversion):
  Bender and Paster on, 92
  -cit., 93
  Benedicton, cit., 94
  Freud on, 7, 56, 86, 94-5, 96
  rejection and, 154
hospitalization, 126, 127
Hug-Hellmuth, 14
hysteria, 78
  cases of, 79

illegitimacy, 140, 184-5
illness:
  child, 170-1, 172, 212
  parental, 145-6, 212
Indians of North America, sexual habits of,
  94
'infantile wanderings', 182-5
inferiority feelings, 76
inhibition, of emotions, 75-6

injuries, 171, 172
Institute for the Scientific Treatment of
  Delinquency, 38
institutions, characteristics of children
  reared in, 128-34
intelligence (I.Q.):
  delinquents',
  -case histories, 243-359 'passim'
  -of paired cases: boys, 240
  —girls, 241
  neurotics',
  -case histories, 360-485 'passim'
  -of paired cases: boys, 240
  —girls, 241
  rating of, of cases for survey, 48
interests and achievements, 195-200, 216
interests and activities, 198-200
irritability, 216
Isaacs, Susan, 14, 32, 33, 133, 187
Ischlondsky, 95

jealousy, 82
Jewish Board of Guardians 38
Judge Baker Foundation Clinic, 12, 38
Jung, 7
juvenile courts, 44, 65, 66
  sexual offences and, 96
Juvenile Delinquency in an English Middle-
  town, 18, 121
Juvenile Psychopathic Institute, 4

Kardiner, 95
Karpman, 16, 17, 21, 26, 91, 107, 117, 120,
  133, 179n, 216
  on 'antisocial grudge', 99-100
  on broken homes, 140
  on conscience and psychopaths, 105
  on delinquents, 158
  on enuresis, 111
Kasanin, on illegitimacy, 140
kindness, Makarenko and, 9
Kirkpatrick, 18, 20, 100
  on stealing, 154
Klein, 14
Kraepelin, 4

Lander, 19, 125
  on 'traumatic environment', 192
Lane, Homer, 187
left-handedness, 89, 111
Leighton, 95
Leves, 23, 121-2, 133, 192
Levinson, 189
Levy, 16, 18, 19, 20, 21, 24, 100, 105, 119,
  124, 147, 154, 160, 192, 214, 216
  on maternal over-protection, 157
  on milieu and aggression in delinquency,
  117
  -cit., 118
  on milieu and neurotic delinquency, 23
  on rejected children, cit., 153

528

INDEX

Pearson, Karl, 57
personality, delinquents (case histories), 243–359 'passim'
neurotics (case histories), 360–485 'passim'
Perth, study of delinquency in, 117n
phobias, *see* fears and phobias
physical conditions, *see* health and physical conditions
pilfering, 63, 68
Poole, 21, 124
Powdermacker, 23, 121–2, 133, 192
Preston:
on normal children, cit., 50n
on psychotics' children, cit., 147
psycho-analysis (psycho-analytic theory):
adaptation to social needs and (institutions), 129
breast-feeding and, 209
conscience and, 19–20, 204
discipline and, 186–7
education and, 187
feeding and, 228
habit-training and, 180, 181
home and family and, 206–7
learning inhibitions and, 55
oral characteristics and, 175–6
plan of research and, 33–4
sexual curiosity and, 96
study and, 201–2
'tough guys' and, 205
traumatic experiences and, 209
treatment by, 10–11, 14–15, 105, 221, 224
White and, 6
Psycho-analytical Approach to Juvenile Delinquency, x, 41n
Psychopaths, 131, 136n, 205
delinquent, 17, 26–7
discipline and, 186
enuresis and, 112
psycho-analysis, conscience and, 105
rejection and, 154
Psychosis, 40, 136
children of psychotics, 147, 149, 150
psychotic delinquents, 27
psychotic parents, 148, 149, 150
sex crimes and, 91
psychotherapy:
delinquents and, 51, 224, 225
length of, 35
punishment, 12, 13
pyloric stenosis, 191

quarrelsomeness, 64
various types of, 71

Ravden, 21, 122, 137, 147, 185, 195
on homes, 125, 140, 212
reading interests, 196–7
reconvictions, Borstal, 28n, 134

Reich, 14, 16, 17, 19, 100, 107, 217
'impulse-ridden character of', 22, 86
on oral characteristics, 175
rejected children, 152–5
research, indications for further, 225–9
research plan, 31–60 'passim'
retardation, in school subjects, 84, 85
Rhodes, 17, 115, 137
on 'tendency or susceptibility to delinquency', 116
survey of young offenders of, 120
Ribble, 174
Riemer, 20
on parents, 147
romancing, 87
Rorschach, experience with delinquents, 21, 98
study of institutional children, 131
tests on enuretics, 112
Rose, 21, 115, 196
Rosenheim, 19, 78–9, 86
on antisocial behaviour, 100
on the rejected child, 153

sado-masochism, 71, 152, 208
'grudge against society' and, 100
Sanford, 189
Saul, 95
Schilder, 19
Schmideberg, 15, 107
Schmidl, 21
cit., 98
school:
adjustment at, 55
attainments, 196, 216
difficulties at, 84–5
record,
–delinquents' (case histories), 243–359 'passim'
–neurotics' (case histories), 360–485 'passim'
Searl, M. N., 14
Sebire, Irene, 174, 177n, 179
self-punishment, statistics, 203
sex, *see also* homosexuality (inversion), *and* masturbation:
behaviour (in general), 90–8
dogs', disturbances in, 95
fantasy and delinquency, 86
Freud on, 7, 29, 56
games, 203
imitation of the opposite, 55–6, 96–7, 216–7, 227–8
offenders, 90–2, 93, 96
perverted, 18, 92
Shaskan, 19
on sex crimes, 91
Shaw, 17, 56, 115, 137, 139, 211n
on delinquency in American cities, cit., 119
on delinquency in Chicago, 116–7

INDEX

NAME INDEX OF DELINQUENT CHILDREN

NAME INDEX OF NEUROTIC CHILDREN